533-8551
6/16

P9-DGN-993

BARRON'S

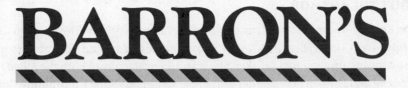

PTCE

Pharmacy Technician Certification Exam

Sacha Koborsi-Tadros, PharmD

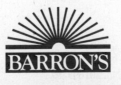

MARY RILEY STYLES PUBLIC LIBRARY
120 NORTH VIRGINIA AVENUE
FALLS CHURCH, VA 22046
(703) 248-5030

BARRON'S

ABOUT THE AUTHOR

Sacha Koborsi-Tadros received her doctorates of pharmacy from The Chicago College of Pharmacy at Midwestern University in Downers Grove, Illinois. She is an educator as well as a pharmacy consultant and professional speaker. She is an adjunct faculty of both the Allied Health department and Social and Human Services department at Columbus State Community College in Columbus, OH. As an educator, Dr. Tadros has instructed dental hygiene students in pharmacology and has participated in professional board review courses. She also instructs pharmacology courses, specializing in substance abuse prevention and treatment. Most recently, she has helped develop and instruct pharmacy technician courses to prepare students for certification. As a consultant, Dr. Tadros has a vital role in promoting pharmacy technicians by serving as a consultant to other colleges in the area. As a professional speaker, she has presented on various topics including herbals, substances of abuse, and pharmacy technician training. She has also received recognition by the PTCB to serve as an advocate educator.

ACKNOWLEDGMENTS

This book is dedicated to my parents who have always encouraged me to follow my dreams. You are forever my inspiration to continue to help others and, without your continued support, I would not be the person I am today. I am forever grateful to you. To my siblings, thank you for being my number one supporters throughout this journey. Thank you to my in-laws for understanding my dreams and ambitions and supporting me in the process. To my loving husband, thank you for understanding my desire to write this book and being my rock in the process. To my dearest children, I hope that you will one day understand why momma needed some time to work away from you. You are my biggest accomplishment, and I will always strive to make you proud. As Khalil Gibran once said, "to understand the heart and mind of a person, look not at what he has already achieved, but at what he aspires to."

Note

While the content of this text was written based on all of the most current information available regarding the pharmacy technician profession and the PTCE exam, readers are still advised to consult with their employers and the Pharmacy Technician Certification Board website (*http://ptcb.org/*) for the latest pharmacy technician standards and guidelines that are applicable to their state.

The presence of knowledge domains in this publication has been determined subjectively by the author. While the author has made every attempt to categorize information by a singular knowledge domain, there may be times when the concepts relate to multiple domains.

The publisher and author have made every effort to ensure that drug selection and dosing information meets current recommendations and guidelines. Information regarding drug therapy and treatment methods requires the independent judgment of a health care professional.

For the purposes of this publication, all trademark symbols have been deleted.

© Copyright 2016 by Barron's Educational Series, Inc.

All rights reserved.
No part of this publication may be reproduced or distributed in any form or
by any means without the written permission of the copyright owner.

All inquiries should be addressed to:
Barron's Educational Series, Inc.
250 Wireless Boulevard
Hauppauge, NY 11788
www.barronseduc.com

ISBN: 978-1-4380-0727-4
Library of Congress Catalog Card No. 2016932976

PRINTED IN THE UNITED STATES OF AMERICA
9 8 7 6 5 4 3 2 1

10%
POST-CONSUMER
WASTE
Paper contains a minimum
of 10% post-consumer
waste (PCW). Paper used
in this book was derived
from certified, sustainable
forestlands.

Contents

PRACTICE TESTS

APPENDIXES

Introduction

1

Pharmacy technicians play a major role in pharmacy practice. Ensuring patient safety and enhancing patient care are only a few of the many valuable contributions made by pharmacy technicians. Pharmacists rely on technicians to help provide patients with the best care possible. Pharmacy technicians who possess a comprehensive understanding of pharmacy practice are well sought after and are a valuable asset in pharmacy practice.

Certification is the process of granting recognition to an individual who has met predetermined qualifications. The CPhT designation is given to an individual with the knowledge, skills, and abilities necessary to function as a pharmacy technician. An individual proves that he/she has the necessary skills by passing either one of two national examinations: the Pharmacy Technician Certification Exam (PTCE) or the Exam for the Certification of Pharmacy Technicians (ExCPT). The PTCE is provided by the Pharmacy Technician Certification Board; the ExCPT is offered by the National Healthcareer Association. This study guide will provide you with a comprehensive review of all the concepts tested on the Pharmacy Technician Certification Exam.

The Pharmacy Technician Certification Board, also known as PTCB®, is a nongovernmental agency that administers the PTCE. In 2012, the Pharmacy Technician Certification Board conducted a job analysis survey to look at the current roles of pharmacy technicians. These results showed a strong need for an update to the exam blueprint. The updated PTCE went into effect on November 1, 2013 and is the format of the test today. The current PTCE exam blueprint assesses knowledge comprehension in 9 knowledge domains; this is a significant change from the previous 3 knowledge domains covered in the past. No changes have been made to the format or length of the test. The PTCE is a 90-question, multiple-choice examination. Within a 2-hour timeframe, 1 hour and 50 minutes are spent taking the test. The remaining 10 minutes are used for a tutorial and for a postexam survey. This review book has been structured to review the content based on these domains. Each chapter focuses on one domain area and contains 10 review questions and answers.

Included with this book is a full-length pretest, two full-length practice tests, and one full-length online exam. The pretest is designed to assess your strengths and weaknesses before beginning your review. The practice tests appear at the end of the book and test what you've learned. The full-length online exam completes your PTCE preparation. These examinations provide an in-depth review of all knowledge domains and are structured to mimic the certification examination. The practice tests assess your knowledge based on all domain areas, and the percentage of each content area is based on the actual PTCE exam structure. For every

---

PTCB® is a registered trademark of the Pharmacy Technician Certification Board.

question, a detailed answer explanation is included that outlines why one choice is correct and why the alternate choices are incorrect.

Use this book to supplement your current pharmacy-related knowledge as you prepare for your certification exam. Determine what you know. Make a list of topics that you need to review further as you continue to prepare for your test. Take the tests to simulate the conditions you will encounter on test day and to practice what you've learned. Congratulations on your journey to embark on a career in pharmacy. Best of luck on your examination!

About the Pharmacy Technician Certification Exam

2

PHARMACY TECHNICIAN CERTIFICATION BOARD

The Pharmacy Technician Certification Board (PTCB) is responsible for ensuring that pharmacy technicians meet predetermined standards that convey competency in the field of pharmacy. These standards include having knowledge and skills pertaining to pharmacy practice. In order to become a certified pharmacy technician, interested candidates need to apply for certification through the PTCB website, *http://ptcb.org/*. In order to qualify for certification, candidates must meet the following criteria:

- Have a high school diploma or an equivalent educational diploma (i.e., a GED or a foreign diploma)
- Provide full disclosure of all criminal actions and all State Board of Pharmacy registration or licensure actions
- Be in compliance with all applicable PTCB certification policies
- Receive a passing score on the Pharmacy Technician Certification Exam (PTCE)

NOTE

Candidates should also check with their State Board of Pharmacy for additional certification requirements.

PHARMACY TECHNICIAN CERTIFICATION EXAM

The Pharmacy Technician Certification Examination (PTCE) is a computer-based, 90-question, multiple-choice examination given over a 2-hour timeframe. Of that time, 1 hour and 50 minutes are allotted for the actual test. The remaining 10 minutes are for a tutorial and a postexam survey. Eighty out of 90 questions are scored questions, and 10 questions are unscored. Test takers will not be able to differentiate between the scored and unscored questions because the unscored questions are randomly distributed throughout the exam.

Scoring

The PTCB uses a scaled scoring system. Candidates receive scores ranging from 1,000 to 1,600. A passing grade is 1,400.

TIP

Since you won't know which questions are scored and which are unscored, do your best on every question!

Test Content

As per the Pharmacy Technician Certification Board, test questions are determined based on nine knowledge domains. Table 2-1 lists these domains.

Table 2-1. PTCE Knowledge Domains and Test Content

Knowledge Domain	Percentage of PTCE Content
1.0—Pharmacology for Technicians	13.75%
2.0—Pharmacy Law and Regulations	12.50%
3.0—Sterile and Non-Sterile Compounding	8.75%
4.0—Medication Safety	12.50%
5.0—Pharmacy Quality Assurance	7.50%
6.0—Medication Order Entry and Fill Process	17.50%
7.0—Pharmacy Inventory Management	8.75%
8.0—Pharmacy Billing and Reimbursement	8.75%
9.0—Pharmacy Information Systems Usage and Application	10.00%

Scheduling Your Exam

The PTCE is administered at Pearson VUE testing centers. Pearson VUE testing centers are available nationwide. They offer computer-based testing (CBT) for a multitude of professions, including the PTCB certification.

Potential CPhT candidates can sign up for a testing slot by following these directions:

1. Go to *http://ptcb.org/*.
2. Click on "Apply for Certification."
3. Create an account or log in to an existing account.
4. Pay the $129 fee.
5. Receive authorization to schedule and take the PTCE. Candidates are sent an authorization to test letter (ATT) via e-mail.
6. Go to *http://pearsonvue.com/ptcb/* or call 866-902-0593 to schedule an appointment.
7. Choose a date, time, and location that works for you to take your exam.

Unofficial preliminary results are available immediately after taking the exam. Official exam results and scores will be posted to your PTCB account 2 to 3 weeks following the examination, and an official certificate will be available for download. Candidates who pass the PTCE will also receive a certification from the Pharmacy Technician Certification Board approximately 4 to 6 weeks after taking the exam. After successfully passing the PTCE examination, candidates will be able to use the certified pharmacy technician (CPhT) designation immediately following their name.

Test-Taking Skills and Strategies Plus Steps for Recertification

3

BEFORE THE TEST

Using this book is an excellent way to review core concepts. However, the PTCB offers other options to help you prepare for the examination.

One option is to visit *http://ptcb.org/* and take a practice test provided by the PTCB:

- The PTCB official practice test is aligned with recent changes to the testing blueprint.
- The format is similar in functionality and mirrors the look of the official examination. The practice test allows candidates to become familiar with the test and the testing environment.
- A fee of $29 dollars is required. You must complete the 90 questions in a maximum of 1 hour and 50 minutes.
- Students will receive a grade and 24 hours of post exam review. No diagnostic information will be provided, and the grade is not scored the same way as the PTCE.
- Only one version of the official practice test is currently available.

Another option allows candidates to become familiar with the testing atmosphere via a testing tutorial:

- Visit *http://www.pearsonvue.com/athena/athena.asp* to download a simulated practice exam and participate in a testing tutorial.
- The computerized testing tutorial allows users to navigate through the testing process. Users will have access to a sample, nonspecific, content-based exam where they can get a feel for the test-taking process.
- The tutorial explains how to answer questions, change answers, and review questions.

Remember these general rules:

- Review the PTCB blueprint to provide yourself with a basis about what you are expected to know.
- Review concepts that you need to understand better.
- Make a study timeline over several weeks or months. Stick to it!
- Test your knowledge by practicing test questions.
- Be confident in your abilities!

TIP

After reviewing the exam material and scheduling your test date, be sure to get adequate sleep the night before the examination!

EXAM DAY

Candidates should arrive 30 minutes prior to the scheduled exam in order to check in. Pearson VUE testing centers require you to bring identification that properly matches the ATT letter. Identification must be valid, unexpired, and government issued. Examples of proper identification can be found on the PTCB website and include:

- A passport
- A government-issued driver's license
- A government-issued driving learner's permit
- An official ID issued by a government agency to nondrivers
- A military ID
- A permanent resident card
- A U.S. Department of Homeland Security-issued employment authorization card

The test center may provide lockers for the storage of personal items; be aware that this varies by location. Items brought to the test center are not allowed in the secure testing area. Examples of personal items include purses, wallets, and cell phones. You may not study in, or bring visitors into, the test center.

After the testing assistant has checked you in and verified your authorization to take the exam, you will be escorted to the testing area. You will be given materials to take notes on or make calculations on as needed and as allowed by the PTCB. A calculator is available to candidates on the computer screen, but a physical calculator may also be requested. You must return all materials to the testing assistant upon completion of your exam. You will then be logged in to the testing computer to begin your exam. Candidates are monitored during the examination and may be recorded.

The PTCE examination has a maximum time allotment of 110 minutes (1 hour and 50 minutes). If you choose to take a break, you must alert the testing assistant by raising your hand. The time will not stop during the unscheduled break, so be aware that time will continue to run down if you do require a break.

AFTER THE EXAM

After completing the exam, you will receive an unofficial score on your computer screen. The test center will also provide you with an unofficial printed copy of the test results. You will have access to your official score report online approximately 1 to 3 weeks following your exam. Scores are not given via e-mail, phone, or U.S. mail.

An official certificate and wallet card will be mailed out approximately 4 to 6 weeks following your exam. You will also have access to an official downloadable certificate by logging in to your account.

You may also request for a test to be hand scored by downloading a "Hand Score Request Form" and submitting a $50 fee to the PTCB. These requests must be completed within 30 days of taking the exam. Results are provided in approximately 4 to 6 weeks.

Candidates are allowed 4 attempts to take the PTCE. They must wait 60 days before applying for the second and third attempt and 6 months before applying for the fourth attempt.

RECERTIFICATION

In order to maintain certification, every CPhT will need to complete a minimum of 20 hours of continuing education (CE) during a 2-year cycle:

- 1 hour of CE must be on pharmacy law (pharmacy technician specific).
- 1 hour of CE must be on patient safety (pharmacy technician specific).
- A maximum of 10 hours may be earned from taking an approved college course and earning a grade of "C" or better.
- A maximum of 5 hours may be earned by completing an in-service project or by training under the direct supervision of a pharmacist. The in-service project or training activity must be outside of the technician's regular responsibilities.
- CE hours do not carry over to the next recertification cycle.

Examples of continuing education providers include:

- Accreditation Council for Pharmacy Education (*https://www.acpe-accredit.org/*)
- American Association of Pharmacy Technicians (*www.pharmacytechnician.com/*)
- American Pharmacists Association® (*www.pharmacist.com/*)
- American Society of Health-System Pharmacists (*www.ashp.org/*)
- Drug Store News (*www.drugstorenews.com/*)
- Drug Topics® (*http://drugtopics.modernmedicine.com/*)
- FreeCE (*www.freece.com/*)
- National Pharmacy Technician Association (*http://www.pharmacytechnician.org/*)
- Pharmacy TechCE (*www.pharmacytechce.org/*)
- Pharmacy Times® (*www.pharmacytimes.com/*)
- U.S. Pharmacist (*www.uspharmacist.com/*)
- State pharmacy associations

Recertification may be completed through your PTCB account via an online application and payment of a $40 recertification fee. Applications for recertification can be made 100 days prior to the certification expiration date but must be submitted at least 30 days prior to the certification expiration date.

In the event that recertification is not completed in time, the pharmacy technician can apply for reinstatement by paying an $80 fee.

ANSWER SHEET
Pretest

1. Ⓐ Ⓑ Ⓒ Ⓓ
2. Ⓐ Ⓑ Ⓒ Ⓓ
3. Ⓐ Ⓑ Ⓒ Ⓓ
4. Ⓐ Ⓑ Ⓒ Ⓓ
5. Ⓐ Ⓑ Ⓒ Ⓓ
6. Ⓐ Ⓑ Ⓒ Ⓓ
7. Ⓐ Ⓑ Ⓒ Ⓓ
8. Ⓐ Ⓑ Ⓒ Ⓓ
9. Ⓐ Ⓑ Ⓒ Ⓓ
10. Ⓐ Ⓑ Ⓒ Ⓓ
11. Ⓐ Ⓑ Ⓒ Ⓓ
12. Ⓐ Ⓑ Ⓒ Ⓓ
13. Ⓐ Ⓑ Ⓒ Ⓓ
14. Ⓐ Ⓑ Ⓒ Ⓓ
15. Ⓐ Ⓑ Ⓒ Ⓓ
16. Ⓐ Ⓑ Ⓒ Ⓓ
17. Ⓐ Ⓑ Ⓒ Ⓓ
18. Ⓐ Ⓑ Ⓒ Ⓓ
19. Ⓐ Ⓑ Ⓒ Ⓓ
20. Ⓐ Ⓑ Ⓒ Ⓓ
21. Ⓐ Ⓑ Ⓒ Ⓓ
22. Ⓐ Ⓑ Ⓒ Ⓓ
23. Ⓐ Ⓑ Ⓒ Ⓓ
24. Ⓐ Ⓑ Ⓒ Ⓓ
25. Ⓐ Ⓑ Ⓒ Ⓓ
26. Ⓐ Ⓑ Ⓒ Ⓓ
27. Ⓐ Ⓑ Ⓒ Ⓓ
28. Ⓐ Ⓑ Ⓒ Ⓓ
29. Ⓐ Ⓑ Ⓒ Ⓓ
30. Ⓐ Ⓑ Ⓒ Ⓓ

31. Ⓐ Ⓑ Ⓒ Ⓓ
32. Ⓐ Ⓑ Ⓒ Ⓓ
33. Ⓐ Ⓑ Ⓒ Ⓓ
34. Ⓐ Ⓑ Ⓒ Ⓓ
35. Ⓐ Ⓑ Ⓒ Ⓓ
36. Ⓐ Ⓑ Ⓒ Ⓓ
37. Ⓐ Ⓑ Ⓒ Ⓓ
38. Ⓐ Ⓑ Ⓒ Ⓓ
39. Ⓐ Ⓑ Ⓒ Ⓓ
40. Ⓐ Ⓑ Ⓒ Ⓓ
41. Ⓐ Ⓑ Ⓒ Ⓓ
42. Ⓐ Ⓑ Ⓒ Ⓓ
43. Ⓐ Ⓑ Ⓒ Ⓓ
44. Ⓐ Ⓑ Ⓒ Ⓓ
45. Ⓐ Ⓑ Ⓒ Ⓓ
46. Ⓐ Ⓑ Ⓒ Ⓓ
47. Ⓐ Ⓑ Ⓒ Ⓓ
48. Ⓐ Ⓑ Ⓒ Ⓓ
49. Ⓐ Ⓑ Ⓒ Ⓓ
50. Ⓐ Ⓑ Ⓒ Ⓓ
51. Ⓐ Ⓑ Ⓒ Ⓓ
52. Ⓐ Ⓑ Ⓒ Ⓓ
53. Ⓐ Ⓑ Ⓒ Ⓓ
54. Ⓐ Ⓑ Ⓒ Ⓓ
55. Ⓐ Ⓑ Ⓒ Ⓓ
56. Ⓐ Ⓑ Ⓒ Ⓓ
57. Ⓐ Ⓑ Ⓒ Ⓓ
58. Ⓐ Ⓑ Ⓒ Ⓓ
59. Ⓐ Ⓑ Ⓒ Ⓓ
60. Ⓐ Ⓑ Ⓒ Ⓓ

61. Ⓐ Ⓑ Ⓒ Ⓓ
62. Ⓐ Ⓑ Ⓒ Ⓓ
63. Ⓐ Ⓑ Ⓒ Ⓓ
64. Ⓐ Ⓑ Ⓒ Ⓓ
65. Ⓐ Ⓑ Ⓒ Ⓓ
66. Ⓐ Ⓑ Ⓒ Ⓓ
67. Ⓐ Ⓑ Ⓒ Ⓓ
68. Ⓐ Ⓑ Ⓒ Ⓓ
69. Ⓐ Ⓑ Ⓒ Ⓓ
70. Ⓐ Ⓑ Ⓒ Ⓓ
71. Ⓐ Ⓑ Ⓒ Ⓓ
72. Ⓐ Ⓑ Ⓒ Ⓓ
73. Ⓐ Ⓑ Ⓒ Ⓓ
74. Ⓐ Ⓑ Ⓒ Ⓓ
75. Ⓐ Ⓑ Ⓒ Ⓓ
76. Ⓐ Ⓑ Ⓒ Ⓓ
77. Ⓐ Ⓑ Ⓒ Ⓓ
78. Ⓐ Ⓑ Ⓒ Ⓓ
79. Ⓐ Ⓑ Ⓒ Ⓓ
80. Ⓐ Ⓑ Ⓒ Ⓓ
81. Ⓐ Ⓑ Ⓒ Ⓓ
82. Ⓐ Ⓑ Ⓒ Ⓓ
83. Ⓐ Ⓑ Ⓒ Ⓓ
84. Ⓐ Ⓑ Ⓒ Ⓓ
85. Ⓐ Ⓑ Ⓒ Ⓓ
86. Ⓐ Ⓑ Ⓒ Ⓓ
87. Ⓐ Ⓑ Ⓒ Ⓓ
88. Ⓐ Ⓑ Ⓒ Ⓓ
89. Ⓐ Ⓑ Ⓒ Ⓓ
90. Ⓐ Ⓑ Ⓒ Ⓓ

Pretest

4

Directions: You will have 1 hour and 50 minutes to complete the following 90 questions. For each question, select the choice that best answers the question, and mark that answer letter on your answer sheet. Remember, this test should be used to help you determine areas that require additional review. Each question represents a particular area of the PTCE blueprint, which can help you pinpoint areas of mastery or concepts that require additional studying. The official PTCE exam uses a scaled score to determine your grade. Only 80 out of 90 questions on the PTCE are scored, and unscored questions are not identified. You should be able to answer about 75 of the questions on this test correctly, averaging an overall percentage of 80% or more on your attempt at this test.

1. For which of the following conditions would a patient receive an inhaler?

   (A) asthma
   (B) diabetes
   (C) hypertension
   (D) gout

2. A patient presents a prescription for Lasix 40 mg, which has been authorized for generic substitution. Which of the following medications may be substituted for Lasix 40 mg?

   (A) metoprolol
   (B) furosemide
   (C) alprazolam
   (D) diltiazem

3. Which of the following is NOT a parenteral route of administration?

   (A) IV
   (B) IM
   (C) SQ
   (D) PO

4. What does the first set of numbers represent in the following National Drug Code (NDC) number?

   00456-012-03

   (A) package size
   (B) manufacturer
   (C) product
   (D) medication indication

5. The laminar flow hood is turned on at 6:00 A.M. What is the earliest time that the technician may use it?

   (A) 6:00 A.M.
   (B) 6:15 A.M.
   (C) 6:30 A.M.
   (D) 7:00 A.M.

6. The following prescription has been received by your pharmacy:

   Prednisone 5 mg #QS
   Sig: 20 mg BID × 2D
   15 mg BID × 2D
   10 mg BID × 2D
   5 mg BID × 2D
   5 mg QD × 2D

   What is the quantity needed to fill this prescription?

   (A) 32 tablets
   (B) 36 tablets
   (C) 42 tablets
   (D) 48 tablets

7. Which of the following auxiliary labels should be included on the label for Augmentin oral suspension?

   (A) "Shake Well Before Using"
   (B) "For The Nose"
   (C) "For External Use Only"
   (D) "Chew Tablets Before Swallowing"

8. A physician orders drug "x" 500 mg BID × 30D. The pharmacy has drug "x" 250 mg in stock. How many 250 mg tablets of drug "x" are needed to fill this order?

   (A) 30 tablets
   (B) 60 tablets
   (C) 90 tablets
   (D) 120 tablets

9. Which of the following medications may NOT have any refills on the same prescription?

   (A) Actos
   (B) Lasix
   (C) Xanax
   (D) Oxycontin

10. How many grams of glucose would you need to make 500 mL of a 10% glucose solution?

    (A) 20 g
    (B) 50 g
    (C) 75 g
    (D) 100 g

11. How many grams of dextrose are contained in a liter of D5W?

    (A) 25 g
    (B) 50 g
    (C) 75 g
    (D) 100 g

12. Which of the following reference books should be used to verify the therapeutic equivalence of products?

    (A) *Physicians' Desk Reference*®
    (B) *Drug Facts and Comparisons*
    (C) *Orange Book*
    (D) *USP-NF*

13. Acyclovir belongs to what drug classification?

    (A) antibiotic
    (B) antiviral
    (C) antiemetic
    (D) antihypertensive

14. Name the type of needle used to prevent glass from entering the final solution when drawing medication from an ampule.

    (A) ampule needle
    (B) universal needle
    (C) curved needle
    (D) filter needle

15. The process of dissolving powder drugs with diluents, such as water or normal saline, is known as _____.

    (A) reconstitution
    (B) levigation
    (C) spatulation
    (D) geometric dilution

16. Which schedule of controlled substances has the highest abuse potential and also an accepted medical use?

    (A) Schedule I
    (B) Schedule II
    (C) Schedule III
    (D) Schedule IV

17. A physician orders amiodarone (Cordarone) 300 mg in 100 mL of D5W to be infused over 30 minutes. Determine the IV flow rate in mL/hour.

    (A) 200 mL/hour
    (B) 100 mL/hour
    (C) 75 mL/hour
    (D) 50 mL/hour

18. Look at the following DEA number:

    BA234567__

    What is the last number in this DEA number sequence?

    (A) 3
    (B) 2
    (C) 4
    (D) 5

19. OBRA '90 requires pharmacists to perform which of the following responsibilities?

    (A) provide prospective drug utilization review and an offer of counseling to discuss the patient's unique therapeutic drug regimen
    (B) lock Schedule II substances in a safe
    (C) provide childproof packaging on prescriptions
    (D) complete an inventory of controlled substances on a biennial basis

20. How many times can a Class III or a Class IV prescription be transferred by pharmacies that do not share the same online database?

    (A) once
    (B) twice
    (C) three times
    (D) never

21. Which of the following would be used to identify a medication in a recall situation?

    (A) lot number and NDC
    (B) drug name and NDC
    (C) drug strength and lot number
    (D) manufacturer and lot number

22. Which of the following dosage forms contains the highest concentration of alcohol?

    (A) solution
    (B) capsule
    (C) suspension
    (D) elixir

23. A laminar flow hood should be cleaned using which of the following methods?

    (A) front to back and bottom to top
    (B) top to bottom and back to front
    (C) side to side and top to bottom
    (D) top to bottom and side to side

24. The markup for a $47.99 bottle of medication is 18%. What is the retail price of this medication?

    (A) $56.63
    (B) $62.99
    (C) $68.25
    (D) $73.49

25. Which of the following clinical decision support systems helps identify problems with medications that are prescribed with the same indication?

    (A) drug-drug interactions
    (B) drug-food interactions
    (C) drug-disease interactions
    (D) therapeutic duplication

26. A(n) _____ agent is used to stabilize a solution against degradation by resisting changes in pH.

    (A) emulsifier
    (B) tonicity agent
    (C) pH buffer
    (D) antioxidant

27. In the absence of stability information, what is the appropriate beyond use date for an oral suspension?

    (A) no later than 6 months
    (B) no later than 14 days
    (C) no later than 30 days
    (D) one year

28. What is the therapeutic classification of clopidogrel?

    (A) inhibitor of platelet aggregation
    (B) antidiabetic
    (C) antihyperlipidemic
    (D) antihypertensive

29. A patient requests a refill for Diazepam 10 mg. After reviewing the patient's profile, the technician discovers that the prescription has been refilled 5 times. The pharmacy technician should _____.

    (A) refill the prescription
    (B) notify a pharmacist because the prescription cannot be refilled
    (C) ask the patient to provide a valid DEA 222 order form
    (D) refuse to fill since the strength of the requested medication is commercially unavailable

30. Which regulatory agency may issue a drug recall?

    (A) DEA
    (B) FDA
    (C) CDC
    (D) USP

31. How is pharmaceutical hazardous waste handled?

    (A) Personnel should consult the medication's MSDS and handle the waste accordingly.
    (B) Personnel can throw hazardous waste into a regular trash bag.
    (C) Personnel should leave the hazardous waste in the compounding area until someone can pick up the hazardous waste and dispose of it.
    (D) Personnel should place the hazardous waste into a sharps container.

32. What is the name of the federal insurance program for patients 65 years and older?

    (A) Medicaid
    (B) Medicare
    (C) PPO
    (D) HMO

33. The Roman numeral CXIV is equal to _____.

    (A) 34
    (B) 54
    (C) 104
    (D) 114

34. PHI is regulated and protected under HIPAA. What does PHI stand for?

    (A) patient health information
    (B) protected health information
    (C) people health information
    (D) personal health information

35. Federal law requires prescriptions to be maintained in the pharmacy for how many years?

    (A) 1 year
    (B) 2 years
    (C) 3 years
    (D) 4 years

36. Which of the following drugs is classified as an antifungal agent?

(A) itraconazole (Sporanox)
(B) oseltamivir (Tamiflu)
(C) clarithromycin (Biaxin)
(D) doxycycline (Vibramycin)

37. Which of the following is NOT an example of a combination drug?

(A) Benzamycin
(B) Atripla
(C) Unasyn
(D) Zyvox

38. Normal saline contains _____ NaCl.

(A) 0.33%
(B) 0.45%
(C) 0.9%
(D) 1.9%

39. Which government agency oversees safety in the workplace?

(A) ASHP
(B) FDA
(C) DEA
(D) OSHA

40. What does "DAW" mean when on a written prescription?

(A) Refills are limited to 5 times within a 6-month period.
(B) The medication should be taken with food.
(C) The brand name medication is to be dispensed as written, with no generic substitution.
(D) The medication is a controlled substance.

41. Nitroglycerin is available as a sublingual tablet, which means that _____.

(A) the tablet should be dissolved under the tongue
(B) the tablet should be swallowed whole, not chewed
(C) the tablet is a sustained, released (long-acting) form
(D) the tablet may be crushed and mixed with applesauce for patients with swallowing problems

42. HEPA stands for _____.

(A) horizontal extraction particulate air filter
(B) high-extraction particle air filter
(C) horizontal efficient parenteral air filter
(D) high-efficiency particulate air filter

43. Which of the following is NOT found on a unit-dose package labeling?

(A) patient's name
(B) expiration date
(C) drug name
(D) strength

44. When a technician receives a rejected claim labeled "invalid person code," this probably means that _____.

(A) the patient is on Medicare
(B) the patient has a mail order program
(C) the person code that was entered does not match the date of birth and/or gender in the insurer's computer
(D) the patient is on Medicaid

45. Visual inspection of parenteral solutions can show the presence of _____ and _____.

(A) particle contamination; precipitation
(B) pH; precipitation
(C) chemical degradation of a drug; osmolarity
(D) pyrogens; precipitation

46. Which of the following OTC medications must be recorded, either electronically or written in a book, before being sold?

    (A) acetaminophen
    (B) cetirizine
    (C) pseudoephedrine
    (D) clotrimazole

47. How many milliliters of 95% (v/v) alcohol and 30% (v/v) alcohol should be mixed to prepare 1,000 mL of a 50% (v/v) solution?

    (A) 502 mL, 498 mL
    (B) 308 mL, 692 mL
    (C) 246 mL, 754 mL
    (D) 130 mL, 870 mL

48. Which disease state is characterized by polyuria, polydipsia, and polyphagia?

    (A) hypertension
    (B) gout
    (C) diabetes
    (D) arthritis

49. How many 30 mg tablets of codeine sulfate should be used in preparing the following prescription?

    Rx: codeine sulfate 15 mg/tsp
        robitussin at 120 mL

    (A) 10 tablets
    (B) 11 tablets
    (C) 12 tablets
    (D) 13 tablets

50. A patient has called in a refill for a selective COX-2 inhibitor. Which of the following drugs should be filled?

    (A) ibuprofen
    (B) naproxen
    (C) celecoxib
    (D) omeprazole

51. Where should a pharmacy store a policy and procedure manual?

    (A) The manual should be in the pharmacy library so it can be checked out.
    (B) The manual should be in the pharmacy manager's office.
    (C) The manual should be in the work area so it is accessible to all personnel.
    (D) A policy and procedure manual is not needed in a pharmacy.

52. Which of the following should NOT be donned by an operator before entering the buffer area?

    (A) gown
    (B) hair cover
    (C) shoe cover
    (D) jewelry

53. The type of drug recall in which the drug may cause serious harm to a patient is called a _____ recall.

    (A) Class I
    (B) Class II
    (C) Class III
    (D) Class IV

54. Which of the following laws protects the privacy rights of the patient?

    (A) OBRA
    (B) HIPAA
    (C) PPPA
    (D) MSDS

55. What is the most important piece of information to verify before filling a patient's prescription?

    (A) the patient's identity
    (B) the patient's insurance
    (C) the patient's address
    (D) the patient's method of payment

56. What word should be used when giving directions for a topical medication?

   (A) take
   (B) insert
   (C) apply
   (D) inhale

57. The abbreviation "a.c." means _____.

   (A) before meals
   (B) after meals
   (C) before bedtime
   (D) before midnight

58. Which of the following safety strategies is used to distinguish medications that have look-alike/sound-alike names?

   (A) short man lettering
   (B) tall man lettering
   (C) colored lettering
   (D) bar codes

59. What volume of a 25 mg/mL solution should be measured to deliver a dose of 40 mg?

   (A) 1.25 mL
   (B) 1.6 mL
   (C) 2.0 mL
   (D) 2.4 mL

60. How many ounces of medication are needed to last 10 days if the dose of medication is one and one half teaspoonfuls twice a day?

   (A) 2 oz
   (B) 3 oz
   (C) 4 oz
   (D) 5 oz

61. A formulary with a limited listing of drugs is called a(n) _____.

   (A) open formulary
   (B) limited formulary
   (C) closed formulary
   (D) restricted formulary

62. What is the name of the label placed onto prescriptions to warn patients and/or provide additional information?

   (A) auxiliary label
   (B) prescription label
   (C) medication guide
   (D) patient package insert

63. Which of the following patient monitoring functions will detect a patient taking a drug that may cause an allergic response?

   (A) drug-drug
   (B) drug-allergy
   (C) drug-food
   (D) therapeutic duplication

64. Which of the following medications does NOT need to be packaged in child-resistant containers?

   (A) metoprolol
   (B) lovastatin
   (C) nitroglycerin sublingual
   (D) penicillin

65. Which of the following is an example of a pair of drugs with look-alike/sound-alike names?

   (A) buspirone/bupropion
   (B) metoprolol/metoclopramide
   (C) penicillin/ampicillin
   (D) omeprazole/ritonavir

66. A patient tells you that he missed his last dose of glyburide. What should you do?

   (A) Tell the patient to take the next dose ASAP.
   (B) Call the pharmacist over to counsel the patient.
   (C) Call the doctor.
   (D) Tell the patient to skip the dose.

67. Convert 15°C to degrees Fahrenheit.

   (A) 55°F
   (B) 57°F
   (C) 59°F
   (D) 61°F

68. What does the last set of numbers of an NDC number indicate?

    (A) manufacturer
    (B) drug
    (C) strength
    (D) package size

69. Single-use container vials _____.

    (A) do not contain preservatives
    (B) contain preservatives
    (C) should not be used for sterile compounding procedures
    (D) contain bacterial endotoxins

70. At what standard time would a patient receive a medication if the military time is 0700 hours?

    (A) 7:00 A.M.
    (B) 7:00 P.M.
    (C) 11:00 A.M.
    (D) 11:00 P.M.

71. Pharmacists are licensed by which agency?

    (A) DEA
    (B) FDA
    (C) ASHP
    (D) State Board of Pharmacy

72. Ativan is the brand name for which drug?

    (A) enalapril
    (B) lorazepam
    (C) lisinopril
    (D) meloxicam

73. Which of the following medications should receive a patient package insert (PPI)?

    (A) Premarin
    (B) amoxicillin
    (C) omeprazole
    (D) lisinopril

74. What should pharmacy counting trays and counters be disinfected with?

    (A) water
    (B) 90% isopropyl alcohol
    (C) 70% isopropyl alcohol
    (D) antibacterial soap

75. What is the maximum weighable amount for a Class A prescription balance?

    (A) 12 g
    (B) 80 g
    (C) 100 g
    (D) 120 g

76. Which of the following dosage forms would be appropriate for a patient who is experiencing nausea and vomiting?

    (A) suppository
    (B) tablet
    (C) suspension
    (D) elixir

77. Inderal is to hypertension as Tazorac is to _____.

    (A) GERD
    (B) BPH
    (C) acne
    (D) psoriasis

78. In a Class 100 environment, the size of the particles per cubic foot of air should not exceed _____ microns and larger.

    (A) 0.3
    (B) 0.4
    (C) 0.5
    (D) 0.6

79. An intravenous medication is administered directly into the _____.

    (A) muscle
    (B) vein
    (C) eye
    (D) skin

80. Where is the volume of an aqueous liquid read on a graduated cylinder?

(A) top surface of the liquid
(B) bottom surface of the liquid
(C) bottom of the meniscus
(D) top of the meniscus

81. A prescription is written for "ProAir HFA #1, Sig: 1–2 puffs q 4–6h prn." If there are 200 doses in one inhaler, what is the day's supply?

(A) 5 days
(B) 16 days
(C) 30 days
(D) 50 days

82. Which of the following DEA forms should be used to surrender out-of-date controlled medications?

(A) DEA Form 222
(B) DEA Form 106
(C) DEA Form 41
(D) DEA Form 224

83. A CPhT must complete 20 hours of continuing education within a 2-year period. How many of those hours must be in patient safety?

(A) 20
(B) 10
(C) 2
(D) 1

84. Which of the following medications should be taken with a glass of water while sitting in an upright position for a minimum of 30 minutes?

(A) alendronate
(B) simvastatin
(C) oxycodone
(D) amoxicillin

85. Which of the following dosage forms bypasses the stomach when ingested?

(A) enteric coated tablet
(B) powder
(C) capsule
(D) suspension

86. Patient assistance programs are offered by which entity?

(A) pharmacy
(B) physician
(C) drug manufacturer
(D) medication distributor

87. Humulin R contains 100 units/mL. How much is needed for a 12-unit dose?

(A) 12 mL
(B) 1.2 mL
(C) 0.12 mL
(D) 1 mL

88. Which of the following is NOT an example of a type of technology that is used in pharmacy information systems?

(A) IVR
(B) reference books
(C) bar codes
(D) touch screens

89. Why are medications rotated on pharmacy shelves?

(A) to move medications that will expire first in front of medications that have a longer shelf life
(B) to prevent dust from accumulating on stock bottles
(C) to consolidate medications for more shelf space
(D) to move newer bottles to the front of the shelf

90. Which of the following is a high-alert medication, as reported by ISMP?

(A) amoxicillin
(B) warfarin
(C) naproxen
(D) lovastatin

PRETEST

1. **A**	31. **A**	61. **C**
2. **B**	32. **B**	62. **A**
3. **D**	33. **D**	63. **B**
4. **B**	34. **B**	64. **C**
5. **C**	35. **B**	65. **A**
6. **C**	36. **A**	66. **B**
7. **A**	37. **D**	67. **C**
8. **D**	38. **C**	68. **D**
9. **D**	39. **D**	69. **A**
10. **B**	40. **C**	70. **A**
11. **B**	41. **A**	71. **D**
12. **C**	42. **D**	72. **B**
13. **B**	43. **A**	73. **A**
14. **D**	44. **C**	74. **C**
15. **A**	45. **A**	75. **D**
16. **B**	46. **C**	76. **A**
17. **A**	47. **B**	77. **C**
18. **B**	48. **C**	78. **C**
19. **A**	49. **C**	79. **B**
20. **A**	50. **C**	80. **C**
21. **A**	51. **C**	81. **B**
22. **D**	52. **D**	82. **C**
23. **B**	53. **A**	83. **D**
24. **A**	54. **B**	84. **A**
25. **D**	55. **A**	85. **A**
26. **C**	56. **C**	86. **C**
27. **B**	57. **A**	87. **C**
28. **A**	58. **B**	88. **B**
29. **B**	59. **B**	89. **A**
30. **B**	60. **D**	90. **B**

ANSWERS EXPLAINED

1. **(A)** Patients who have asthma experience trouble breathing and require the use of an inhaler to open their airways, allowing for the passage of oxygen to their lungs more freely. Patients with type 1 or type 2 diabetes have high blood glucose levels and require the use of insulin and/or an oral hypoglycemic to correct one of the following: insulin resistance, insulin deficiency, or increased hepatic glucose output. Hypertensive patients experience high blood pressure. Treatment includes aerobic exercise, salt intake reduction, lifestyle changes, weight reduction, and antihypertensives. Gout is a condition that results when the body lacks the ability to process uric acid, resulting in increased levels of uric acid in the body. (*Knowledge Domain 1.6*)

2. **(B)** Furosemide is the generic equivalent for Lasix. Metoprolol is the generic equivalent for Toprol XL. Alprazolam is the generic equivalent for Xanax. Diltiazem is the generic equivalent for Cardizem. (*Knowledge Domain 1.1*)

3. **(D)** PO, or per oral, is an enteral route of administration, meaning that it requires absorption through the gastrointestinal tract before reaching the bloodstream. IV (intravenous), IM (intramuscular), and SQ (subcutaneous) are all parenteral routes of administration that are not absorbed through the gastrointestinal tract. (*Knowledge Domain 1.4*)

4. **(B)** The manufacturer, or labeler, is indicated by the first set of numbers in the NDC. The package size is indicated by the last set of numbers in the NDC. The product is indicated by the second, or middle, set of numbers in the NDC. The medication indication is not represented by the NDC. (*Knowledge Domain 5.1*)

5. **(C)** The laminar flow hood should be turned on for a minimum of 30 minutes before use. (*Knowledge Domain 3.5*)

6. **(C)** 20 mg BID × 2D = (4 tablets × 2) × 2 = 16 tablets
   15 mg BID × 2D = (3 tablets × 2) × 2 = 12 tablets
   10 mg BID × 2D = (2 tablets × 2) × 2 = 8 tablets
   5 mg BID × 2D = (1 tablet × 2) × 2 = 4 tablets
   5 mg QD × 2D = (1 tablet × 1) × 2 = 2 tablets
   16 + 12 + 8 + 4 + 2 = 42 tablets (*Knowledge Domain 6.3*)

7. **(A)** The label "Shake Well Before Using" is commonly placed on suspensions because they contain undissolved particles in a liquid solvent. "For The Nose" and "For External Use Only" are not appropriate auxiliary labels for an oral medication. "Chew Tablets Before Swallowing" is not an appropriate auxiliary label for an oral suspension. (*Knowledge Domain 6.5*)

8. **(D)** The prescription is written for 500 mg BID × 30D. The pharmacy has 250 mg BID × 30D. You will need 2 of the 250 mg tablets to equal 1 of the 500 mg tablets; (2 × 2) × 30 = 120 tablets. (*Knowledge Domain 6.3*)

9. **(D)** Oxycontin is a Class II substance. No refills are allowed for this substance (as per federal law). Actos and Lasix are both noncontrolled substances. These medications do not have limitations on the amount of refills unless expressly written on the prescription. Xanax is a Class IV substance. Per federal law, up to 5 refills in 6 months are allowed for this substance. (*Knowledge Domain 6.2*)

10. **(B)** Set up a proportion:

$$\frac{10 \text{ g}}{100 \text{ mL}} = \frac{x}{500 \text{ mL}}$$

$x = 50$ g (*Knowledge Domain 3.6*)

11. **(B)** Set up a proportion:

$$\frac{5 \text{ g}}{100 \text{ mL}} = \frac{x}{1,000 \text{ mL}}$$

$x = 50$ g (*Knowledge Domain 3.6*)

12. **(C)** The *Orange Book* provides a comprehensive listing of approved drug products and their therapeutic equivalences. The *Physicians' Desk Reference*® is a publication providing information pertaining to health care for both health professionals and consumers. The *Drug Facts and Comparisons* publication provides detailed information for both prescription and OTC drugs. The *USP-NF* provides information on drug purity and quality, including official monographs of drugs. (*Knowledge Domain 2.15*)

13. **(B)** Acyclovir is classified as an antiviral. (*Knowledge Domain 1.6*)

14. **(D)** A filter needle is used when withdrawing medication from an ampule. (*Knowledge Domain 3.5*)

15. **(A)** Reconstitution is the process of mixing a powder with diluents prior to administration. Levigation is the process of grinding a powder by incorporating a liquid. Spatulation is the process of using a spatula to mix ingredients in a plastic bag, on ointment paper, or on another medium. Geometric dilution is the process used when mixing two or more ingredients of different quantities to achieve a homogenous mixture. (*Knowledge Domain 3.7*)

16. **(B)** Schedule II medications have a high potential for abuse and an accepted medical use in the United States. Schedule I medications have a high potential for abuse but do not have a currently accepted medical use in the United States. Schedule III medications have a potential for abuse that is less than Schedules I and II medications. Schedule IV medications contain a potential for abuse that is less than that of Schedule III medications. (*Knowledge Domain 2.4*)

17. **(A)** IV flow rate is determined using the following formula:

$$\frac{\text{volume (mL)}}{\text{time (min)}} \times \frac{60 \text{ min}}{1 \text{ hour}} = \text{IV flow rate} \left(\frac{\text{mL}}{\text{hr}}\right)$$

$$\frac{100 \text{ mL}}{30 \text{ min}} \times \frac{60 \text{ min}}{1 \text{ hour}} = \text{IV flow rate} \left(\frac{\text{mL}}{\text{hr}}\right)$$

$$\frac{200 \text{ mL}}{1 \text{ hr}} = \text{IV flow rate} \ (\textit{Knowledge Domain 3.3})$$

18. **(B)** The following formula can be used to determine the validity of a DEA number and to check the DEA number:

STEP 1 Add together the 1st, 3rd, and 5th numbers.

$$2 + 4 + 6 = 12$$

STEP 2 Add together the 2nd, 4th, and 6th numbers. Then double the total.

$$(3 + 5 + 7) \times 2 = 15 \times 2 = 30$$

(STEP 3) Add the two totals together.

$$12 + 30 = 4\underline{2}$$

The second number should match the last number in the DEA number sequence. (*Knowledge Domain 2.5*)

19. **(A)** OBRA '90 mandates that pharmacists provide prospective drug utilization review and an offer of counseling to discuss the patient's unique therapeutic drug regimen. The DEA mandates that pharmacists lock Schedule II substances in a safe. The Poison Prevention Packaging Act requires manufacturers to provide childproof packaging on prescriptions. Federal law mandates that an inventory of controlled substances be completed on a biennial basis. (*Knowledge Domain 2.9*)

20. **(A)** Controlled substances may be transferred only once if different online databases are used. (*Knowledge Domain 2.3*)

21. **(A)** The medication lot number and the NDC are used to identify a medication. The lot number is a production number used to track a product. (*Knowledge Domain 2.1*)

22. **(D)** Elixirs are hydroalcoholic liquids with an alcohol content range of 5–40% (10–80 proof). Solutions, capsules, and suspensions do not contain alcohol. (*Knowledge Domain 1.4*)

23. **(B)** Laminar flow hoods are cleaned from top to bottom and from back to front to eliminate contamination. (*Knowledge Domain 2.11*)

24. **(A)** $47.99 × 0.18 = $8.64
    $47.99 + $8.64 = $56.63 (*Knowledge Domain 8.2*)

25. **(D)** Therapeutic duplication monitoring is used to identify medications with the same indication or pharmacological drug class. Drug-drug interactions are used to identify medications that may cause problems if taken simultaneously. Drug-food interactions are used to identify medications that may cause allergies for the patient. Drug-disease interactions are used to identify medications that may cause problems with a patient's medical condition, age, weight, or other physiological factors. (*Knowledge Domain 9.1*)

26. **(C)** pH buffers help stabilize solutions against degradation by resisting changes in pH when quantities of acid or base are added. Emulsifiers are used to create a uniform concentration of an active drug in solution. Tonicity agents are used to help adjust the formulation to an appropriate isotonic range. Antioxidants prevent degradation against the component drug. (*Knowledge Domain 3.5*)

27. **(B)** Suspensions, oral solutions containing water, have a beyond use date of no later than 14 days from the reconstitution date. (*Knowledge Domain 3.4*)

28. **(A)** Plavix (clopidogrel) inhibits the aggregation of platelets, which is thought to be the primary mechanism of blood clotting. (*Knowledge Domain 1.6*)

29. **(B)** Prescriptions of Schedule III, IV, and V drugs cannot be refilled more than 5 times. A patient must bring in a new prescription after the last refill is executed. Prescriptions older than 6 months require a new prescription in order to be filled. (*Knowledge Domain 2.3*)

30. **(B)** The FDA may issue a drug recall. (*Knowledge Domain 5.4*)

31. **(A)** OSHA requires that Material Safety Data Sheets (MSDS) be maintained for all hazardous chemicals. Proper handling procedures may be found in each chemical's MSDS. (*Knowledge Domain 3.2*)

32. **(B)** Medicare is a national insurance program for people ages 65 years and older. Medicaid is a state funded insurance program for individuals who meet certain income guidelines. PPO and HMO are two types of private insurance. (*Knowledge Domain 8.1*)

33. **(D)** CXIV = 100 + 10 + 4 = 114 (*Knowledge Domain 6.1*)

34. **(B)** The acronym PHI stands for protected health information. (*Knowledge Domain 2.8*)

35. **(B)** Federal law mandates that prescriptions be maintained in the pharmacy for a period of 2 years. (*Knowledge Domain 2.6*)

36. **(A)** Itraconazole (Sporanox) is classified as an antifungal agent. Oseltamivir (Tamiflu) is classified as an antiviral agent. Clarithromycin (Biaxin) is classified as a macrolide antibiotic. Doxycycline (Vibramycin) is classified as a tetracycline antibiotic. (*Knowledge Domain 1.6*)

37. **(D)** Zyvox is an antibiotic containing the ingredient linezolid. Benzamycin is a combination acne drug containing erythromycin and benzoyl peroxide. Atripla is a combination antiretroviral drug containing efavirenz, emtricitabine, and tenofovir. Unasyn is a combination penicillin antibiotic containing ampicillin and sulbactam. (*Knowledge Domain 1.1*)

38. **(C)** Normal saline is a parenteral solution containing 0.9% NaCl. (*Knowledge Domain 3.5*)

39. **(D)** The OSHA oversees safety in the workplace. The ASHP is an organization that oversees the accreditation of pharmacy technician training programs. The FDA oversees the marketing and approval of drugs. The DEA implements the Controlled Substances Act. (*Knowledge Domain 2.11*)

40. **(C)** "DAW" is an acronym for "dispense as written." It indicates that the brand name drug should be dispensed. (*Knowledge Domain 6.2*)

41. **(A)** The word sublingual means "under the tongue." Therefore, nitroglycerin should be placed under the tongue. (*Knowledge Domain 1.4*)

42. **(D)** HEPA stands for high-efficiency particulate air filter. (*Knowledge Domain 3.5*)

43. **(A)** Unit-dose packaging is a method of preparing individual doses of medication. The container is not reusable, and it does not contain any patient identifying information. (*Knowledge Domain 3.3*)

44. **(C)** An "invalid person code" rejection error message is provided by the third-party reimburser as an indication that the person's date of birth or gender is missing or incorrect. (*Knowledge Domain 3.2*)

45. **(A)** Visual inspection of a parenteral preparation could indicate changes in color, the formation of precipitants, or the presence of contaminants in the solution. Changes in pH,

osmolarity, and the presence of pyrogens may not be visible to the naked eye. (*Knowledge Domain 5.3*)

46. **(C)** The Combat Methamphetamine Epidemic Act of 2005 places limitations on the amount of pseudoephedrine- and ephedrine-containing products that may be purchased. (*Knowledge Domain 2.7*)

47. **(B)**

> STEP 1 Set up an alligation (like the one pictured below), placing 95 in the top left corner and 30 in the bottom left corner. The final preparation concentration is placed in the middle. The "H" next to the "95" means that this is the highest concentration of alcohol. The "L" next to the "30" means that this is the lowest concentration of alcohol. The "P" next to the "50" means that this is the concentration of the final preparation.

95 (H)		20 (P − L)
	50 (P)	
30 (L)		45 (H − P)

> STEP 2 Determine the number of parts by subtracting as indicated above in the right column.

> STEP 3 Add the number of parts in the right column together to determine the total number of parts.

$$20 + 45 = 65 \text{ total parts}$$

> STEP 4 Set up a proportion to determine the quantity needed of each solution.

$$95\%: \frac{20}{65} = \frac{x}{1,000 \text{ mL}}$$

$$x = 308 \text{ mL}$$

$$30\%: \frac{45}{65} = \frac{x}{1,000 \text{ mL}}$$

$$x = 692 \text{ mL}$$

The answer is 308 mL, 692 mL. (*Knowledge Domain 3.6*)

48. **(C)** Polyuria (increased urine output), polydipsia (increased thirst), and polyphagia (excessive hunger) are all symptoms of diabetes. (*Knowledge Domain 1.5*)

49. **(C)**

> STEP 1 Set up a proportion to solve for the volume of robitussin needed for 30 mg of codeine sulfate.

$$\frac{15 \text{ mg}}{5 \text{ mL}} = \frac{30 \text{ mg}}{x}$$

$$x = 10 \text{ mL}$$

(STEP 2) Determine the amount of 30 mg tablets needed to produce 120 mL.

$$\frac{120 \text{ mL}}{10 \text{ mL}} = 12 \text{ tablets}$$

The answer is 12 tablets. (*Knowledge Domain 3.7*)

50. **(C)** Celecoxib is a selective COX-2 inhibitor. Ibuprofen and naproxen are both nonselective inhibitors of both COX-1 and COX-2. Omeprazole is a proton pump inhibitor (PPI). (*Knowledge Domain 1.1*)

51. **(C)** Policy and procedure manuals should be kept in an accessible work area. (*Knowledge Domain 2.15*)

52. **(D)** Prior to entering the buffer area, the operator should remove all jewelry, cosmetics, and outerwear. The operator should don appropriate PPE, including shoe and hair covers and a gown. (*Knowledge Domain 3.1*)

53. **(A)** A Class I recall involves violative products that are likely to cause serious adverse health consequences or death. A Class II recall involves violative products that may cause temporary health issues or the probability of serious adverse health consequence is remote. A Class III recall involves violative products that are not likely to cause adverse health consequences. There are no Class IV recalls. (*Knowledge Domain 2.10*)

54. **(B)** The Health Insurance Portability and Accountability Act (HIPAA) protects patient information. The Omnibus Budget Reconciliation Act (OBRA) mandates counseling for all Medicaid patients. The Poison Prevention Packaging Act (PPPA) requires safety caps for over-the-counter and prescription medications. Material Safety Data Sheets (MSDS) are provided by the manufacturer and provide information about hazardous chemicals, including handling and disposal procedures. (*Knowledge Domain 2.8*)

55. **(A)** The patient's identity is the most important piece of information to verify. Do this by confirming the patient's date of birth, address, and phone number. (*Knowledge Domain 6.1*)

56. **(C)** "Apply" is used for medications that will be applied topically. "Take" is used for medications that will be ingested orally. "Insert" is used for medications that will be inserted vaginally or rectally. "Inhale" is used for medications that will be breathed or inhaled through the mouth. (*Knowledge Domain 6.5*)

57. **(A)** The abbreviation "a.c" means "before meals" and indicates that the patient should take the medication before eating. (*Knowledge Domain 6.2*)

58. **(B)** Tall man lettering is a strategy used to distinguish the parts of similar words that are different. (*Knowledge Domain 4.6*)

59. **(B)**

$$\frac{25 \text{ mg}}{1 \text{ mL}} = \frac{40 \text{ mg}}{x}$$
$$x = 1.6 \text{ mL}$$

The answer is 1.6 mL. (*Knowledge Domain 6.3*)

60. **(D)** Remember that one and one half teaspoonfuls = 7.5 mL.

$$7.5 \text{ mL} \times 2 = 15 \text{ mL a day}$$

$$15 \text{ mL} \times 10 = 150 \text{ mL}$$

$$\frac{30 \text{ mL}}{1 \text{ oz}} = \frac{150 \text{ mL}}{x}$$

$$x = 5 \text{ oz}$$

The answer is 5 oz. (*Knowledge Domain 6.3*)

61. **(C)** A closed formulary places limits on the amount of drugs that are covered by the Pharmacy Benefits Manager. (*Knowledge Domain 7.2*)

62. **(A)** Auxiliary labels are labels that contain warnings or instructions for administration. Prescription labels contain the drug name, dose, instructions for use, quantity, expiration date, patient's name, physician's name, pharmacy name and address, and pharmacist's name or initials. The medication guide is a paper handout that addresses issues that are specific to certain drugs. The patient package insert is a paper handout supplied with medications to provide additional pharmacological information. (*Knowledge Domain 6.4*)

63. **(B)** A drug-allergy interaction will identify a drug that has been identified as a drug allergy in the patient's profile. A drug-drug interaction will identify potential interactions or problems that may occur if two drugs are taken together. A drug-food interaction will identify a drug that may cause problems or be affected if taken with a specific food. A therapeutic duplication will identify drugs in the same therapeutic category. (*Knowledge Domain 9.1*)

64. **(C)** Nitroglycerin sublingual is a tablet used for angina. It should be readily accessible to the patient in case of anginal pain. (*Knowledge Domain 6.6*)

65. **(A)** Buspirone/bupropion is an example of a pair of drugs that have similar-sounding names. (*Knowledge Domain 4.4*)

66. **(B)** The pharmacy technician should never counsel the patient. Instead, he or she should call over the pharmacist to address the situation. (*Knowledge Domain 4.3*)

67. **(C)**

$$°F = \left(°C \times \frac{9}{5}\right) + 32$$

$$°F = \left(15 \times \frac{9}{5}\right) + 32$$

$$°F = 59$$

The answer is 59°F. (*Knowledge Domain 3.7*)

68. **(D)** The package size is indicated by the last set of numbers of the NDC. (*Knowledge Domain 7.1*)

69. **(A)** Single-use container vials do not contain preservatives and are not reusable. (*Knowledge Domain 3.5*)

70. **(A)** 0700 means 7 hours after midnight, which is 7:00 A.M. (*Knowledge Domain 3.6*)

71. **(D)** Pharmacists are licensed by the State Board of Pharmacy. (*Knowledge Domain 2.13*)

72. **(B)** Lorazepam is the generic drug name for Ativan. Enalapril is the generic drug name for Vasotec. Lisinopril is the generic drug name for Prinivil. Meloxicam is the generic drug name for Mobic. (*Knowledge Domain 1.2*)

73. **(A)** The FDA mandates that the benefits and risks of all estrogen-containing drugs, including Premarin, must be communicated to the patient in the form of a patient package insert. (*Knowledge Domain 4.2*)

74. **(C)** 70% isopropyl alcohol is used as a disinfectant to clean counting trays, counters, and laminar flow hoods. (*Knowledge Domain 2.11*)

75. **(D)** A Class A prescription balance has a maximum weighable amount of 120 g. (*Knowledge Domain 3.5*)

76. **(A)** A suppository is inserted rectally or vaginally and bypasses the stomach (where nausea occurs), making it ideal for patients who have nausea and/or vomiting. (*Knowledge Domain 1.4*)

77. **(C)** Inderal is the brand name for the drug propranolol, which is a beta blocker indicated for hypertension. Tazoroc is the brand name for the drug tazarotene, which is used for acne. (*Knowledge Domain 1.1*)

78. **(C)** *USP* <797> states that all Class 100 environments should not contain particles per cubic foot of air that are 0.5 microns and larger. (*Knowledge Domain 2.11*)

79. **(B)** Intravenous refers to an injection made into a vein. Intramuscular means an injection made into a muscle. Intraocular is an injection made into the eye. Intradermal is an injection made into the skin. (*Knowledge Domain 3.5*)

80. **(C)** The meniscus is the curved surface at the top of a column of liquid. The most accurate place to read the volume is at the bottom of the meniscus. (*Knowledge Domain 3.7*)

81. **(B)** When reading a prescription for an inhaler, it must be assumed that the patient will take the maximum amount of the drug. In the Rx described in the question, "1–2 puffs q 4–6h prn" means that the patient can take up to 2 puffs 6 times a day for a total of 12 puffs a day: $\frac{200}{12} = 16.66$. The day's supply for this medication is 16 days. Do not round up because the medication would not last a full 17 days. A higher day's supply could potentially leave the patient without an inhaler. (*Knowledge Domain 6.2*)

82. **(C)** DEA Form 41 is used for outdated or damaged controlled substances that are to be surrendered or destroyed. (*Knowledge Domain 2.3*)

83. **(D)** Within every 2-year period, 20 hours of CE are required for recertification. Out of those 20 hours, 1 hour must be completed in pharmacy law and 1 hour must be completed in patient safety. (*Knowledge Domain 2.13*)

84. **(A)** Alendronate is a medication used for the treatment of osteoporosis. Due to adverse effects, including stomach ulceration, it is best to take this medication with a full glass of water and sit in an upright position for 30 minutes afterward. (*Knowledge Domain 1.5*)

85. **(A)** The outer coating of an enteric coated tablet prevents dissolution in the stomach. As a result, the tablet breaks down in the intestines. (*Knowledge Domain 1.6*)

86. **(C)** The drug manufacturer offers patient assistance programs directly. (*Knowledge Domain 8.3*)

87. **(C)**

$$\frac{100 \text{ units}}{1 \text{ mL}} = \frac{12 \text{ units}}{x}$$

$$x = 0.12 \text{ mL}$$

The answer is 0.12 mL. (*Knowledge Domain 6.2*)

88. **(B)** Pharmacy reference books can be found in a pharmacy, but they are not examples of a type of technology. Several pharmacology databases, however, are integrated in the pharmacy computer system that require the use of technology. (*Knowledge Domain 9.1*)

89. **(A)** Stock with the closest expiration date is moved to the front of the pharmacy shelf to ensure that it is used before expiring. (*Knowledge Domain 7.3*)

90. **(B)** Warfarin is an example of an anticoagulant medication on ISMP's List of High-Alert Medications in Community/Ambulatory Health Care. (*Knowledge Domain 4.5*)

Pharmacology for Technicians

5

KNOWLEDGE DOMAIN 1.0

Pharmacology for Technicians　　　　　　　　　　　　　　　　**13.75%**
→ Knowledge Area 1.1: Generic and brand names of pharmaceuticals
→ Knowledge Area 1.2: Therapeutic equivalence
→ Knowledge Area 1.3: Drug interactions (e.g., drug-disease, drug-drug, drug-dietary supplement, drug-OTC, drug-laboratory, drug-nutrient)
→ Knowledge Area 1.4: Strengths/dose, dosage forms, physical appearance, routes of administration, and duration of drug therapy
→ Knowledge Area 1.5: Common and severe side or adverse effects, allergies, and therapeutic contraindications associated with medications
→ Knowledge Area 1.6: Dosage and indication of legend, OTC medications, herbal and dietary supplements

LEARNING OBJECTIVES

☐ Define terms associated with pharmacology.
☐ Be familiar with common terms used to describe drug interactions.
☐ Identify brand and generic drug names of medications in each pharmaceutical classification.
☐ Identify common dosage forms, routes of administration, and the duration of drug therapy for each pharmaceutical agent.
☐ Identify common available doses of each pharmaceutical agent.
☐ Identify common side effects and therapeutic contraindications of frequently prescribed agents.
☐ List common indications associated with each pharmaceutical agent.

A 2014 Gallup survey of consumers rated pharmacists as the second most trusted profession. This profession consistently ranks high in both honesty and ethical standards annually. As a pharmacy technician, it is important to uphold those same standards. This starts with having a basic understanding of medications and being able to identify them.

The pharmacy contains thousands of medications that serve a wide range of indications and age ranges to help treat, prevent, or cure diseases. Pharmacy technicians should be able to classify drugs by major therapeutic categories, and they should be able to identify main indications (the therapeutic use of a drug). It is also essential for technicians to identify common brand and generic drug names. Look for commonly used drug prefixes and suffixes, dubbed "stems" as noted by the United States Approved Names (USAN) Council, throughout

NOTE

Make sure to test
your knowledge
of the top brand
name drugs
by reviewing
Appendix A and
Appendix B in
this book!

this chapter. A stem refers to a unique pharmacological or chemical relationship between drugs and can be used to help recall a medication or a classification.

IMPORTANT TERMS TO KNOW

- **PHARMACOLOGY:** Derived from the Greek words "pharmakon," meaning *remedy*, and "logos," meaning *knowledge*, the word *pharmacology* loosely translates to "the knowledge of drugs."
- **PHARMACOKINETICS:** A branch of pharmacology referring to the rate of drug absorption, distribution, metabolism, and excretion (ADME).
- **PHARMACODYNAMICS:** A branch of pharmacology referring to the biological and physical effects of the drug on the body.
- **BRAND NAME:** A proprietary name protected by a patent. This is often referred to as the manufacturer's trademarked name. The first letter of a brand name is always capitalized.
- **GENERIC NAME:** A nonproprietary name approved by the United States Adopted Name Council (USAN). The generic drug must have the same active ingredient, dosage strength, and formulation as the brand name drug, but it may have different inactive ingredients. The first letter of a generic name is not capitalized.
- **CHEMICAL NAME:** A name given to a drug during the initial clinical investigation, referring to its atomic or molecular structure.
- **DOSAGE FORM:** The physical manifestation of the drug or how the drug is supplied. Table 5-1 lists the usual dosage forms.

TIP

Remember
the difference:
Pharmacokinetics
is what the body
does to the drug.
Pharmacodynamics
can be remembered
as what the drug
does to the body.

Table 5-1. Dosage Forms

Form	Definition	Example
aerosol spray	A solution containing an active ingredient with a propellant that is meant to carry the drug to the site of action	benzocaine aerosol spray
Caplet	A tablet shaped like a capsule, containing a solid inside	erythromycin caplet
Capsule	A dosage form containing powder or liquid in a gelatin coating	Nexium capsule
Cream	An oil-in-water emulsion for external use	hydrocortisone cream
Elixir	A flavored, sweetened hydroalcoholic solution	phenobarbital elixir
Emulsion	A dosage form made by the dispersion of one liquid into another that is immiscible	estradiol emulsion
Extract	A potent dosage form containing a powder, ointment-like form, or a solid produced by the evaporation of the aqueous solvent	peppermint extract
Gel	A dosage formed from ultrafine particles in a liquid	lidocaine gel
Intradermal implant, pellet	A dosage form placed under the skin via minor surgery, allowing the drug to be released slowly	Implanon
Lotion	A liquid suspension that is used for topical administration, containing insoluble dispersed solids	calamine lotion

Form	Definition	Example
Lozenge, pastilles, troches	A dosage form made with flavored or sweetened ingredients; generally designed to be dissolved in the mouth for a local effect	Over-the-counter (OTC) cough drops
Micropump	A system of 5,000 to 10,000 microparticles contained within a tablet or capsule; each microparticle is released in the stomach and is able to deliver a drug over an extended period of time	Coreg CR
Ointment	A water-in-oil semisolid preparation for external use	lanolin ointment
Solution	A homogenous liquid dosage form containing one or more solutes dissolved in a solvent	lactulose solution
Spirit	An alcoholic or hydroalcoholic solution containing volatile aromatic compounds	peppermint spirit, aromatic ammonia spirit
Suppository	A solid formulation intended for rectal or vaginal administration	promethazine suppository
Suspension	A dispersion containing an insoluble solid in a liquid	amoxicillin suspension
Syrup	An aqueous solution containing sugar	lithium citrate syrup
Tablet	A molded or compressed dosage form containing active ingredient(s) along with inert binder (inactive ingredients)	levothyroxine tablet
Tincture	An alcoholic or hydroalcoholic solution	Belladona tincture, iodine tincture
Transdermal patch	A percutaneous delivery system consisting of a permeable polymer membrane, backing, drug reservoir, adhesive layer, and protective strip	fentanyl patch, nicotine patch

- **DRUG CLASSIFICATION:** Drugs are grouped by their common actions and effects on the body (e.g., anti-infective, anxiolytic, analgesic).
- **THERAPEUTIC EQUIVALENCE:** This classification is given to drugs that meet certain criteria. The drugs must be proven to be safe and effective, and they must be deemed as pharmaceutically equivalent. This means that identical amounts of active drug are present. The dosage form and route must also be the same. Standards of strength, purity, and quality must be met. Bioequivalence must also be proven. According to the FDA, this is completed through testing to prove the drugs have similar rates of absorption under similar conditions and dosage parameters. Therapeutic equivalence can be checked by looking at the *Approved Drug Products with Therapeutic Equivalence Evaluations*, which is commonly referred to as the *Orange Book*. This publication is the U. S. Food and Drug Administration's (FDA) official listing for prescription, over-the-counter, biologic, military, discontinued, or otherwise never-marketed drugs.
- **SIDE EFFECTS:** Secondary effects of the drug other than the primary therapeutic effect it was originally intended for.

■ **DRUG INTERACTIONS:** A desirable or an undesirable effect that can occur when the effect of one drug is altered by the action of another drug or substance. This phenomenon can produce undesirable effects, resulting in a lack of efficacy or even toxicity. Factors contributing to an increased number of drug interactions include multiple prescribers, poor patient compliance, taking multiple drugs, advanced age, and comorbidity. There are several different types of drug interactions.

Drug-drug interactions occur when a drug interacts with or interferes with another drug. This interaction may be additive, synergistic, potentiated, or antagonistic. An **additive** interaction results when two drugs given in combination have an effect equal to the sum of the individual effects. A **synergistic** interaction results when drugs given in combination produce an effect greater than the sum of the individual effects. A **potentiated** interaction occurs when one drug intensifies the activity of another drug. An **antagonistic** interaction occurs when drugs given in combination cause a decreased, or diminished, effect in one or more drugs.

Drug-food interactions occur when a drug reacts with a food. An example of this is when drinking grapefruit juice causes an increase in the serum concentration of the antihyperlipidemic drug lovastatin (Mevacor).

Drug-disease interactions may occur when a prescription or an over-the-counter medication interacts or interferes with an existing medical condition. For example, a drug-disease interaction occurs when an individual with hypertension takes pseudo-ephedrine.

Drug-nutritional supplement interactions occur when a drug affects vitamin absorption or metabolism. For example, anticonvulsants, such as phenytoin, can cause vitamin D deficiency.

Drug-laboratory interactions occur when a drug or a substance alters the concentrations of substances in the body. For example, potassium-sparing diuretics, such as triamterene, increase serum potassium levels. In addition, the H_2 blocker cimetidine can elevate serum creatinine levels.

Drug-nutrient interactions occur when a drug affects the use of a nutrient in the body. The drug may affect the nutrient's absorption, the use of the nutrient by the body, or the excretion of the nutrient. For example, antihyperlipidemic agents, such as cholestyramine, can decrease the absorption of the fat-soluble vitamins (vitamins A, D, E, and K).

The FDA's Center for Drug Evaluation and Research (CDER) oversees clinical trial investigations used to explore the safety and effectiveness of medications, safety devices, and medical strategies for humans. Figure 5-1 provides more information about the process of drug approval.

	Discovery/ Preclinical Testing		Phase 1	Phase 2	Phase 3		FDA	Phase 4
Years	6.5		1.5	2	3.5		1.5	
Test Population	Laboratory and animal studies	File IND at FDA	20 to 100 healthy volunteers	100 to 500 patient volunteers	1,000 to 5,000 patient volunteers	File NDA at FDA		
Purpose	Assess safety, biological activity, and formulations		Determine safety and dosage	Evaluate effectiveness, look for side effects	Confirm effectiveness, monitor adverse reactions from long-term use		Review process/ approval	Additional postmarketing testing required by FDA
Success Rate	5,000 compounds evaluated		5 enter trials				1 approved	

Figure 5-1. Clinical trials

On average, a drug takes 12 years to go from laboratory testing to the pharmacy shelf. During its development, the drug sponsor requests a **patent** to protect the company's interest in having an exclusive right to the drug. The patent excludes other companies from marketing, developing, or using the drug while the patent is valid. The term of a patent is 20 years from the initial filing date submitted with the IND application. A patent extension may be granted and is determined on an individual basis.

ANTIANXIETY, ANTIEPILEPTIC, ANTIDEPRESSANT, AND SEDATIVE AGENTS

You should familiarize yourself with the USAN stems for antianxiety, antiepileptic, antidepressant, and sedative agents, as outlined in Table 5-2.

NOTE

Antidepressants work by altering the levels of chemicals known as neurotransmitters in the brain. Generally, these agents may take 4-6 weeks to become effective.

Table 5-2. USAN Stems for Antianxiety, Antiepileptic, Antidepressant, and Sedative Agents

Stem	Description	Example
-azepam	Benzodiazepine anxiolytic	temazepam
-pidem	Zolpidem-type sedative/hypnotic	zolpidem
-plon	Nonbenzodiazepine anxiolytic	zaleplon

Table 5-3 lists vital information about common antianxiety, antiepileptic, antidepressant, and sedative agents, including common strengths/dosages, dosage forms, routes, and indications.

Table 5-3. Antianxiety, Antiepileptic, Antidepressant, and Sedative Agents

Generic Name	Brand Name	Common Strengths/ Dosages	Dosage Forms	Route	Indication
alprazolam	Xanax	0.25 mg, 0.5 mg, 1 mg, 2 mg, 3 mg, 1 mg/mL	Tablet, liquid solution	PO	Treatment of anxiety (C-IV)
chlordiazepoxide	Librium	5 mg, 10 mg, 25 mg, 100 mg	Tablet, parenteral	IV, PO, IM	Treatment of anxiety (C-IV)
clonazepam	Klonopin	0.125 mg, 0.25 mg, 0.5 mg, 1 mg, 2 mg	Tablet	PO	Treatment of anxiety (C-IV)
clorazepate	Tranxene	3.75 mg, 7.5 mg, 15 mg	Tablet	PO	Treatment of anxiety (C-IV)
diazepam	Valium	2 mg, 5 mg, 10 mg, 5 mg/mL	Tablet, oral solution, parenteral	PO, IV, IM	Treatment of anxiety (C-IV)
lorazepam	Ativan	0.5 mg, 1 mg, 2 mg, 2 mg/mL	Tablet, oral concentration, parenteral	PO, IV	Treatment of anxiety (C-IV)
meprobamate	Equanil	200 mg, 400 mg	Tablet	PO	Treatment of anxiety (C-IV)
oxazepam	Serax	10 mg, 15 mg, 30 mg	Capsule	PO	Treatment of anxiety (C-IV)
buspirone	Buspar	5 mg, 7.5 mg, 10 mg, 15 mg, 30 mg	Tablet	PO	Treatment of anxiety
carbamazepine	Tegretol	100 mg, 200 mg, 300 mg, 400 mg, 100 mg/5 mL	Tablet, capsule, oral suspension	PO	Treatment of epilepsy
divalproex sodium	Depakote	125 mg, 250 mg, 500 mg, 100 mg/mL	Tablet, capsule	PO	Treatment of epilepsy
ethosuximide	Zarontin	250 mg, 250 mg/mL	Capsule, oral suspension	PO	Treatment of epilepsy
gabapentin	Neurontin	100 mg, 300 mg, 400 mg, 600 mg, 800 mg, 250 mg/mL	Tablet, capsule, oral solution	PO	Treatment of epilepsy
lamotrigine	Lamictal	2 mg, 5 mg, 25 mg, 100 mg, 150 mg, 200 mg	Tablet	PO	Treatment of epilepsy
levetiracetam	Keppra	250 mg, 500 mg, 750 mg, 1,000 mg, 100 mg/mL	Tablet, oral solution	PO	Treatment of epilepsy
oxcarbazepine	Trileptal	150 mg, 300 mg, 600 mg, 300 mg/5 mL	Tablet, oral suspension	PO	Treatment of epilepsy
phenytoin	Dilantin	50 mg, 125 mg/5 mL	Tablet, capsule, oral solution, parenteral	PO, IV, IM	Treatment of epilepsy
pregabalin	Lyrica	50 mg, 75 mg, 100 mg, 150 mg, 200 mg, 225 mg, 20 mg/mL	Capsule, oral solution	PO	Treatment of epilepsy
tiagabine	Gabitril	2 mg, 4 mg, 12 mg, 16 mg	Tablet	PO	Treatment of epilepsy
topiramate	Topamax	15 mg, 25 mg, 50 mg, 100 mg, 200 mg	Tablet, capsule	PO	Treatment of epilepsy

Generic Name	Brand Name	Common Strengths/ Dosages	Dosage Forms	Route	Indication
valproic acid	Depakene	250 mg, 250 mg/5 mL	Capsule, oral solution	PO	Treatment of epilepsy
zonisamide	Zonegran	25 mg, 50 mg, 100 mg	Capsule	PO	Treatment of epilepsy
amitriptyline	Elavil	10 mg, 25 mg, 50 mg, 75 mg, 100 mg, 150 mg	Tablet	PO	Treatment of depression
buproprion	Wellbutrin	75 mg, 100 mg, 150 mg, 200 mg, 300 mg	Tablet	PO	Treatment of depression
citalopram	Celexa	10 mg, 20 mg, 40 mg, 10 mg/5 mL	Tablet, oral solution	PO	Treatment of depression
desipramine	Norpramin	25 mg, 50 mg, 75 mg, 100 mg, 150 mg	Tablet	PO	Treatment of depression
doxepin	Sinequan	10 mg, 25 mg, 50 mg, 75 mg, 100 mg, 150 mg, 10 mg/mL	Tablet, oral solution	PO	Treatment of depression
duloxetine	Cymbalta	20 mg, 30 mg, 60 mg	Capsule	PO	Treatment of depression
escitalopram	Lexapro	5 mg, 10 mg, 20 mg, 5 mg/5 mL	Tablet, oral solution	PO	Treatment of depression
fluoxetine	Prozac	10 mg, 20 mg, 40 mg, 90 mg	Capsule	PO	Treatment of depression
fluvoxamine	Luvox	25 mg, 50 mg, 100 mg	Tablet	PO	Treatment of depression
imipramine	Tofranil	10 mg, 25 mg, 50 mg, 75 mg, 100 mg, 125 mg, 150 mg	Tablet, capsule	PO	Treatment of depression
iscocarboxazid	Marplan	10 mg	Tablet	PO	Treatment of depression
maprotiline	Ludiomil	25 mg, 50 mg, 75 mg	Tablet	PO	Treatment of depression
mirtazapine	Remeron	15 mg, 30 mg, 45 mg	Tablet	PO	Treatment of depression
nefazodone	Serzone	50 mg, 100 mg, 150 mg, 200 mg, 250 mg	Tablet	PO	Treatment of depression
nortriptyline	Pamelor	10 mg, 25 mg, 50 mg, 75 mg	Tablet	PO	Treatment of depression
paroxetine	Paxil	10 mg, 12.5 mg, 20 mg, 25 mg, 30 mg, 37.5 mg, 40 mg	Tablet	PO	Treatment of depression
phenelzine	Nardil	15 mg	Tablet	PO	Treatment of depression
sertraline	Zoloft	25 mg, 50 mg, 100 mg, 20 mg/mL	Tablet, oral solution	PO	Treatment of depression
trazodone	Desyrel	50 mg, 100 mg, 150 mg, 300 mg	Tablet	PO	Treatment of depression

Generic Name	Brand Name	Common Strengths/ Dosages	Dosage Forms	Route	Indication
venlafaxine	Effexor	25 mg, 37.5 mg, 50 mg, 75 mg, 100 mg, 150 mg	Tablet, capsule	PO	Treatment of depression
eszopiclone	Lunesta	1 mg, 2 mg, 3 mg	Tablet	PO	Treatment of insomnia (C-IV)
temazepam	Restoril	7.5 mg, 15 mg, 22.5 mg, 30 mg	Capsule	PO	Treatment of insomnia (C-IV)
triazolam	Halcion	0.125 mg, 0.25 mg	Tablet	PO	Treatment of insomnia (C-IV)
zaleplon	Sonata	5 mg, 10 mg	Capsule	PO	Treatment of insomnia (C-IV)
zolpidem	Ambien	5 mg, 6.25 mg, 10 mg, 12.5 mg	Tablet	PO	Treatment of insomnia (C-IV)
ramelteon	Rozerem	8 mg	Tablet	PO	Treatment of insomnia

ANTI-INFECTIVE AGENTS

Refer to Table 5-4 for the USAN stems for anti-infective agents that you should know.

Table 5-4. USAN Stems for Anti-Infective Agents

TIP

Oral antibiotic agents may need to be reconstituted. These agents are mixed by the pharmacist or technician upon dispensing due to their short shelf life. Oral syringes or dosing spoons should also be dispensed with pediatric oral medications.

Stem	Description	Example
-bactam	Beta-lactamase	sulbactam
cef-	Cephalosporins	cefepime
-cillin	Penicillins	piperacillin
-conazole	Miconazole-type antifungal	itraconazole
-cycline	Tetracyclines	doxycycline
-ezolid	Oxazolidone antibiotics	linezolid
-oxacin	Quinolones	levofloxacin
-vir	Antivirals (general undefined)	acyclovir

Anti-infective agents, or antimicrobials, are agents that either kill microorganisms or slow the spread by inhibiting growth. These agents are classified as either bactericidal (kill the microorganisms) or bacteriostatic (inhibit the growth of the microorganisms). Antibiotics are agents produced by microorganisms and, at low concentrations, kill or inhibit the growth of bacteria.

Microorganisms most commonly include bacteria (antibacterial) and viruses (antiviral) but could also refer to fungi (antifungal) and protozoa (antiprotozoal). Selection of an agent depends on the following:

- Pathogen—determined via previous acquisition, antimicrobial testing, or from a disease state
- Drug—attributes to be considered include pharmacokinetics, pharmacodynamics, and toxicity
- Cost—low cost vs. high cost, insurance, and so on
- Administration—oral vs. I.V., hospital or home infusion, and so on
- Host—variables that must be considered include age, liver and/or kidney function, and immune status

Antibacterial agents are categorized by the spectrum of activity (gram-positive and/or gram-negative), bacterial effect (bactericidal or bacteriostatic), and mode of action.

Tables 5-5 to 5-12 provide information on the most commonly prescribed anti-infective drug classifications. Each table provides information on drug classifications, modes of action, bacterial effects, spectrums of action, common indications and side effects, and the duration of therapy.

Table 5-5. Penicillins

Classification: penicillin
Mode of Action: inhibitor of cell wall synthesis
Bacterial Effect: bactericidal
Spectrum of Action: usually gram-positive
Common Indications: prophylaxis, respiratory infections, otitis media, pneumonia, meningitis
Common Side Effects: stomach upset, diarrhea, and allergic reactions (i.e., rash, hives, edema, and anaphylactic shock)
Typical Duration: 3-, 7-, or 10-day therapy

Generic Name	Brand Name	Common Strengths	Dosage Forms	Route
amoxicillin	Amoxil, Moxatag, Trimox	250 mg, 500 mg, 125 mg/5 ml, 200 mg/5 mL, 250 mg/5 mL, 400 mg/5 mL	Capsule, powder for suspension, chewable tablet, extended-release tablet, tablet	PO
amoxicillin and clavulanate	Augmentin	250 mg, 500 mg, 875 mg, 125 mg/5 mL, 200 mg/5 mL, 250 mg/5 mL, 400 mg/5 mL, 600 mg/5 mL	Tablet, powder for suspension, extended-release tablet	PO
ampicillin	Omnipen	125 mg, 250 mg, 125 mg/5 mL, 250 mg/5 mL	Capsule, oral suspension	PO
ampicillin and sulbactam	Unasyn	150 mg, 300 mg, 1.5 g, 3 g	Parenteral	IV, IM
dicloxacillin	Dynapen	250 mg, 500 mg	Capsule	PO

Generic Name	Brand Name	Common Strengths	Dosage Forms	Route
penicillin G	Bicillin-LA	600,000 units/ 1 mL, 1.2 million units/2 mL, 2.4 million units	Parenteral	IV, IM
penicillin V potassium	Penicillin VK, Pen Vee K, Penicillin V, Veetids	250 mg, 500 mg, 125 mg/5 mL, 250 mg/5 mL	Tablet, liquid	PO
piperacillin and tazobactam	Zosyn	2.25 g, 3.375 g, 4.5 g	Parenteral	IV
ticarcillin and clavulanate	Timentin	3.1 g	Parenteral	IV

Table 5-6. Cephalosporins

Classification: cephalosporin
Mode of Action: inhibitor of cell wall synthesis
Bacterial Effect: bactericidal
Spectrum of Action: gram-positive and some gram-negative
Common Indications: prophylaxis, respiratory infections, pneumonia, dental procedures, genitourinary tract infections
Common Side Effects: upset stomach, diarrhea, and allergic reactions (i.e., rash, hives, edema, and anaphylactic shock)
Contraindications: hypersensitivity to penicillin, renal impairment
Special Considerations: 1–3% cross-sensitivity to penicillin
Typical Duration: 7–14 day therapy

Generic Name	Brand Name	Common Strengths	Dosage Forms	Route
cefaclor	Ceclor	250 mg, 500 mg, 125 mg/5 mL, 250 mg/5 mL, 375 mg/5 mL	Capsule, tablet, suspension	PO
cefadroxil	Duricef	250 mg, 500 mg, 250 mg/5 mL, 500 mg/5 mL, 1 g	Capsule, suspension, tablet	PO
cefazolin	Ancef	500 mg, 1 g	Parenteral	IV
cefdinir	Omnicef	300 mg, 125 mg/5 mL, 250 mg/5 mL	Capsule, suspension	PO
cefepime	Maxipime	500 mg, 1 g, 2 g	Parenteral	IV
cefixime	Suprax	400 mg, 100 mg/5 mL, 200 mg/5 mL, 500 mg/5 mL	Tablet, suspension	PO
cefproxil	Cefzil	250 mg, 500 mg, 125 mg/5 mL, 250 mg/5 mL	Tablet, suspension	PO
ceftazidime	Fortaz	1 g, 2 g, 6 g	Parenteral	IV

Generic Name	Brand Name	Common Strengths	Dosage Forms	Route
ceftriaxone	Rocephin	250 mg, 500 mg, 1 g, 2 g	Parenteral	IV
cefuroxime	Ceftin	250 mg, 500 mg, 125 mg/5 mL, 250 mg/5 mL	Tablet, suspension	PO
cephalexin	Keflex	250 mg, 500 mg, 750 g, 125 mg/5 mL, 250 mg/5 mL	Capsule, suspension	PO

Table 5-7. Macrolides

Classification: macrolide
Mode of Action: inhibitor of protein synthesis
Bacterial Effect: bacteriostatic
Spectrum of Action: mostly gram-positive and some gram-negative
Common Indications: respiratory infections, skin infections, pneumonia, chlamydia, sinusitis
Common Side Effects: upset stomach, diarrhea
Contraindications: QT elongation, hepatic impairment, renal impairment
Special Considerations: intensifies the effect of warfarin, digoxin, and cyclosporine; take on an empty stomach; potential ototoxicity after IV administration of erythromycin
Typical Duration: 7–14 day therapy

Generic Name	Brand Name	Common Strengths	Dosage Forms	Route
azithromycin	Zithromax, Zmax	250 mg, 500 mg, 600 mg, 100 mg/5 mL, 200 mg/5 mL, 1 g	Tablet, suspension, parenteral, powder	IV, PO
clarithromycin	Biaxin	250 mg, 500 mg, 125 mg/5 mL, 250 mg/5 mL	Tablet, suspension	PO
erythromycin base	Ery-tab, PCE Dispertab	250 mg, 500 mg, 1 g	Tablet, capsule	PO

Table 5-8. Tetracyclines

Classification: tetracycline
Mode of Action: inhibitor of protein synthesis
Bacterial Effect: bacteriostatic
Spectrum of Action: gram-positive and gram-negative
Common Indications: acne, chronic bronchitis
Common Side Effects: upset stomach
Contraindications: children, pregnancy, renal impairment, hepatic impairment
Special Considerations: photosensitivity resulting in sunburn and rashes; may stain teeth; antacids and dairy products should be taken several hours before or after tetracycline therapy (will decrease the effectiveness of the antibiotic); ingesting expired tetracycline can result in kidney damage; expired tetracycline should be discarded appropriately
Typical Duration: Daily; up to 14 days

Generic Name	Brand Name	Common Strengths	Dosage Forms	Route
doxycycline	Vibramycin	50 mg, 75 mg, 100 mg, 25 mg/5 mL	Parenteral, tablet, capsule, suspension	IV, PO
minocycline	Minocin	50 mg, 75 mg, 100 mg	Parenteral, capsule	IV, PO
tetracycline	Sumycin	250 mg, 500 mg	Capsule	PO

Table 5-9. Quinolones

Classification: quinolone
Mode of Action: inhibit bacterial DNA synthesis
Bacterial Effect: bactericidal
Spectrum of Action: gram-positive and gram-negative
Common Indications: pneumonia, sinusitis, respiratory infections, urinary tract infections, chronic bronchitis
Common Side Effects: nausea, vomiting, joint swelling
Contraindications: myasthenia gravis, patients < 18 years and patients > 60 years
Special Considerations: black box warning: increased risk of tendinitis and tendon rupture; phototoxicity; antacids should be avoided or taken several hours before or after tetracycline therapy (may interfere with absorprtion)
Typical Duration: 3–7 day therapy

Generic Name	Brand Name	Common Strengths	Dosage Forms	Route
ciprofloxacin	Cipro	250 mg, 500 mg, 250 mg/5 mL, 500 mg/5 mL	Tablet, parenteral	IV, PO
levofloxacin	Levaquin	250 mg, 500 mg, 750 mg, 250 mg/10 mL, 25 mg/mL, 0.5%	Tablet, parenteral, solution, ophthalmic drops	IV, PO, ophthalmic
moxifloxacin	Avelox, Vigamox	400 g, 0.5%	Tablet, ophthalmic drops	PO, ophthalmic
norfloxacin	Noroxin	400 mg	Tablet	PO
ofloxacin	Floxin	400 mg, 0.3%	Tablet, ophthalmic, otic	PO, ophthalmic, otic

Table 5-10. Ketolide

Classification: ketolide
Mode of Action: inhibit protein synthesis
Bacterial Effect: bacteriostatic
Spectrum of Action: gram-positive, gram-negative, atypicals
Common Indications: community acquired pneumonia
Common Side Effects: blurred vision, upset stomach, diarrhea
Contraindications: QT elongation, hepatic impairment, renal impairment
Special Considerations: life-threatening respiratory failure seen in patients with myasthenia gravis
Typical Duration: 7–10 days

Generic Name	Brand Name	Common Strengths	Dosage Forms	Route
telithromycin	Ketek	400 mg	Tablet	PO

Table 5-11. Aminoglycosides

Classification: aminoglycoside
Mode of Action: inhibit bacterial protein synthesis
Bacterial Effect: bactericidal
Spectrum of Action: broad gram-negative activity
Common Indications: endocarditis, sepsis, immune-compromised patients
Common Side Effects: renal toxicity, neurotoxicity (vestibular and auditory toxicity)
Contraindications: neuromuscular blockage, neurotoxicity
Special Considerations: may prolong the activity of neuromuscular blockers
Typical Duration: dosed every 8–12 hours

Generic Name	Brand Name	Common Strengths	Dosage Forms	Route
amikacin	Amikin	500 mg/2 mL, 1,000 mg/4 mL	Parenteral	IV, IM
gentamicin	Gentak	0.1%, 0.3%, 40 mg/mL	Cream ointment, ophthalmic cream, ophthalmic drops, parenteral	Topical, IV
streptomycin*		1 g	Parenteral	IM
tobramycin	Tobrex	28 mg, 300 mg, 3 mg/mL, 300 mg/4 mL, 300 mg/5 mL, 0.3%	Solution, inhalation, capsule, ophthalmic solution, ophthalmic ointment	IV, ophthalmic, inhaler

*No brand name formulation is currently available.

Table 5-12. Carbapenems and Monobactams

Classification: carbapenem and monobactam	
Mode of Action: inhibit bacterial cell wall synthesis	
Bacterial Effect: bactericidal	
Spectrum of Action: gram-positive and gram-negative	
Common Indications: community-acquired pneumonia, complicated UTI, complicated skin infections, complicated intra-abdominal infections	
Common Side Effects: upset stomach, diarrhea	
Contraindications: history of seizures, CNS disorders	
Special Considerations: sensitivity to beta-lactams or ertapenem	
Typical Duration: 7–14 days	

Generic Name	Brand Name	Common Strengths	Dosage Forms	Route
aztreonam	Azactam	1 g, 2 g	Parenteral	IV
ertapenem	Invanz	1 g	Parenteral	IV, IM
imipenem and cilastin	Primaxin	250 mg, 500 mg, 1 g	Parenteral	IV
meropenem	Merrem	1 g	Parenteral	IV

Miscellaneous Anti-Infective Agents

These agents, as outlined in Table 5-13, are used to treat a variety of infections. Proper selection of an agent is determined by an initial accurate diagnosis, the duration of therapy, the need for cost-effective agents, and individual host characteristics, including state of mind. Appropriate selection can maximize the effect of treatment while minimizing side effects and unintended consequences, such as microbial resistance.

Table 5-13. Miscellaneous Anti-Infective Agents

Generic Name	Brand Name	Common Strengths	Dosage Form & Route	Spectrum of Activity	Indication	Mode of Action
clindamycin	Cleocin	1%, 2%, 100 mg, 150 mg, 300 mg, 600 mg/4 mL, 900 mg/ 6 mL	Gel, solution, suppository, capsule, parenteral, topical, rectal, PO, IV	Gram + aerobes, gram + anaerobes, gram – anaerobes	Acne, dental prophylaxis, anaerobic infections, bone infections	Inhibit protein synthesis
daptomycin	Cubicin	500 mg	Parenteral, IV	Gram +	Skin infections, complicated gram + infections, endocarditis	Inhibit DNA and RNA synthesis
linezolid	Zyvox	600 mg, 100 mg/5 mL, 200 mg/100 mL, 600 mg/300 mL	Capsule, parenteral	Gram +, some gram –, and anaerobes	Treatment of methicillin-resistant *S. aureus* (MRSA) and vancomycin-resistant *E. faecium*	Inhibit bacterial protein synthesis
nitrofurantoin	Macro-dantin, Macrobid	25 mg/5 mL, 50 mg, 100 mg	Suspension, capsule, oral	Gram –, some gram +	Urinary tract infection	Interfere with metabolism and cell wall synthesis
quinupristin, dalfopristin	Synercid	500 mg	Parenteral, IV	Gram +	Complicated skin infections, vancomycin-resistant *E. faecium*	Inhibit protein synthesis at the bacterial ribosome
trimethoprim, sulfamethoxazole	Bactrim, Septra	400–80 mg, 800–160 mg, 200–40/5 mL	Tablet, PO	Gram +, gram –	Sulfonamide antibiotic	Inhibit enzyme systems involved in the synthesis of tetra-hydrofolic acid
vancomycin	Vancocin	125 mg, 250 mg, 1,000 mg, 5 g, 10 g	Capsule, parenteral, PO, IV	Gram + aerobes, gram + anaerobes	Pseudomem-branous colitis, endocarditis	Interfere with bacterial cell wall formation

ANTIFUNGAL AGENTS

Antifungal agents, listed in Table 5-14, are used to treat fungal infections, such as athlete's foot and candidiasis (thrush). They can also be used to treat more complicated conditions such as aspergillosis and blastomycosis. Some antifungal drugs are found over-the-counter, while others require prescriptions. Long-term antifungal use requires monitoring of the liver functions and enzymes due to the potential for liver toxicity. Patients with CHF should not use itraconazole due to enzyme inhibition. Therapy may last a few weeks to several months depending on the type of fungal infection.

Table 5-14. Antifungal Agents

Generic Name	Brand Name	Common Strengths/ Dosages	Dosage Forms	Route
amphotericin b	AmBisome, Amphocin, Fungizone	50 mg, 100 mg	Parenteral	IV
butenafine	Mentax	1%	Cream	Topical
caspofungin	Cancidas	50 mg, 70 mg	Parenteral	IV
ciclopirox	Loprox, Penlac	0.77%, 1%, 8%	Gel, cream, shampoo	Topical
clotrimazole	Lotrimin *OTC formulation available	10 mg, 1%	Troche, lozenge, cream	Topical, vaginal
fluconazole	Diflucan	50 mg, 100 mg, 150 mg, 200 mg, 10 mg/mL, 40 mg/mL	Tablet, liquid, parenteral	PO, IV
itraconazole	Sporanox	100 mg, 10 mg/mL	Capsule, liquid	PO
ketoconazole	Nizoral	200 mg, 400 mg, 1%, 2%	Tablet, cream, shampoo	PO, topical
miconazole	Monistat 1, Monistat 3, Monistat 7 *OTC formulation available	100 mg, 200 mg, 1,200 mg	Cream	Vaginal
nystatin	Mycostatin	100,000 U	Liquid, topical	PO, topical
terbinafine	Lamisil *OTC formulation available	250 mg, 500 mg	Cream	Topical
terconazole	Terazol	0.4%, 0.8%	Cream	Topical
voriconazole	Vfend	200 mg, 200 mg/5 mL	Tablet, parenteral, suspension	IV, oral

ANTIVIRAL AGENTS

Antiviral drugs, described in Table 5-15, are used to treat viral infections. These drugs prevent the growth of the offending pathogen by inhibiting replication (acyclovir, famciclovir, ganciclovir, valacyclovir), stopping the release of the virus from the cell (oseltamivir, zanamivir), preventing DNA synthesis (cidofivir), or preventing the virus from affecting the cell (palivizumab). Antivirals can be used to treat herpes simplex virus, respiratory syncytial virus (RSV), influenza, HIV, herpes zoster (shingles), and varicella zoster (chickenpox). The length of therapy varies. Patients may require medication daily, for a few weeks, or for months.

Table 5-15. Antiviral Agents

Generic Name	Brand Name	Common Strengths/ Dosages	Dosage Forms	Route
acyclovir	Zovirax	200 mg, 400 mg, 800 mg, 5%, 200 mg/5 mL	Capsule, tablet, ointment, suspension	Oral, topical
amantadine	Symmetrel	100 mg, 50 mg/5 mL	Tablet, capsule, solution	Oral
cidofovir	Vistide	75 mg/mL	Parenteral	IV
famciclovir	Fosvir	125 mg, 250 mg, 500 mg	Tablet	Oral
ganciclovir	Cytovene, Zirgan	500 mg, 0.15%	Parenteral, gel	IV, topical
oseltamivir	Tamiflu	30 mg, 45 mg, 75 mg, 6 mg/mL	Capsule, suspension	Oral
palivizumab	Synagis	100 mg/mL	Parenteral	IV
valacyclovir	Valtrex	500 mg, 1,000 mg	Tablet	Oral
zanamivir	Relenza	5 mg	Diskhaler	Inhalation

ANTIRETROVIRAL AGENTS

Antiretroviral agents, listed in Table 5-16, are used for the treatment of the human immunodeficiency virus (HIV) and are categorized based on their reaction with HIV replication. Nucleoside (NRTIs)/nucleotide (NtRTI) reverse transcriptase inhibitors stop HIV DNA synthesis by attaching to the HIV DNA chain. Side effects of NRTIs and NtRTIs may include anemia, hepatotoxicity, lactic acidosis, lipodystrophy (fat redistribution), and skin rash. Non-nucleoside reverse-transcriptase inhibitors (NNRTIs) inhibit the conversion of HIV RNA to HIV DNA. These agents may have adverse effects, including hepatotoxicity, lipodystrophy, and skin rash. Protease inhibitors (PI) exert their action by interfering with protease, an enzyme that breaks the HIV virus into small segments. Side effects of protease inhibitors include hepatotoxicity, hyperglycemia, hyperlipidemia, lipodystrophy, osteonecrosis (bone death), and skin rash. A C-C motif chemoreceptor 5 (CCR5) inhibitor interferes with the HIV virus's ability to bind to the outer surface of a cell. This class of drug may cause hepatotoxicity. Integrase inhibitors block the HIV enzyme integrase; the virus uses the enzyme to help transfer its genetic material into the DNA of infected cells. Fusion inhibitors prevent HIV from entering a cell by interfering with the virus's ability to fuse with the cell membrane.

Table 5-16. Antiretroviral Agents

Drug Class and Indication	Generic Name	Brand Name	Common Strengths/ Dosages	Dosage Forms	Route
Nucleoside/nucleotide reverse transcriptase inhibitors (NRTI); human immunodeficiency virus (HIV)	abacavir	Ziagen	300 mg, 20 mg/mL	Tablet, oral solution	PO
	didanosine	Videx, Videx EC	125 mg, 200 mg, 250 mg, 400 mg, 10 mg/mL	Capsule, powder for oral solution	PO
	emtricitabine	Emtriva	200 mg, 10 mg/mL	Capsule, oral solution	PO
	lamivudine	Epivir, Epivir HBV	100 mg, 150 mg, 300 mg, 5 mg/mL, 10 mg/mL	Tablet, oral solution	PO
	stavudine	Zerit	15 mg, 20 mg, 30 mg, 40 mg, 1 mg/mL	Capsule, oral solution	PO
	zidovudine	Retrovir	100 mg, 300 mg, 10 mg/mL	Tablet, capsule	PO
Non-nucleoside reverse-transcriptase inhibitors (NNRTI); human immunodeficiency virus (HIV)	efavirenz	Sustiva	50 mg, 200 mg, 600 mg	Tablet, capsule	PO
	etravirine	Intelence	100 mg, 200 mg	Tablet	PO
	nevirapine	Viramune	200 mg, 400 mg, 50 mg/5 mL	Tablet, oral suspension	PO
Protease inhibitor (PI)	atazanavir	Reyataz	50 mg, 150 mg, 200 mg, 300 mg	Capsule, oral powder	PO
	darunavir	Prezista	150 mg, 400 mg, 600 mg, 800 mg	Tablet	PO
	fosamprenavir	Lexiva	700 mg, 50 mg/mL	Tablet, oral suspension	PO
	indinavir	Crixivan	200 mg, 400 mg	Capsule	PO
	lopinavir, ritonavir	Kaletra	100 mg/25 mg, 200 mg/50 mg, 400 mg/100 mg/5 mL	Tablet, oral solution	PO
	nelfinavir	Viracept	250 mg, 625 mg	Tablet	PO
	saquinavir	Invirase	200 mg, 500 mg	Tablet, capsule	PO
	tipranavir	Aptivus	250 mg, 100 mg/mL	Capsule, oral solution	PO
C-C motif chemoreceptor 5 (CCR5) inhibitor; human immunodeficiency virus (HIV)	maraviroc	Selzentry	150 mg, 300 mg	Tablet	PO
Integrase inhibitor; human immunodeficiency virus (HIV)	raltegravir	Isentress	100 mg, 400 mg	Tablet, powder for oral solution	PO
Fusion inhibitor; human immunodeficiency virus (HIV)	enfuvirtide	Fuzeon	90 mg	Parenteral	PO

CARDIOVASCULAR AGENTS

Table 5-17 reviews commonly used USAN stems for cardiovascular agents.

Table 5-17. USAN Stems for Cardiovascular Agents

Stem	Description	Example
-arone	Antiarrhythmics	amiodarone
-azosin	Prazosin-type antihypertensive	terazosin
-dralazine	Hydrazine-phthalazine-type antihypertensive	hydralazine
-olol	Beta blockers	metoprolol
-pril	ACE inhibitor–type hypertensive	lisinopril
-sartan	Angiotensin II receptor antagonist	losartan
-teplase	Plasminogen activator	reteplase
-vastatin	HMG-CoA reductase inhibitor–type antihyperlipidemics	simvastatin

NOTE

Sublingual nitroglycerin should be kept in the original container and at room temperature away from heat, light, and moisture. Pharmacy technicians may be required to label the medication container along with the prescription vial. Make sure to check with your pharmacist for state-specific requirements.

The ACE (angiotensin-converting enzyme) inhibitors prevent the conversion of angiotensin I to angiotensin II. This inhibition results in vasodilation and indirectly inhibits the increase of fluid from aldosterone. Medications in this class end in the suffix "-pril" and include lisinopril (Prinivil, Zestril). Common side effects include hyperkalemia (an increase in serum potassium), a dry hacking cough, rash, and hypotension.

Beta blockers, such as atenolol (Tenormin), block the stimulatory effects of epinephrine by exerting antagonist effects on beta-1 and beta-2 receptors. Medications such as atenolol (Tenormin) are used as antihypertensive agents to reduce the workload of the heart and to reduce blood pressure. Common side effects include drowsiness, weakness, and dry mouth. Caution should be observed in patients with diabetes because these agents have been found to mask symptoms of hypoglycemia.

Calcium channel blockers (CCB) block the entry of calcium into the heart muscle and vessel walls. The conduction of electrical signals depends on the movement of calcium into the cell. A blockage of calcium results in relaxation of the vessel wall, causing dilation of the arteries. The relaxed vessels allow blood to flow easier, thereby lowering blood pressure. Medications that reduce the strength and rate of the heart's contraction include diltiazem (Cardizem) and verapamil (Isoptin, Calan). These drugs are primarily used as antiarrhythmics. Amlodipine (Norvasc) is recommended for the treatment of heart failure due to its vasodilatory effects. CCB side effects include edema, rash, hypotension, and gingivitis. Patients should be advised to avoid concomitant consumption of grapefruit juice to avoid increased serum concentrations of the CCB.

Diuretic agents promote the excretion of salt and water from the kidneys, thus, resulting in an increase in urine production. These agents are generally used to treat hypertension and CHF (congestive heart failure). Loop diuretics, including furosemide (Lasix), prevent the reabsorption of chloride and sodium in the loop of Henle. Both thiazide and potassium-sparing diuretics exert effects on the distal convoluted tubules. Thiazide diuretics, such as hydrochlorothiazide (Microzide), prevent the reabsorption of sodium, whereas potassium-sparing diuretics prevent an excessive loss of sodium ions. Thiazide diuretics may cause photosensitivity, dizziness, blurred vision, and hypokalemia. Potassium-sparing diuretics may cause

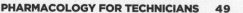

hyperkalemia, diarrhea, rash, edema, and—in some cases—gynecomastia (an enlargement of breasts in males).

Statins are a class of antihyperlipidemics that inhibit the enzyme HMG-CoA reductase, resulting in decreased cholesterol production. This class includes agents such as atorvastatin (Lipitor) and simvastatin (Zocor). These agents are commonly taken at night when the body produces endogenous cholesterol. Side effects may include muscle pain, hyperglycemia, rash, flushing, and liver damage.

Thrombolytic drugs are also called plasminogen activators or fibrinolytic drugs due to mechanisms used to dissolve blood clots. These agents activate plasminogen, forming a product called plasmin. This resulting compound is an enzyme that breaks cross-links between fibrin molecules, resulting in the compromised structural integrity of a blood clot.

Table 5-18. Cardiovascular Agents

Drug Class and Indication	Generic Name	Brand Name	Common Strengths/ Dosages	Dosage Forms	Route
ACE inhibitor; antihypertensive	benazepril	Lotensin	5 mg, 10 mg, 20 mg, 40 mg	Tablet	PO
	captopril	Capoten	12.5 mg, 25 mg, 50 mg, 100 mg	Tablet	PO
	enalapril	Vasotec, Epaned	2.5 mg, 5 mg, 10 mg, 20 mg, 1 mg/mL	Tablet, oral solution	PO
	fosinopril	Monopril	10 mg, 20 mg, 40 mg	Tablet	PO
	lisinopril	Prinivil, Zestril	2.5 mg, 5 mg, 10 mg, 20 mg, 30 mg, 40 mg	Tablet	PO
	moexipril	Univasc	7.5 mg, 15 mg	Tablet	PO
	perindopril	Aceon	2 mg, 4 mg, 8 mg	Tablet	PO
	quinapril	Accupril	5 mg, 10 mg, 20 mg, 40 mg	Tablet	PO
	ramipril	Altace	1.25 mg, 2.5 mg, 5 mg, 10 mg	Capsule	PO
	trandolapril	Mavik	1 mg, 2 mg, 4 mg	Tablet	PO
Angiotensin II receptor antagonist (ARB); antihypertensive	candesartan	Atacand	4 mg, 8 mg, 16 mg, 32 mg	Tablet	PO
	eprosartan	Teveten	400 mg, 600 mg	Tablet	PO
	irbesartan	Avapro	75 mg, 150 mg, 300 mg	Tablet	PO
	losartan	Cozaar	50 mg, 75 mg, 100 mg	Tablet	PO
	olmesartan	Benicar	5 mg, 20 mg, 40 mg	Tablet	PO
	telmisartan	Micardis	20 mg, 40 mg, 80 mg	Tablet	PO
	valsartan	Diovan	40 mg, 80 mg, 160 mg, 320 mg	Tablet	PO
Antiarrhythmic	amiodarone	Cordarone, Pacerone	100 mg, 200 mg, 400 mg, 50 mg/mL	Tablet, parenteral	PO, IV
	digoxin	Lanoxin	125 mcg, 250 mcg, 50 mcg/mL, 100 mcg/mL, 250 mcg/mL	Tablet, parenteral	PO, IV

Drug Class and Indication	Generic Name	Brand Name	Common Strengths/ Dosages	Dosage Forms	Route
Beta blocker (BB); antihypertensive	acebutolol	Sectral	200 mg, 400 mg	Capsule	PO
	atenolol	Tenormin	25 mg, 50 mg, 100 mg	Tablet	PO
	bisoprolol fumerate	Monocor, Zebeta	5 mg, 10 mg	Tablet	PO
	carvedilol	Coreg	3.125 mg, 6.25 mg, 12.5 mg, 25 mg,	Tablet	PO
	labetalol	Trandate	100 mg, 200 mg, 300 mg, 5 mg/mL	Tablet, parenteral	PO, IV
	metoprolol succinate	Toprol XL	25 mg, 50 mg, 100 mg, 200 mg	Tablet	PO
	metoprolol tartrate	Lopressor	5 mg, 50 mg, 100 mg	Tablet, solution	PO, IV
	nadolol	Corgard	20 mg, 40 mg, 80 mg	Tablet	PO
	nebivolol	Bystolic	2.5 mg, 5 mg, 10 mg, 20 mg	Tablet	PO
Calcium channel blocker (CCB); antihypertensive, antianginal, antiarrhythmic	amlodipine	Norvasc	2.5 mg, 5 mg, 10 mg	Tablet	PO
	diltiazem	Cardizem, Cardizem SR, Cardizem LA	30 mg, 60 mg, 90 mg, 120 mg, 180 mg, 240 mg, 300 mg, 360 mg, 420 mg, 5 mg/mL	Tablet, capsule, parenteral	PO, IV
	felodipine	Plendil	2.5 mg, 5 mg, 10 mg	Tablet	PO
	nifedipine	Adalat CC, Procardia, Procardia XL	10 mg, 20 mg, 30 mg, 60 mg, 90 mg	Tablet, capsule	PO
	nisoldipine	Sular	8.5 mg, 17 mg, 20 mg, 25.5 mg, 30 mg, 34 mg, 40 mg	Tablet	PO
	propranolol	Inderal LA, Inderal XL	10 mg, 20 mg, 40 mg, 60 mg, 80 mg, 120 mg, 160 mg, 1 mg/mL	Tablet, capsule, parenteral	PO, IV
	sotalol	Betapace, Sotylize	80 mg, 120 mg, 160 mg, 240 mg, 5 mg/mL, 15 mg/mL	Tablet, oral solution, parenteral	PO, IV
	verapamil	Isoptin, Isoptin SR, Calan, Calan SR	40 mg, 80 mg, 100 mg, 120 mg, 180 mg, 200 mg, 240 mg, 300 mg, 360 mg, 2.5 mg/mL	Tablet, capsule, parenteral	PO, IV

Drug Class and Indication	Generic Name	Brand Name	Common Strengths/Dosages	Dosage Forms	Route
Diuretic; antihypertensives	bumetanide	Bumex	0.5 mg, 1 mg, 2 mg, 0.25 mg/mL	Tablet, parenteral	PO, IV, IM
	chlorthalidone	Hygroton	25 mg, 50 mg	Tablet	PO
	furosemide	Lasix	20 mg, 40 mg, 80 mg, 10 mg/mL, 40 mg/5 mL	Tablet, oral solution, parenteral	PO, IV, IM
	hydrochloro-thiazide	Hydrodiuril, Microzide	12.5 mg, 25 mg, 50 mg	Tablet, capsule	PO
	indapamide	Lozol	1.25 mg, 2.5 mg	Tablet	PO
	metolazone	Zaroxolyn	2.5 mg, 5 mg, 10 mg	Tablet	PO
	spironolactone	Aldactone	25 mg, 50 mg, 100 mg,	Tablet	PO
	torsemide	Demadex	5 mg, 10 mg, 20 mg, 100 mg	Tablet	PO
	triamterene	Dyrenium	50 mg, 100 mg	Capsule	PO
Alpha blocker antihypertensives	doxazosin	Cardura	1 mg, 2 mg, 4 mg, 8 mg	Tablet	PO
	prazosin	Minipress	1 mg, 2 mg, 5 mg	Capsule	PO
	terazosin	Hytrin	1 mg, 2 mg, 5 mg, 10 mg	Capsule	PO
Miscellaneous antihypertensives	alsikiren	Tekturna	150 mg, 300 mg	Tablet	PO
	clonidine	Catapres	0.1 mg/24 hr, 0.2 mg/24 hr, 0.3 mg/24 hr	Patch	Topical
	hydralazine	Apresoline	10 mg, 25 mg, 50 mg, 100 mg, 20 mg/mL	Tablet, parenteral	PO, IV, IM
HMG-CoA reductase inhibitor; antihyperlipidemics	atorvastatin	Lipitor	10 mg, 20 mg, 40 mg, 80 mg	Tablet	PO
	fluvastatin	Lescol, Lescol XL	20 mg, 40 mg, 80 mg	Tablet, capsule	PO
	lovastatin	Mevacor, Altoprev	10 mg, 20 mg, 40 mg, 60 mg	Tablet	PO
	pitavastatin	Livalo	1 mg, 2 mg, 4 mg	Tablet	PO
	pravastatin	Pravachol	10 mg, 20 mg, 40 mg, 80 mg	Tablet	PO
	rosuvastatin	Crestor	5 mg, 10 mg, 20 mg, 40 mg	Tablet	PO
	simvastatin	Zocor	5 mg, 10 mg, 20 mg, 40 mg, 80 mg	Tablet	PO

Drug Class and Indication	Generic Name	Brand Name	Common Strengths/ Dosages	Dosage Forms	Route
Miscellaneous antihyperlipidemics	cholestyramine	Prevalite, Questran, Questran light	5 mg, 9 mg	Powder	PO
	ezetimibe	Zetia	10 mg	Tablet	PO
	fenofibrate	TriCor, Lofibra	40 mg, 50 mg, 54 mg, 67 mg, 120 mg, 134 mg, 150 mg, 160 mg, 200 mg	Tablet, capsule	PO
	gemfibrozil	Lopid	600 mg	Tablet	PO
	niacin	Niaspan	100 mg, 250 mg, 500 mg, 750 mg, 1,000 mg	Tablet, capsule	PO
	omega-3-carboxylic acids	Epanova	1,000 mg	Capsule	PO
Thrombolytic agents	alteplase	Activase, Cathflo Activase	1 mg, 100 mg	Parenteral	IV
	reteplase	Retavase	50 mg, 100 mg	Parenteral	IV
	streptokinase	Streptase	250,000 IU, 750,000 IU, 1,500,000 IU	Parenteral	IV
	tenecteplase	TNKase, TNK TpA	50 mg	Parenteral	IV
	urokinase	Abbokinase	1.5 mg	Parenteral	IV
Miscellaneous agents used to prevent or reduce the risk of blood clot formation	heparin	Hep-Lock	10 U/mL, 100 U/mL, 1,000 IU, 5,000 IU, 10,000 IU, 20,000 IU	Parenteral	IV, SQ
	warfarin	Coumadin, Jantoven	1 mg, 2 mg, 2.5 mg, 3 mg, 4 mg, 5 mg, 6 mg, 7.5 mg, 10 mg	Tablet	PO
Miscellaneous agents used to prevent heart attacks and strokes or for the prevention or treatment of chest pain	acetylsalicylic acid	Bayer aspirin *Available OTC	81 mg, 325 mg, 500 mg, 650 mg	Tablet, capsule, caplet, gelcap	PO
	clopidogrel	Plavix	75 mg	Tablet	PO
	dipyridamole	Persantine	25 mg, 50 mg, 75 mg, 5 mg/mL	Tablet	PO, IV
	prasugrel	Effient	5 mg, 10 mg	Tablet	PO
	ticlopidine	Ticlid	250 mg	Tablet	PO
Miscellaneous agents used to prevent angina	isosorbide dinitrate	Isordil	5 mg, 10 mg, 20 mg, 30 mg, 40 mg	Tablet	PO
	isosorbide mononitrate	Imdur	10 mg, 20 mg, 30 mg, 60 mg, 120 mg	Tablet	PO
	nitroglycerin	Nitro-Bid ointment, Nitro-Dur, Nitrolingual	0.1 mg/hr, 0.2 mg/hr, 0.4 mg/hr, 0.6 mg/hr, 0.3 mg, 0.4 mg, 0.6 mg	Ointment, patch, spray	Topical, sublin-gual

DERMATOLOGICAL AGENTS

Dermatological agents may be identified by recognizing prefixes and suffixes used in USAN stem names. Table 5-19 lists commonly used stems for dermatological agents that are recognized by the USAN council.

Table 5-19. USAN Stems for Dermatological Agents

Stem	Description	Example
-cort	Cortisone derivative	hydrocortisone
-olone	Steroids	triamcinolone
-onide	Steroids	flucinonide
sulfa	Antimicrobial (sulfonamide derivative)	silver sulfadiazine
-vir	Antiviral	acyclovir

Dermatological agents, such as those listed in Table 5-20, are used to treat a variety of skin conditions, including acne, burns, itching, infections, rashes, and psoriasis. Most agents can be applied topically to the site of the irritation or condition. Topical agents have fewer side effects because they are not absorbed systemically. The effect of the topical agent is contained to the application site. Potential side effects include irritation, dryness, and redness. The drug isotretinoin is an oral acne agent that is reserved for the treatment of cystic acne. It is also a Risk Evaluation and Mitigation Strategies (REMS) agent that has restricted prescribing due to the teratogenic effects of the drug. The patient, prescriber, and pharmacy must be registered through the iPLEDGE program, which requires the patient to follow monthly precautions and guidelines.

Table 5-20. Dermatological Agents

Generic Name	Brand Name	Common Strengths/ Dosages	Dosage Forms	Route	Indication
adapalene	Differin	0.1 %	Cream, solution, gel	Topical	Treatment of acne
benzoyl peroxide	Benoxyl, Benzac AC	2.5–10%	Lotion, cream, gel	Topical	Treatment of acne
clindamycin	Cleocin	1%	Gel, lotion	Topical	Treatment of acne
clindamycin and benzoyl peroxide	Benzaclin, Duac	1%, 5%	Gel	Topical	Treatment of acne
erythromycin and benzoyl peroxide	Benzamycin	3%, 5%	Gel	Topical	Treatment of acne
isotretinoin	Clavaris, Amnesteem, Absorbica, Myorisan	10 mg, 20 mg, 30 mg, 40 mg	Capsule	PO	Treatment of acne
tazarotene	Tazorac	0.05%, 0.1%	Cream, gel	Topical	Treatment of acne
tretinoin	Retin-A	0.025%, 0.04%, 0.05%, 0.1%	Cream, gel	Topical	Treatment of acne
betamethasone dipropionate, clotrimazole	Lotrisone	0.05%, 1%	Cream, lotion	Topical	Treatment of minor skin redness, itching, and swelling

Generic Name	Brand Name	Common Strengths/ Dosages	Dosage Forms	Route	Indication
clobetasol propionate	Temovate	0.05%	Cream, ointment	Topical	Treatment of minor skin irritations, rashes, and itching
desoxymetasone	Topicort	0.25%	Cream	Topical	Treatment of minor skin irritations, rashes, and itching
flucinonide	Lidex	0.2%	Cream, ointment	Topical	Treatment of minor skin irritations, rashes, and itching
fluticasone proprionate	Cutivate	0.005%, 0.05%	Cream, ointment	Topical	Treatment of minor skin irritations, rashes, and itching
hydrocortisone	Cortaid *Available OTC	0.5%, 1%, 2.5%	Cream	Topical	Treatment of minor skin irritations, rashes, and itching
mometasone furoate	Elocon	0.1%	Cream, ointment	Topical	Treatment of minor skin irritations, rashes, and itching
triamcinolone	Kenalog	0.025%, 0.1%, 0.5%	Cream, ointment	Topical	Treatment of minor skin irritations, rashes, and itching
bacitracin	Baciguent *Available OTC	500 iU/g	Ointment	Topical	Treatment or prevention of an infection of minor skin wounds
mupirocin	Bactroban	2%	Ointment	Topical	Treatment or prevention of an infection of minor skin wounds
neomycin, polymyxin, bacitracin	Neosporin *Available OTC	3.5 mg/5,000 U/ 400 U/1g	Ointment	Topical	Treatment or prevention of an infection of minor skin wounds
acyclovir	Zovirax	5%	Ointment	Topical	Treatment of cold sores
docosanol	Abreva *Available OTC	10%	Cream	Topical	Treatment of cold sores
pyrithione zinc	Head and Shoulders *Available OTC	1%	Shampoo	Topical	Treatment of dandruff
selenium disulfide	Selsun Blue	1%	Shampoo	Topical	Treatment of dandruff
ketoconazole	Nizoral *Available OTC	2%	Cream, shampoo	Topical	Treatment of fungal infections

Generic Name	Brand Name	Common Strengths/ Dosages	Dosage Forms	Route	Indication
terbinafine	Lamisil *Available OTC	1%	Cream	Topical	Treatment of fungal infections
acitretin	Soriatane	10 mg, 17.5 mg, 22.5 mg, 25 mg	Capsule	PO	Treatment of psoriasis
calcipotriene	Dovonex	0.005%	Cream, ointment	Topical	Treatment of psoriasis
pimecrolimus	Elidel	1%	Cream	Topical	Treatment of psoriasis
diphenhydramine	Benadryl *Available OTC	1% (OTC), 2%	Ointment	Topical	Used as an antihistamine for the treatment of rashes, itches, or skin irritations
imiquimod	Aldara	5%	Cream	Topical	Used to treat actinic keratosis
silver sulfadiazine	Silvadene	1%	Cream	Topical	Treatment of infections due to second- and third-degree burns

EARS, EYES, NOSE, AND THROAT AGENTS

Medications in this category treat a variety of conditions and are sometimes referred to as medications pertaining to the senses. Use Table 5-21 to help you recognize common stems used by the USAN council.

TIP

A pharmacy technician should pay attention to the package quantity input in the pharmacy computer when transcribing the script. Most pharmacy systems ask for the total package size (e.g., 1 g or 5 mL), not the number of units (e.g., 1 box or 1 bottle). Make sure to check with the pharmacist before proceeding.

Table 5-21. USAN Stems for Ears, Eyes, Nose, and Throat Agents

Stem	Description	Example
-astine	H1 receptor	azelastine
-olol	Beta antagonists	betaxolol
-onide	Corticosteroid	budesonide

Ears, eyes, nose, and throat agents are used to treat a variety of disease states and symptoms (see Table 5-22). Varying formulations within routes are also available. Proper selection is based on the condition treated. Ophthalmic (eye) and otic (ear) formulations include drops and ointments. Medications for these routes may have anti-infective properties such as ciprofloxacin (Ciloxan), may act as histamine blockers like oloptadine (Pataday, Patanol), or may be used to decrease ocular pressure like brimonidine (Alphagen P). Treatment may last a few days for conditions like redness or ear pain. In contrast, infections may require a 7–10 day course of therapy. Patients who have chronic conditions, including glaucoma, must continue medications long term. Medications for the nose are used to treat allergy symptoms or nasal congestion. These medications may be taken long term, seasonally, or for a few days.

Oxymetazoline (Afrin, Vicks Sinex) is an alpha-adrenergic agonist used to produce vasoconstriction in the nasal arteries, therefore, increasing airflow and reducing nasal congestion. These agents should not be used for more than three to five days because of the possibility of causing rebound congestion. Medications for the throat have anesthetic properties used as needed to treat pain in the oral mucosa and throat.

Table 5-22. Ears, Eyes, Nose, and Throat Agents

Generic Name	Brand Name	Common Strengths/ Dosages	Dosage Forms	Route	Indication
azelastine	Astelin, Astepro	0.1%, 0.15%	Nasal spray	Intranasal	Treatment of allergic rhinitis
beclomethasone	Beconase AQ	168 mcg	Nasal spray	Intranasal	Treatment of allergic rhinitis
budesonide	Rhinocort Aqua	32 mcg	Nasal spray	Intranasal	Treatment of allergic rhinitis
ciclesonide	Omnaris, Zetonna	37 mcg, 50 mcg	Nasal spray	Intranasal	Treatment of allergic rhinitis
mometasone	Nasonex	50 mcg	Nasal spray	Intranasal	Treatment of allergic rhinitis
triamcinolone	Nasacort *Available OTC	110 mcg	Nasal spray	Intranasal	Treatment of allergic rhinitis
fluticasone	Flonase *OTC formulation available	27.5 mcg, 50 mcg	Nasal spray	Intranasal	Treatment of nonallergic rhinitis
oxymetazoline	Afrin, Vicks Sinex *Available OTC	0.05%	Nasal spray	Intranasal	Treatment of nasal congestion
sodium chloride	Ayr, Ocean, Simply Saline *Available OTC	0.65%	Nasal spray	Intranasal	Treatment of nasal congestion
azelastine	Optivar	0.05%	Eyedrop	Ophthalmic	Treatment of allergic conjunctivitis
ketorolac	Acular	0.4%, 0.5%	Eyedrop	Ophthalmic	Treatment of allergic conjunctivitis
ketotifen fumarate	Alaway, Zaditor *Available OTC	0.025%	Eyedrop	Ophthalmic	Treatment of allergic conjunctivitis
loteprednol	Alrex, Lotemax	0.2%, 0.5%	Eyedrop	Ophthalmic	Treatment of allergic conjunctivitis
olopatadine	Pataday, Patanol, Pateo	0.1%, 0.2%, 0.7%	Eyedrop	Ophthalmic	Treatment of allergic conjunctivitis

Generic Name	Brand Name	Common Strengths/ Dosages	Dosage Forms	Route	Indication
lodoxamide	Alomide	0.1%	Eyedrop	Ophthalmic	Treatment of conjunctivitis
naphazoline	Naphcon-A, Opcon-A, Visine-A	0.025%	Eyedrop	Ophthalmic	Treatment of decongestion, ocular vasoconstrictor
betaxolol	Betoptic, Betoptic S	0.25%, 0.5%	Eyedrop	Ophthalmic	Treatment of glaucoma
bimatoprost	Lumigan	0.03%	Eyedrop	Ophthalmic	Treatment of glaucoma
brimonidine	Alphagen P	0.1%, 0.15%	Eyedrop	Ophthalmic	Treatment of glaucoma
brinzolamide	Azopt	1%	Eyedrop	Ophthalmic	Treatment of glaucoma
dorzolamide	Trusopt	2%	Eyedrop	Ophthalmic	Treatment of glaucoma
erythromycin	Ilotycin Ophthalmic	0.5%	Ointment	Ophthalmic	Treatment of glaucoma
gatifloxacin	Zymar, Zymaxin	0.3%	Eyedrop	Ophthalmic	Treatment of glaucoma
gentamicin	Gentak, Garamycin Ophthalmic	0.3%	Eyedrop	Ophthalmic	Treatment of glaucoma
latanoprost	Xalatan	0.005%	Eyedrop	Ophthalmic	Treatment of glaucoma
pilocarpine	IsoptoCarpine	1%, 2%, 4%	Eyedrop	Ophthalmic	Treatment of glaucoma
timolol	Timoptic	0.25%, 0.5%	Eyedrop, gel	Ophthalmic	Treatment of glaucoma
travoprost	Travatan, Travatan Z	0.004%	Eyedrop	Ophthalmic	Treatment of glaucoma
ciprofloxacin	Ciloxan	0.3%	Eyedrop, ointment	Ophthalmic	Treatment of bacterial conjunctivitis
moxifloxacin	Moxeza, Vigamox	0.5%	Eyedrop	Ophthalmic	Treatment of bacterial conjunctivitis
sulfacetamide	Bleph-10	10%	Eyedrop	Ophthalmic	Treatment of bacterial conjunctivitis
tobramycin	Tobrex, AK-Tob	0.3%	Eyedrop, ointment	Ophthalmic	Treatment of bacterial conjunctivitis
trimethoprim, polymixin B	Polytrim Ophthalmic	1 mg/ 10,000 U	Eyedrop	Ophthalmic	Treatment of bacterial conjunctivitis
neomycin, polymixin B, dexamethasone	Dexasporin, Maxitrol	3.5 mg/ 10,000 U/0.1%	Eyedrop, ointment	Ophthalmic	Treatment of ocular infections

Generic Name	Brand Name	Common Strengths/ Dosages	Dosage Forms	Route	Indication
fluorometholone	FML, FML Forte	0.1%	Eyedrop, ointment	Ophthalmic	Treatment of ocular inflammation
prednisolone	Pred Forte, Pred Mild	0.12%, 1%	Eyedrop	Ophthalmic	Treatment of ocular inflammation
ciprofloxacin, dexamethasone	Ciprodex	0.3%/0.1%	Eardrop	Otic	Treatment of acute otitis externa
ciprofloxacin, hydrocortisone	Cipro HC otic	0.2%/0.1%	Eardrop	Otic	Treatment of acute otitis externa
ofloxacin	Floxin otic	0.3%	Eardrop	Otic	Treatment of otitis media
acetic acid, hydrocortisone	Acetasol, VoSol HC	1%/2%	Eardrop	Otic	Treatment of external ear infections
hydrocortisone, neomycin, polymyxin B	Cortisporin otic	3.5 mg/ 10,000 U/1 mg	Eardrop	Otic	Treatment of external ear infections
acetic acid	VoSol	2%	Eardrop	Otic	Removal of wax and debris from the ear
benzocaine	Anbesol, Orabase, Orajel *Available OTC	7.5%, 10%, 20%	Cream, gel	Oral mucosa	Treatment of pain
benzocaine, menthol	Cepacol *Available OTC	10%/2 mg	Lozenge	Throat	Treatment of pain and sore throat
phenol	Chloraseptic	1.4%	Spray	Throat	Treatment of pain and sore throat

ENDOCRINE AGENTS

Review endocrine USAN stems by looking at Table 5-23. These stems identify the most commonly prescribed medications used to treat diabetes mellitus.

NOTE

Insulin is stored in the pharmacy refrigerator prior to being dispensed.

Table 5-23. USAN Stems for Encodrine Agents

Stem	Description	Example
-formin	Hypoglycemic	metformin
-glinide	Meglitinide	repaglinide
-gliptin	Dipeptidyl peptidase-4 inhibitor	saxagliptin
-glitazone	Thiazolidene derivative	rosiglitazone

Diabetes mellitus is a chronic condition resulting from abnormally high levels of glucose. This may be due to an inadequate production of insulin by the pancreas or an inability for the cells to react to the activity of insulin. Diabetes mellitus can be further subdivided into two categories based on these mechanisms. Type I diabetes is an autoimmune disease occurring when there is little to no production of insulin. Treatment for this type of diabetes is based solely on the use of exogenous insulin. In type II diabetes, insulin is present, but the cells are not sensitive to its action. This type of diabetes is treated with oral medications with insulin therapy and other injectables reserved for chronic resistance. Acute complications include hyperglycemia (high blood glucose levels) and hypoglycemia (low blood glucose levels). Patients should perform daily glucose testing. Their practitioner should also screen for HbA1C (a test to check for the presence of glycated hemoglobin) to assess average blood sugar over a period of three months.

Sulfonylureases, like glimepiride (Amaryl), are used to stimulate insulin secretion from beta cells. This class of medications is noted to cause hypoglycemia and weight gain. α-glucosidase inhibitors, including acarbose (Precose), prevent the digestion of carbohydrates that are turned into simple sugars. Serious side effects include severe stomach pain, constipation, and easy bruising. Rapid insulin secretors, such as repaglinide (Prandin), increase the sensitivity of beta cells to elevated blood glucose levels. This class of medications is taken immediately before a meal to reduce postprandial hyperglycemia. Insulin-sensitizing agents, such as the thiazolidinediones and biguanides, are also used in the treatment of type II diabetes. These include medications such as pioglitazone (Actos) and metformin (Glucophage), respectively. Dipeptidyl peptidase-IV (DPP-IV) inhibitors, such as saxagliptin (Onglyza), are used in addition to diet and exercise and have been shown to improve glucose tolerance and HbA1C. Canagliflozin (Invokana) belongs to a new class of selective sodium-glucose transporter-2 (SGLT2) inhibitors indicated as adjunct therapy to diet and exercise.

Hypothyroidism is an endocrine disorder resulting from a deficiency in the production of a thyroid hormone from the thyroid gland. Thyroid levels can be examined by checking T4 (thyroxine tetraiodothyronine) and T3 (triiodothyronine). T4 is actively converted to T3, which accounts for most of the metabolic activity. A deficiency in one or more of these hormones may warrant the initiation of medication. Medications used to treat hypothyroidism target either T4 (e.g., levothyroxine) or T3 (e.g., liothyronine sodium) production. Generally, medications targeting T4 are used because of their longer half-life, leading to once-a-day dosing and the conversion to T3 in the bloodstream. These medications are taken in the morning, 30 minutes before eating. Antacids and medications containing iron should be avoided because they may interfere with absorption.

Hyperthyroidism is a result of an excess of thyroid hormones due to an overactive thyroid gland. TRH (thyrotropin-releasing hormone) is released from the hypothalamus, which in turn sends a signal to the pituitary gland to release TSH (thyroid-stimulating hormone). This, in turn, signals the thyroid gland to release thyroid hormones T4 and T3. Overactivity of these glands may result in an increase in and potential excessive production of thyroid hormones. The antithyroid medications methimazole (Tapazole) and propylthiouracil (PTU) are used to block the production of thyroid hormones. Patients are monitored for potential agranulocytosis, a condition that occurs due to the suppression of white blood cell production. Table 5-24 lists numerous endocrine agents.

Table 5-24. Encodrine Agents

Generic Name	Brand Name	Common Strengths/Dosages	Dosage Forms	Route	Indication
acarbose	Precose	25 mg, 50 mg, 100 mg	Tablet	PO	Treatment of diabetes mellitus
alogliptin	Nesina	25 mg	Tablet	PO	Treatment of diabetes mellitus
alogliptin, metformin	Kazano	12.5 mg/500 mg, 12.5 mg/1,000 mg	Tablet	PO	Treatment of diabetes mellitus
alogliptin, pioglitazone	Oseni	25 mg/15 mg, 25 mg/30 mg, 25 mg/45 mg	Tablet	PO	Treatment of diabetes mellitus
canagliflozin	Invokana	100 mg, 300 mg	Tablet	PO	Treatment of diabetes mellitus
exenatide	Byetta	5 mcg, 10 mcg	Parenteral	SQ	Treatment of diabetes mellitus
glimepiride	Amaryl	1 mg, 2 mg, 4 mg	Tablet	PO	Treatment of diabetes mellitus
glipizide	Glucotrol	2.5 mg, 5 mg, 10 mg	Tablet	PO	Treatment of diabetes mellitus
glyburide	Diabeta, Micronase	1.25 mg, 1.5 mg, 2.5 mg, 3 mg, 5 mg, 6 mg	Tablet	PO	Treatment of diabetes mellitus
llraglutide	Victoza	0.6 mg, 1.2 mg, 1.8 mg	Parenteral	SQ	Treatment of diabetes mellitus
metformin	Glucophage	500 mg, 750 mg, 850 mg, 1,000 mg	Tablet	PO	Treatment of diabetes mellitus
metformin, glipizide	Metaglip	2.5 mg/250 mg, 2.5 mg/500 mg, 5 mg/500 mg	Tablet	PO	Treatment of diabetes mellitus
metformin, glyburide	Glucovance	1.25 mg/250 mg, 2.5 mg/500 mg, 5 mg/500 mg	Tablet	PO	Treatment of diabetes mellitus
miglitol	Glyset	25 mg, 50 mg, 100 mg	Tablet	PO	Treatment of diabetes mellitus
nateglinide	Starlix	60 mg, 120 mg	Tablet	PO	Treatment of diabetes mellitus
pioglitazone	Actos	15 mg, 30 mg, 45 mg	Tablet	PO	Treatment of diabetes mellitus
pramlintide	Symlin	60 mcg	Parenteral	SQ	Treatment of diabetes mellitus
repaglinide	Prandin	0.5 mg, 1 mg, 2 mg	Tablet	PO	Treatment of diabetes mellitus
rosiglitazone	Avandia	2 mg, 4 mg, 8 mg	Tablet	PO	Treatment of diabetes mellitus
rosiglitazone, metformin	Avandamet	1 mg/500 mg, 2 mg/500 mg, 4 mg/500 mg	Tablet	PO	Treatment of diabetes mellitus
saxagliptin	Onglyza	2.5 mg, 5 mg	Tablet	PO	Treatment of diabetes mellitus

Generic Name	Brand Name	Common Strengths/Dosages	Dosage Forms	Route	Indication
sitagliptin	Januvia	25 mg, 50 mg, 100 mg	Tablet	PO	Treatment of diabetes mellitus
sitagliptin, metformin	Janumet	50 mg/500 mg, 50 mg/1,000 mg	Tablet	PO	Treatment of diabetes mellitus
levothyroxine	Levoxyl, Synthroid, Tirosint	13 mcg, 25 mcg, 50 mcg, 75 mcg, 88 mcg, 100 mcg, 112 mcg, 125 mcg, 137 mcg, 150 mcg, 175 mcg, 200 mcg, 300 mcg, 500 mcg	Tablet, capsule, parenteral	PO, IV, IM	Treatment of hypothyroidism
liothyronine sodium	Cytomel	5 mcg, 10 mcg, 25 mcg, 50 mcg	Tablet, parenteral	PO, IV	Treatment of hypothyroidism
methimazole	Tapazole	5 mg, 10 mg	Tablet	PO	Treatment of hyperthyroidism
propylthiouracil	PTU	50 mg	Tablet	PO	Treatment of hyperthyroidism

Insulin is used in the treatment of diabetes. Patients with type I diabetes mellitus are unable to produce insulin due to the autoimmune destruction of beta cells in the pancreas. A lack of insulin production leads to a dangerous increase in glucose levels. Exogenous insulin is used to provide glycemic control, reducing microvascular complications and cardiovascular events and also decreasing mortality. A diagnosis of type II diabetes may also warrant the use of insulin to supplement oral antidiabetic therapy (see Table 5-25). Insulin regimens may include a basal (long-acting) insulin given with preprandial (premeal) short or rapid-acting insulin.

Table 5-25. Insulin

Type	Generic Name	Brand Name	Dosage Form	Route
Rapid acting	insulin aspart	Humalog	Parenteral	SQ
	insulin glulisine	Apidra	Parenteral	SQ
	insulin human	Afrezza	Oral inhalation	Inhalation
	insulin lispro	Novolog	Parenteral	SQ
Short acting	regular insulin	Humulin R, Novolin R	Parenteral	SQ
Intermediate acting	NPH insulin	Humulin N, Novolin N	Parenteral	SQ
Long acting	insulin degludec	Tresiba	Parenteral	SQ
	insulin detemir	Levemir	Parenteral	SQ
	insulin glargine	Lantus, Toujeo	Parenteral	SQ

GASTROINTESTINAL AGENTS

Test yourself on gastrointestinal USAN stem names by covering the descriptions in Table 5-26 with your hand. Review the stems that you do not recognize right away before proceeding.

Table 5-26. USAN Stems for Gastrointestinal Agents

Stem	Description	Example
-prazole	Antiulcer agents (bezimidazole derivatives)	lansoprazole
-setron	Serotonin 5-HT3 antagonists	ondansetron
-tidine	H2-receptor antagonists	famotidine

Gastrointestinal agents are used to treat conditions of the GI tract, including constipation, diarrhea, gastroesophageal reflux (GERD), heartburn, indigestion, nausea, spasms, ulcers, and vomiting. Ulcers can be caused by excess acid production, chronic use of nonsteroidal anti-inflammatory agents, or by the bacteria *Helicobacter pylori*. The most effective way to treat ulcers caused by *H. pylori* is to use drug combinations that include acid-reducing agents and antibiotics. Although most of these medications can be taken orally, intravenous, topical, and rectal formulations are available for patients who require alternative routes (see Table 5-27). Common side effects of the gastrointestinal agents include upset stomach, nausea and vomiting, and headaches.

> **TIP**
>
> Some medications used to treat gastroesophageal reflux are available without a prescription. The pharmacy technician should inform the patient of any OTC medications as noted on their prescription. OTC medications may be covered by insurance; coverage should be verified before filling the prescription.

Table 5-27. Gastrointestinal Agents

Generic Name	Brand Name	Common Strengths/Dosages	Dosage Forms	Route	Indication
aluminum hydroxide, magnesium hydroxide	Maalox *Available OTC	200 mg/200 mg/5 mL	Liquid	PO	Treatment of heartburn and indigestion
aluminum hydroxide, magnesium hydroxide, simethicone	Maalox Advanced, Mylanta *Available OTC	200 mg/200 mg/20 mg/5 mL	Liquid	PO	Treatment of heartburn and indigestion
calcium carbonate	Tums *Available OTC	500 mg, 750 mg, 1,000 mg	Tablet	PO	Treatment of heartburn and indigestion
calcium carbonate, magnesium hydroxide	Rolaids *Available OTC	550 mg/110 mg	Tablet	PO	Treatment of heartburn and indigestion
cimetidine	Tagamet-HB, Tagamet *Available OTC	200 mg, 300 mg, 400 mg, 800 mg, 300 mg/5 mL	Tablet, liquid	PO	Treatment of heartburn, indigestion, and ulcers
famotidine	Pepcid-AC, Pepcid *OTC formulation available	10 mg, 20 mg, 40 mg	Tablet	PO	Treatment of heartburn, indigestion, and ulcers

Generic Name	Brand Name	Common Strengths/Dosages	Dosage Forms	Route	Indication
nizatidine	Axid-AR, Axid *Available OTC	75 mg, 150 mg, 300 mg, 15 mg/mL	Tablet, capsule, liquid	PO	Treatment of heartburn, indigestion, and ulcers
ranitidine	Zantac-75, Zantac-150, Zantac *Available OTC	75 mg, 150 mg, 300 mg, 15 mg/mL, 25 mg/mL	Tablet, liquid, parenteral	PO	Treatment of heartburn, indigestion, and ulcers
metoclopramide	Reglan	5 mg, 10 mg, 5 mg/5 mL, 5 mg/mL	Tablet, solution, parenteral	PO, IV	Treatment of GERD and treatment of chemotherapy-induced nausea/vomiting
dexlansoprazole	Dexilant	30 mg, 60 mg	Tablet	PO	Treatment of GERD and ulcers
esomeprazole	Nexium-24HR, Nexium *Available OTC	20 mg, 40 mg	Capsule, granule for oral suspension, powder for parenteral administration	PO	Treatment of GERD and ulcers
lansoprazole	Prevacid-24HR, Prevacid *Available OTC	15 mg, 30 mg	Capsule, powder for parenteral administration	PO, IV	Treatment of GERD and ulcers
omeprazole	Prilosec OTC, Prilosec *Available OTC	20 mg, 40 mg	Tablet, capsule	PO	Treatment of GERD and ulcers
pantroprazole	Protonix	20 mg, 40 mg	Tablet, granule for oral suspension, powder for parenteral administration	PO, IV	Treatment of GERD and ulcers
rabeprazole	Aciphex	20 mg	Tablet	PO	Treatment of GERD and ulcers
sucralfate	Carafate	1 g, 1 g/10 mL	Tablet, liquid	PO	Treatment of active duodenal ulcer
mesalamine	Apriso, Asacol, Canasa, Pentasa, Rowasa	250 mg, 375 mg, 400 mg, 1,000 mg, 4 g/60 mL	Tablet, capsule, suppository	PO, rectal	Treatment of ulcerative colitis
sulfasalazine	Azulfidine	500 mg	Tablet	PO	Treatment of ulcerative colitis
bismuth subcitrate potassium, metronidazole, tetracycline	Pylera	140 mg/125 mg/ 125 mg	Capsule	PO	Treatment of ulcers due to the bacteria *H. pylori*

Generic Name	Brand Name	Common Strengths/Dosages	Dosage Forms	Route	Indication
bismuth subsalicylate, metronidazole, tetracycline	Helidac	262.4 mg/250 mg/ 500 mg	Tablet, capsule	PO	Treatment of ulcers due to the bacteria *H. pylori*
lansoprazole, amoxicillin, clarithromycin	Prevpac	30 mg/1 g/500 mg	Tablet, capsule	PO	Treatment of ulcers due to the bacteria *H. pylori*
misoprostol	Cytotec	100 mcg, 200 mcg	Tablet	PO	Treatment of NSAID-induced ulcers
dicyclomine	Bentyl	10 mg, 20 mg, 10 mg/5 mL, 10 mg/mL	Capsule, tablet, solution, parenteral	PO, IV	Treatment of irritable bowel syndrome
hyoscyamine	Levbid, Levsin, Anaspaz, Cytospaz, Nulev	0.125 mg, 0.375 mg, 0.125 mg/5 mL, 0.5 mg/mL	Tablet, elixir, parenteral	PO, IV	Treatment of gastrointestinal disorders, including spasms
meclizine	Antivert, Bonine *Available OTC	12.5 mg, 25 mg	Tablet	PO	Treatment of motion sickness
dolasetron	Anzemet	50 mg, 100 mg, 20 mg/mL	Tablet, parenteral	PO, IV	Treatment of nausea and vomiting
granisetron	Kytril, Sancuso	1 mg, 3.1 mg/24 hr, 2 mg/10 mL, 1 mg/mL	Tablet, solution, patch, parenteral	PO, topical, IV	Treatment of nausea and vomiting
ondansetron	Zofran, Zofran ODT	4 mg/8 mg	Tablet, film, parenteral	PO, parenteral	Treatment of nausea and vomiting
prochlorperazine	Compazine	5 mg, 10 mg, 25 mg	Tablet, suppository	PO, rectal	Treatment of nausea and vomiting
promethazine	Phenergan, Promethegan	12.5 mg, 25 mg, 50 mg, 6.25 mg/5 mL, 25 mg/mL, 50 mg/mL	Tablet, syrup, suppository, parenteral	PO, rectal, parenteral	Treatment of nausea and vomiting
polyethylene glycol 3350	Miralax *Available OTC	17 g	Powder for solution	PO	Osmotic laxative
polyethylene glycol electrolyte solution	GoLyte/ GoLytely	2 L, 4 L	Liquid	PO	Bowel preparation
polyethylene glycol electrolyte solution and bisacodyl	HalfLytely	2 L, 5 mg	Liquid	PO	Bowel preparation
docusate	Colace *Available OTC	50 mg, 100 mg	Tablet, capsule	PO	Stool softener

Generic Name	Brand Name	Common Strengths/Dosages	Dosage Forms	Route	Indication
bisacodyl	Dulcolax *Available OTC	5 mg, 10 mg	Tablet, suppository	PO, rectal	Treatment of constipation
lactulose	Enulose, Kristalose	10 mg/10 mg/15 mL	Powder packet, solution	PO	Treatment of constipation
psyllium	Metamucil *Available OTC	500 mg, 0.52 g, 3.5 g, 4.1 g	Capsule, powder	PO	Treatment of constipation
senna	Senokot, SennaGen *Available OTC	8.6 mg, 15 mg, 25 mg, 8.8 mg/5 mL	Tablet, syrup	PO	Treatment of constipation
attapulgite	Kaopectate	600 mg/15 mL, 750 mg/15 mL	Liquid	PO	Treatment of diarrhea
loperamide	Imodium, Imodium-AD *Available OTC	2 mg, 1 mg/5 mL	Tablet, caplet, liquid	PO	Treatment of diarrhea
loperamide, simethicone	Imodium Advanced *Available OTC	2 mg/125 mL	Tablet, caplet	PO	Treatment of diarrhea
diphenoxylate, atropine	Lomotil	2.5 mg/0.025 mg, 2.5 mg/0.025 mg/ 5 mL	Tablet, solution	PO	Treatment of diarrhea (C-V)

NOTE

Medications that are used to treat pain are highly regulated. Some states may require double counting procedures, and others may have restrictions on who may count narcotics. Check your state regulations to ensure that you are meeting all requirements.

MUSCULAR, SKELETAL, AND OSTEOPOROSIS MEDICATIONS

Use Table 5-28 to test your knowledge of the USAN stem names for common muscular, skeletal, and osteoporosis medications.

Table 5-28. USAN Stems for Muscular, Skeletal, and Osteoporosis Medications

Stem	Description	Example
-ac	Anti-inflammatory agents (acetic acid derivatives)	diclofenac
-caine	Local anesthetics	lidocaine
-coxib	COX-2 inhibitor	celecoxib
-dronate	Bisphosphonates	ibandronate
-icam	Anti-inflammatory agents (isoxicam type)	piroxicam

Medications in this group treat a wide range of symptoms and diseases (see Table 5-29). Medications for pain are grouped based on their ability to relieve pain, their abuse potential, and their effect (e.g., anti-inflammatory).

Opioid-based medications are scheduled under the Controlled Substances Act. Most of the controlled pain agents are C-II or C-V and are indicated for moderate-to-severe pain. These agents exert their action by binding and interacting with mu (μ) receptors. Dosing schedules for these medications vary and depend on the indication and duration of treatment. The opioid-based agents (e.g., oxycodone, hydrocodone) can cause CNS depression and constipation. The non-narcotic opioids are indicated for mild-to-moderate pain. They have anti-inflammatory effects like the NSAIDS (e.g., Nonselective COX inhibitors target COX-I and COX-II and include the drugs ibuprofen or naproxen. Selective COX inhibitors target COX-II and include the drug Celebrex.). Adverse effects for these agents include gastrointestinal upset, cramping, ulcers, and headaches.

Medications for the treatment of rheumatoid arthritis can be taken daily, weekly, or monthly. They work by preventing synovial infection due to the inactivation of Tumor Necrosis Factor (TNF). A risk for serious infection is possible while taking agents with a parenteral formulation. Oral rheumatoid arthritis agents can cause gastrointestinal side effects such as nausea, cramping, and diarrhea. Muscle relaxants relieve local skeletal muscle spasms and, in return, can make the user feel drowsy, dizzy, or confused. Drugs that treat osteoporosis can cause stomach ulcers. Patients may be told to take their medication with a full glass of water and remain upright for 30 minutes to lessen the risk of developing a stomach ulcer.

Bisphosphonates are first-line pharmacological agents indicated for the treatment of osteoporosis due to osteoclast-mediated bone loss. They are also prescribed for conditions such as low bone density, multiple myeloma, and Paget's disease. These agents indirectly increase bone density by inhibiting bone resorption. These agents should be taken in the morning, 60 minutes before eating or drinking. When taking these agents, the patient should sit in an upright position, drink a full glass of water, and remain in the upright position for 60 minutes as a precaution to avoid esophageal and gastrointestinal side effects. Bisphosphonates are available in daily, weekly, or monthly dosage regimens.

Table 5-29. Muscular, Skeletal, and Osteoporosis Medications

Generic Name	Brand Name	Common Strengths/Dosages	Dosage Forms	Routes	Indication
fentanyl	Actiq, Duragesic, Sublimaze, Onsolls, Fentora	400 mcg, 600 mcg, 800 mcg, 1,200 mcg, 1,600 mcg, 12.5 mcg/hr, 25 mcg/hr, 50 mcg/hr, 75 mcg/hr, 100 mcg/hr	Lozenge, patch, parenteral, buccal film, buccal tablet	PO, transdermal, IV, IM, buccal	Treatment of moderate to severe pain (C-II)
hydrocodone, acetaminophen	Vicodin, Lorcet, Lortab	5 mg/300 mg, 7.5 mg/300 mg, 10 mg/300 mg	Tablet	PO	Treatment of moderate to severe pain (C-II)
hydrocodone, ibuprofen	Vicoprofen	2.5 mg/200 mg, 5 mg/200 mg, 7.5 mg/200 mg, 10 mg/200 mg	Tablet	PO	Treatment of moderate to severe pain (C-II)
hydromorphone	Dilaudid	2 mg, 4 mg, 8 mg, 12 mg, 16 mg, 24 mg, 32 mg, 1 mg/mL, 2 mg/mL, 4 mg/mL, 10 mg/mL	Tablet, capsule, liquid, parenteral	PO, IV, IM	Treatment of moderate to severe pain (C-II)
meperidine	Demorol	50 mg, 100 mg, 50 mg/5 mL, 25 mg/mL, 50 mg/mL, 75 mg/mL, 100 mg/mL	Tablet, solution, parenteral	PO, IV, IM	Treatment of moderate to severe pain (C-II)

Generic Name	Brand Name	Common Strengths/Dosages	Dosage Forms	Routes	Indication
methadone	Dolophine	5 mg, 10 mg, 40 mg, 5 mg/5 mL, 10 mg/5 mL, 10 mg/mL	Tablet, solution, parenteral	PO, IV, IM	Treatment of moderate to severe pain (C-II)
morphine	Roxanol	15 mg, 30 mg, 10 mg/5 mL, 20 mg/5 mL, 1 mg/mL, 5 mg/mL, 10 mg/mL, 50 mg/mL	Tablet, solution, parenteral	PO, IV, IM	Treatment of moderate to severe pain (C-II)
morphine ER	MS Contin, Kadian, Avinza	15 mg, 30 mg, 50 mg, 60 mg, 90 mg, 100 mg, 120 mg, 200 mg	Tablet, capsule	PO	Treatment of moderate to severe pain (C-II)
oxycodone	Oxy IR	5 mg, 10 mg, 15 mg, 20 mg, 30 mg, 5 mg/5 mL	Tablet, capsule	PO	Treatment of moderate to severe pain (C-II)
oxycodone ER	Oxycontin	10 mg, 15 mg, 20 mg, 30 mg, 40 mg, 60 mg, 80 mg	Tablet	PO	Treatment of moderate to severe pain (C-II)
oxycodone, acetaminophen	Percocet, Roxicet, Endocet	2.5 mg/325 mg, 5 mg/325 mg, 5 mg/500 mg, 7.4 mg/500 mg, 7.5 mg/325 mg, 10 mg/325 mg, 10 mg/650 mg	Tablet	PO	Treatment of moderate to severe pain (C-II)
oxycodone, aspirin	Percodan	4.8355 mg/325 mg	Tablet	PO	Treatment of moderate to severe pain (C-II)
butorphanol	Stadol	1 mg/mL, 2 mg/mL, 10 mg/mL	Nasal spray, parenteral	Nasal, IV, IM	Treatment of moderate to severe pain (C-IV)
pentazocine, naloxone	Talwin NX	50 mg/0.5 mg	Tablet	PO	Treatment of moderate to severe pain (C-IV)
tramadol	Ultram	50 mg, 100 mg, 200 mg, 300 mg	Tablet	PO	Treatment of moderate to severe pain (C-IV)
baclofen	Liorsal	10 mg, 20 mg	Tablet	PO	Muscle relaxant
cyclobenzaprine	Flexeril	5 mg, 7.5 mg, 10 mg, 15 mg	Tablet, capsule	PO	Muscle relaxant
metaxalone	Skelaxin	800 mg	Tablet	PO	Muscle relaxant

Generic Name	Brand Name	Common Strengths/Dosages	Dosage Forms	Routes	Indication
methocarbamol	Robaxin	500 mg, 750 mg, 100 mg/mL	Tablet, parenteral	PO, IV, IM	Muscle relaxant
orphenadrine	Norflex	100 mg, 30 mg/mL	Tablet, parenteral	PO, IV, IM	Muscle relaxant
tizanidine	Zanaflex	4 mg, 5 mg	Parenteral	IV	Muscle relaxant
carisoprodol	Soma	250 mg, 350 mg	Tablet	PO	Muscle relaxant (C-IV)
acetaminophen	Tylenol	80 mg, 120 mg, 160 mg, 325 mg, 500 mg, 650 mg, 160 mg/5 mL, 80 mg/0.8 mL	Tablet, capsule, suppository, solution	PO, rectal	Treatment of mild to moderate pain
celecoxib	Celebrex	100 mg, 200 mg	Tablet	PO	Treatment of pain and inflammation
diclofenac	Voltaren, Solaraze	25 mg, 50 mg, 75 mg, 100 mg, 1%, 3%	Tablet, gel	PO	Treatment of pain and inflammation
etodolac	Lodine	200 mg, 300 mg, 400 mg, 500 mg, 600 mg	Tablet	PO	Treatment of pain and inflammation
ibuprofen	Motrin, Aleve *OTC formulation available	200 mg, 400 mg, 600 mg, 800 mg, 100 mg/5 mL, 400 mg/5 mL	Tablet, capsule, liquid	PO	Treatment of pain and inflammation
indomethacin	Indocin	25 mg, 50 mg, 75 mg, 25 mg/5 mL	Capsule, suspension, suppository	PO, rectal	Treatment of pain and inflammation
ketorolac	Toradol	10 mg, 15 mg/mL, 30 mg/mL	Tablet, parenteral	PO, IV	Treatment of pain and inflammation
meloxicam	Mobic	7.5 mg, 15 mg, 7.5 mg/mL	Tablet, suspension	PO	Treatment of pain and inflammation
nabumetone	Relafen	500 mg, 750 mg	Tablet	PO	Treatment of mild to moderate pain and inflammation
naproxen	Aleve, Naprosyn *OTC formulation available	250 mg, 375 mg, 500 mg, 125 mg/5 mL	Tablet, suspension	PO	Treatment of mild to moderate pain and inflammation
piroxicam	Feldene	10 mg, 20 mg	Capsule	PO	Treatment of mild to moderate pain and inflammation

Generic Name	Brand Name	Common Strengths/Dosages	Dosage Forms	Routes	Indication
dexamethasone	Decadron	0.5 mg, 0.75 mg, 1 mg, 1.5 mg, 2 mg, 4 mg, 6 mg, 0.5 mg/5 mL	Tablet, suspension, elixir	PO	Treatment of inflammation
methylprednisolone	Medrol	2 mg, 4 mg, 8 mg, 16 mg, 32 mg	Tablet	PO	Treatment of inflammation
prednisone	Deltasone, Orasone	2.5 mg, 5 mg, 10 mg, 20 mg, 5 mg/5 mL	Tablet, solution	PO	Treatment of inflammation
adalimumab	Humira	40 mg	Parenteral	SQ	Treatment of rheumatoid arthritis
anakinra	Kineret	100 mg	Parenteral	SQ	Treatment of rheumatoid arthritis
etanercept	Enbrel	50 mg/mL	Parenteral	SQ	Treatment of rheumatoid arthritis
infliximab	Remicade	100 mg	Parenteral	SQ	Treatment of rheumatoid arthritis
leflunomide	Arava	10 mg, 20 mg	Tablet	PO	Treatment of rheumatoid arthritis
methotrexate	Rheumatrex	2.5 mg, 5 mg, 7.5 mg, 10 mg, 15 mg, 25 mg/mL	Tablet, parenteral	PO, IM	Treatment of rheumatoid arthritis
sulfasalazine	Azulfidine	500 mg	Tablet	PO	Treatment of rheumatoid arthritis
lidocaine	Lidoderm	5%	Patch	Topical	Treatment of pain
alendronate	Fosamax	5 mg, 10 mg, 35 mg, 70 mg, 70 mg/75 mL	Tablet, solution	PO	Treatment and prevention of osteoporosis
alendronate, Vitamin D	Fosamax D	70 mg/2,800 U, 70 mg/5,600 U	Tablet	PO	Treatment and prevention of osteoporosis
calcitonin	Fortical, Miacalcin	200 U	Nasal spray	Nasal	Treatment and prevention of osteoporosis
ibandronate	Boniva	2.5 mg, 150 mg	Tablet	PO	Treatment and prevention of osteoporosis
risedronate	Actonel	5 mg, 30 mg, 35 mg, 150 mg	Tablet	PO	Treatment and prevention of osteoporosis

Generic Name	Brand Name	Common Strengths/Dosages	Dosage Forms	Routes	Indication
raloxifene	Evista	60 mg	Tablet	PO	Treatment and prevention of osteoporosis in postmenopausal women
teriparatide	Forteo	20 mcg	Parenteral	SQ	Treatment of osteoporosis

REPRODUCTIVE AGENTS

Table 5-30 includes the most common USAN stem name used for reproductive agents. The USAN stem "estr-" indicates that the pharmaceutical agent contains the hormone estrogen. Recall this USAN stem name when identifying hormones used in reproductive agents.

Table 5-30. USAN Stem for Reproductive Agents

Stem	Description	Example
estr-	Estrogens	estradiol

Reproductive agents are most commonly associated with hormone therapy (see Table 5-31). Women are prescribed agents that contain a form of progestin (e.g., medroxyprogesterone) and estrogen (e.g., estradiol) or a combination of both. The progestins are used to treat conditions such as abnormal vaginal bleeding or an overgrowth of the uterus lining. Estrogens, on the other hand, are typically prescribed to regulate hormonal imbalances. Estrogens can be used to treat symptoms of menopause in the treatment of certain breast cancers. Testosterone is prescribed to men to treat symptoms of low testosterone. Typical side effects for reproductive agents include headaches, mood disorders, anxiety, fluid retention, weight gain, and menstrual irregularities.

NOTE

Oral contraceptives comes in quantities of 21 or 28 tablets. Typically, packages that have 21 tablets contain 21 active tablets. Packages that have 28 tablets contain 21 active tablets and 7 placebo tablets. The manufacturer adds the 7 placebo tablets so the consumer remembers to start a new pack after 28 days.

Table 5-31. Reproductive Agents

Generic Name	Brand Name	Common Strengths/Dosages	Dosage Forms	Route	Indication
conjugated equine estrogens	Premarin, Premarin Vaginal Cream, Premphase	0.3 mg, 0.45 mg, 0.625 mg, 0.9 mg, 1.25 mg, 0.625 mg/5 mg, 0.625 mg/g	Tablet, cream	PO, intravaginal	Hormone replacement
conjugated equine estrogens, medroxyprogesterone	Prempro	0.3 mg,/1.5 mg, 0.45 mg/1.5 mg, 0.625 mg/2.5 mg, 0.625 mg/5 mg	Tablet	PO	Hormone replacement
estradiol	Estrace Vaginal Cream, Estrace Vaginal Ring	0.1 mg/g, 2 mg	Cream, ring	PO, intravaginal	Hormone replacement
estradiol	Alora, Climara, Estraderm, Vivelle Dot	0.025 mg/24 hr, 0.0375 mg/hr 0.05 mg/24 hr, 0.06 mg/hr, 0.075 mg/24 hr, 0.1 mg/24 hr	Patch	Transdermal	Hormone replacement
estradiol	Vagifem	10 mg, 25 mg	Tablet	Intravaginal	Hormone replacement
estradiol, norethindrone	Activella, Combipatch	0.5 mg/0.1 mg, 1 mg/0.5 mg	Tablet, patch	PO, transdermal	Hormone replacement
estradiol, norgestimate	Ortho-Prefest	1 mg, 1 mg/0.09 mg	Tablet	PO	Hormone replacement
ethinyl estradiol, norethindrone	Femhrt	2.5 mcg, 0.5 mg, 5 mcg/1 mg	Tablet	PO	Hormone replacement
etonogestrel and ethinyl estradiol vaginal ring	NuvaRing	0.12–0.15 mg/24 hr	Ring	Intravaginal	Hormone replacement
medroxyprogesterone	DepoProvera, Depo-SubQ	2.5 mg, 5 mg, 10 mg, 104 mg/0.65 mL, 150 mg/mL	Tablet	PO	Hormone replacement
micronized estradiol	Estrace	0.5 mg, 1 mg, 2 mg	Tablet, solution, suspension	PO, IM, SC	Hormone replacement
synthetic conjugated estrogens	Cenestin	0.3 mg, 0.45 mg, 0.625 mg, 0.9 mg, 1.25 mg	Tablet	PO	Hormone replacement
testosterone	Testim, Androgel, Depo-testosterone	1%, 100 mg/mL	Gel, parenteral	Topical, IM	Hormone replacement

Common Oral Contraceptives

Oral contraceptives contain varying amounts of estrogen and progestin. Use Table 5-32 below to familiarize yourself with these commonly prescribed agents.

Table 5-32. Common Oral Contraceptives

Active Ingredients	Generic Name	Brand Name
Ethinyl estradiol and desogestrel	apri	Desogen
	kariva	Mircette
	velivet	Cyclessa
Ethinyl estradiol and drospirenone	gianvi	Yaz
	ocella	Yasmin
Ethinyl estradiol and levonorgestrel	aviane	Alesse
	enpresse	Trivora
	jolessa	Seasonale
	levora	Nordette
	quasense	Seasonale
	portia	Nordette
Ethinyl estradiol and norethindrone	balziva	Ovcon 35
	junel FE	Loestrin FE
	nortrel 7/7/7	Ortho Novum
Ethinyl estradiol and norgestrel	cryselle	Low-Ogestrel

RESPIRATORY AGENTS

Use Table 5-33 to review common USAN stems for respiratory agents.

Table 5-33. USAN Stems for Respiratory Agents

Stem	Description	Example
-ast	Antiasthmatics/antiallergics	montelukast
-astine	H1 receptor antagonists	azelastine
-(a)tadine	H1 receptor antagonists (loratadine derivatives)	loratadine
-terol	Bronchodilators	albuterol

NOTE

Cough medications containing codeine are often scheduled as C-V and may have refill limitations, dispensing restrictions, and record-keeping requirements. These laws vary by state.

Respiratory agents (see Table 5-34) are used to treat many conditions, including asthma, chronic obstructive pulmonary disorder (COPD), emphysema, colds, and allergies. Medications associated with asthma are given via inhalation through an inhaler or nebulizer. These medications may work by causing bronchodilation (used to expand the airway) like salmeterol. These inhalers may be used as "rescue inhalers" to treat acute respiratory distress. Other inhalers are used as maintenance medications to prevent breathing difficulties from occurring. Leukotriene inhibitors, like montelukast, stop inflammatory responses by blocking leukotrienes. Corticosteroids inhibit inflammatory mediators and are available in both oral and inhalation dosage forms. Inhaled corticosteroids may cause oral candidiasis (thrush), and patients should be instructed to swish and spit after inhaling the medication. Oral corticosteroids may cause weight gain, an increase in facial hair, or even breast development in men with chronic use. Cough and cold agents treat a variety of symptoms. Expectorants are used to thin mucus associated with coughs and colds. Decongestants are used to treat congestion. Antitussives are used in cough and cold products to relieve dry coughs. These agents are often used in combination to treat multicold symptoms.

Table 5-34. Respiratory Agents

Generic Name	Brand Name	Common Strengths/Dosages	Dosage Forms	Route	Indication
montelukast	Singulair	4 mg, 10 mg	Tablet	PO	Prophylaxis and long-term management of asthma
zafirlukast	Accolate	10 mg, 20 mg	Tablet	PO	Prophylaxis and long-term management of asthma
zileuton	Zyflo-CR	600 mg	Tablet	PO	Prophylaxis and long-term management of asthma
beclomethasone	Beconase, Qvar	40 mcg, 80 mcg, 168 mcg,	Nasal spray, inhaler	Nasal, inhalation	Treatment of allergies, including rhinitis and inflammation
budesonide	Rhinocort	32 mcg	Nasal spray	Nasal	Treatment of allergies, including rhinitis and inflammation
ciclesonide	Omnaris, Alvesco	37.50 mg, 50 mg, 80 mcg, 160 mcg	Nasal spray, inhaler	Nasal, inhalation	Treatment of allergies, including rhinitis and inflammation
fluticasone	Flonase, Veramyst *OTC formulation available	27.5 mcg, 50 mcg	Nasal spray	Nasal	Treatment of allergies, including rhinitis and inflammation
mometasone	Nasonex, Asmanex	100 mcg, 220 mcg	Nasal spray, inhaler	Nasal, inhalation	Treatment of allergies, including rhinitis and inflammation
triamcinolone	Nasacort *OTC formulation available	110 mcg	Nasal spray	Nasal	Treatment of allergies, including rhinitis and inflammation
budenoside, formoterol	Symbicort	80 mcg, 160 mcg	Inhaler	Inhalation	Treatment of allergies and inflammation, bronchodilator
fluticoasone, salmeterol	Advair Diskus	100-50 mcg, 250-50 mcg, 500-50 mcg	Inhaler	Inhalation	Treatment of allergies and inflammation, bronchodilator

Generic Name	Brand Name	Common Strengths/Dosages	Dosage Forms	Route	Indication
dexamethasone	Decadron, Dexamethasone intensol	0.5 mg, 0.75 mg, 1 mg, 1.5 mg, 4 mg, 6 mg, 0.5 mg/5 mL	Tablet	PO	Treatment of inflammation
methylprednisolone	Medrol	4 mg	Tablet	PO	Treatment of inflammation
prednisolone	Orapred, Pediapred	15 mg/5 mL	Solution	PO	Treatment of inflammation
prednisone	(The brand name for prednisone is no longer available in the U.S.)	1 mg, 2.5 mg, 5 mg, 10 mg, 20 mg, 5 mg/5 mL, 5 mg/mL	Tablet, solution	PO	Treatment of inflammation
azelastine	Astelin	137 mcg	Nasal spray	Nasal	Treatment of allergies, antihistamine
cetirizine	Zyrtec *OTC formulation available	10 mg, 1 mg/mL	Tablet, solution	PO	Treatment of allergies, antihistamine
chlorpheniramine	Chlor-Trimeton *OTC formulation available	4 mg	Tablet	PO	Treatment of allergies, antihistamine
desloratadine	Clarinex	5 mg	Tablet	PO	Treatment of allergies, antihistamine
diphenhydramine	Benadryl *OTC formulation available	25 mg	Capsule, tablet, solution, parenteral	PO, IV	Treatment of allergies, antihistamine
fexofenadine	Allegra *OTC formulation available	60 mg, 180 mg	Tablet	PO	Treatment of allergies, antihistamine
hydroxyzine	Vistaril	10 mg, 25 mg, 50 mg, 25 mg/mL, 50 mg/mL	Capsule, parenteral	PO, IV	Treatment of allergies, antihistamine
levocetirizine	Xyzal	5 mg	Tablet	PO	Treatment of allergies, antihistamine
loratadine	Claritin, Alavert *OTC formulation available	10 mg	Tablet	PO	Treatment of allergies, antihistamine
epinephrine	EpiPen, Auvi-Q	0.15 mg/0.15 mL, 0.15 mg/0.3 mL, 0.3 mg/0.3 mL, 2.25%	Parenteral	IM, SQ	Treatment of anaphylactic shock, bronchodilator
aminophylline	Amoline, Aminophyllin	25 mg/mL, 50 mg/mL	Parenteral	IV	Treatment of asthma, bronchodilator

Generic Name	Brand Name	Common Strengths/Dosages	Dosage Forms	Route	Indication
theophylline	Theo-24, Theophylline	100 mg, 200 mg, 300 mg, 400 mg, 800 mg	Capsule, parenteral	PO, IV	Treatment of asthma, bronchodilator
flunisolide	Aerospan HFA	80 mcg	Inhaler	Inhalation	Treatment of asthma, corticosteroid
albuterol	ProAir HFA, Proventil HFA, Ventolin HFA, AccuNeb	90 mcg, 0.63 mg, 1.25 mg	Inhaler, solution	Inhalation	Treatment of asthma, COPD, bronchodilator
formoterol	Foradil	12 mcg	Inhaler	Inhalation	Treatment of asthma, COPD, bronchodilator
levalbuterol	Xopenex, Xopenex HFA	0.31 mg, 0.63 mg, 1.25 mg, 45 mcg	Solution, inhaler	Inhalation	Treatment of asthma, COPD, bronchodilator
salmeterol	Serevent	50 mcg	Inhaler	Inhalation	Treatment of asthma, COPD, bronchodilator
ipratropium	Atrovent	18 mcg	Inhaler	Inhalation	Treatment of COPD, bronchodilator
ipratroprium, albuterol	Combivent	103–18 mcg	Inhaler	Inhalation	Treatment of COPD, bronchodilator
tiotropium	Spiriva	18 mcg	Inhaler	Inhalation	Treatment of COPD, bronchodilator
guaifenesin	Robitussin, Mucinex *OTC formulation available	200 mg, 400 mg, 600 mg, 1,200 mg	Solution, tablet	PO	Treatment of cough, expectorant
benzonatate	Tessalon	100 mg, 200 mg	Capsule	PO	Treatment of cough, antitussive
dextromethorphan	Delsym *OTC formulation available	30 mg	Solution	PO	Treatment of cough, antitussive
oxymetazoline	Afrin	0.05%	Nasal spray	Nasal	Treatment of nasal decongestion
phenylephrine	Sudafed-PE *OTC formulation available	10 mg	Tablet	PO	Decongestant
pseudoephedrine	Sudafed *Available OTC **Kept behind the pharmacy counter	30 mg	Tablet	PO	Decongestant

URINARY SYSTEM AGENTS

Urinary system agents are used to treat a variety of conditions ranging from painful urination to the treatment of benign prostatic hyperplasia (BPH). Use Table 5-35 to identify common USAN stem names used in treating these conditions.

Women who are pregnant or are of childbearing age should not handle any testosterone reductase agents, including dutasteride and finasteride. Absorption of testosterone reductase agents through the skin may cause fetal abnormalities.

Table 5-35. USAN Stems for Urinary Agents

Stem	Description	Example
-afil	PDE inhibitors	sildenafil
-steride	Testosterone reductase inhibitors	dutasteride

The urinary system performs functions related to the removal of waste products and fluid balance maintenance, including electrolyte and pH balances. Medications in this category can be prescribed to relieve urinary difficulty or to treat painful urination (see Table 5-36). Antimuscarinic agents (e.g., tolterodine) prevent bladder contractions and are used to treat overactive bladders and urinary incontinence. Phosphodiesterase (PDE) inhibitors (e.g., sildenafil) are used to treat male impotence. They increase blood flow to the penis following sexual stimulation. Patients on PDE inhibitors may experience headaches and should be cautioned of a potential adverse effect called priapism (painful and persistent erection), which constitutes a medical emergency. Men over the age of 50 may experience symptoms of an enlarged prostate, commonly known as benign prostatic hyperplasia (BPH). Symptoms of BPH include painful or limited urination, incomplete bladder emptying, and urgency. Patients may be prescribed an alpha blocker (e.g., tamsulosin), which works by relaxing the muscles of the prostate and bladder.

Table 5-36. Urinary Agents

Generic Name	Brand Name	Common Strengths/Dosages	Dosage Forms	Route	Indication
avanafil	Stendra	50 mg, 100 mg, 200 mg	Tablet	PO	Erectile dysfunction
sildenafil	Viagra	25 mg, 50 mg, 100 mg	Tablet	PO	Erectile dysfunction
tadalafil	Cialis	5 mg, 10 mg, 20 mg	Tablet	PO	Erectile dysfunction
vardenafil	Levitra, Staxyn	2.5 mg, 5 mg, 10 mg, 20 mg	Tablet, orally disintegrating tablet	PO	Erectile dysfunction
alfuzosin	Uroxatral	10 mg	Tablet	PO	Treatment of benign prostatic hyperplasia (BPH)
doxazosin	Cardura	1 mg, 2 mg, 4 mg, 8 mg	Tablet	PO	Treatment of benign prostatic hyperplasia (BPH)
dutasteride	Avodart	0.5 mg	Capsule	PO	Treatment of benign prostatic hyperplasia (BPH)
finasteride	Proscar	5 mg	Tablet	PO	Treatment of benign prostatic hyperplasia (BPH)

Generic Name	Brand Name	Common Strengths/Dosages	Dosage Forms	Route	Indication
tamsulosin	Flomax	0.4 mg	Capsule	PO	Treatment of benign prostatic hyperplasia (BPH)
terazosin	Hytrin	1 mg, 2 mg, 5 mg, 10 mg	Capsule	PO	Treatment of benign prostatic hyperplasia (BPH)
darifenacin	Enablex	7.5 mg, 15 mg	Tablet	PO	Treatment of overactive bladder
oxybutynin	Ditropan, Ditropan XL, Gelnique, Oxytrol	3.9 mg, 5 mg, 10 mg, 15 mg, 10%	Tablet, gel, transdermal patch	PO, trans-dermal, topical	Treatment of overactive bladder
solifenacin	Vesicare	5 mg, 10 mg	Tablet	PO	Treatment of overactive bladder
tolterodine	Detrol, Detrol LA	1 mg, 2 mg, 4 mg	Tablet, capsule	PO	Treatment of overactive bladder
phenazopyri-dine	Azo-Standard, pyridium *OTC formula-tion available	95 mg, 100 mg, 200 mg	Tablet	PO	Treatment of painful urination

MISCELLANEOUS MEDICATIONS

Table 5-37 provides additional information on the medications used to treat Alzheimer's disease and Parkinson's disease.

Alzheimer's disease is a progressive disorder affecting memory and cognition. Pharmaceutical drug therapy is focused on two main neurotransmitters: acetylcholine and glutamate, both of which are associated with memory and learning. Medications are aimed at inhibiting the breakdown of acetylcholine in order to improve patient symptoms and outcomes or aimed at inhibiting the buildup of glutamate. The medications used to treat Alzheimer's disease exert their therapeutic effect by enhancing cholinergic activity (donepezil, rivastigmine, tacrine), by inhibiting acytelcholinesterase (galantamine), by acting as antagonists for the N-methyl-D-aspartate (NMDA) receptor associated with glutamate production (memantine), or by using a combination of pathways to improve cholinergic activity. Common side effects for these agents include dizziness, confusion, diarrhea or constipation, fatigue, and headaches. Alzheimer's medications are indicated for long-term control and treatment.

Parkinson's disease is a progressive neurological disorder affecting movement. Early symptoms include tremors, stiffness, and slowness of movement. They are due to inactivity or a decrease in the neurotransmitter dopamine. Medications used for Parkinson's are aimed at increasing the free levels of dopamine in the body by one of three mechanisms: acting as dopamine agonists (pramipexole, ropinirole), introducing exogenous dopamine (levodopa), or prolonging the effect of levodopa by acting as a catechol-O-methyltransferase (COMT) inhibitor (entacapone). Side effects of these agents may include nausea, orthostatic hypotension, and, in some cases, dyskinesia (involuntary movements resulting from the administration of large doses of levodopa). Patients are slowly weaned off these medications. Medication therapy is long term.

Table 5-37. Alzheimer's Disease and Parkinson's Disease

Generic Name	Brand Name	Common Strengths/Dosages	Dosage Forms	Route	Indication
donepezil	Aricept	5 mg, 10 mg	Tablet	PO	Treatment of Alzheimer's disease
galantamine	Razadyne	4 mg, 8 mg, 12 mg, 16 mg, 24 mg	Tablet, capsule	PO	Treatment of Alzheimer's disease
memantine	Namenda	5 mg, 10 mg	Tablet	PO	Treatment of Alzheimer's disease
memantine extended-release, donepezil	Namzaric	14 mg/10 mg, 28 mg/10 mg	Capsule	PO	Treatment of Alzheimer's disease
rivastigmine	Exelon	1.5 mg, 2.5 mg, 3 mg, 6 mg, 4.6 mg/24 hr, 9.5 mg/24 hr	Capsule, patch	PO, transdermal	Treatment of Alzheimer's disease
tacrine	Cognex	10 mg, 20 mg, 30 mg, 40 mg	Capsule	PO	Treatment of Alzheimer's disease
benztropine	Cogentin	0.5 mg, 1 mg, 2 mg, 1 mg/mL	Tablet, parenteral	PO, IV	Treatment of Parkinson's disease
carbidopa, levodopa	Sinemet	10 mg/100 mg, 25 mg/100 mg, 25 mg/250 mg, 50 mg/200 mg	Tablet	PO	Treatment of Parkinson's disease
entacapone	Comtan	200 mg	Tablet	PO	Treatment of Parkinson's disease
pramipexole	Mirapex	0.125 mg, 0.25 mg, 0.375 mg, 0.5 mg, 0.75 mg, 1 mg, 1.5 mg, 2.25 mg, 3.75 mg, 4.5 mg	Tablet	PO	Treatment of Parkinson's disease
ropinirole	Requip	0.25 mg, 0.5 mg, 1 mg, 2 mg, 3 mg, 4 mg, 5 mg	Tablet	PO	Treatment of Parkinson's disease
rotigotine	Neupro	1 mg/24 hr, 2 mg/24 hr, 3 mg/24 hr, 4 mg/24 hr, 6 mg/24 hr, 8 mg/24 hr	Patch	Transdermal	Treatment of Parkinson's disease

Attention deficit hyperactivity disorder (ADHD), as discussed in Table 5-38, is a chronic condition affecting attention and resulting in hyperactivity and impulsivity. Medications in this category are either classified as stimulants or as nonstimulants. Stimulant drugs (e.g., lisdexamfetamine, dexmethylphenidate) increase the levels of dopamine, which is a neurotransmitter associated with mood, motivation, pleasure, and attention. These agents may cause restlessness, insomnia, loss of appetite, personality changes, and mood swings. There is also a potential for abuse and psychiatric problems, including depression and paranoia.

Nonstimulant agents work to increase the levels of the neurotransmitter norepinephrine (atomoxetine). Atomoxetine (Straterra) may cause somnolence, mood swings, and, in some cases, suicidal ideations.

Table 5-38. Attention Deficit Hyperactivity Disorder (ADHD)

Generic Name	Brand Name	Common Strengths/Dosages	Dosage Forms	Route	Indication
atomoxetine	Straterra	10 mg, 18 mg, 25 mg, 40 mg, 60 mg, 100 mg	Capsule	PO	Treatment of ADHD
guanfacine	Intuiv	1 mg, 2 mg, 3 mg, 4 mg	Tablet	PO	Treatment of ADHD
dexmethylphenidate	Focalin, Focalin XR	2.5 mg, 5 mg, 10 mg, 20 mg	Tablet, capsule	PO	Treatment of ADHD (C-II)
dextroamphetamine	Adderall, Adderall XR	5 mg, 7.5 mg, 10 mg, 12.5 mg, 15 mg, 20 mg, 30 mg	Tablet, capsule	PO	Treatment of ADHD (C-II)
lisdexamfetamine	Vyvanse	20 mg, 30 mg, 40 mg, 50 mg, 70 mg	Capsule	PO	Treatment of ADHD (C-II)
methylphenidate	Concerta, Daytrana, Focalin, Metadate CD, Ritalin, Ritalin LA, Ritalin SR	5 mg, 10 mg, 18 mg, 20 mg, 27 mg, 30 mg, 36 mg, 50 mg, 54 mg, 10 mg/9 hr, 15 mg/9 hr, 20 mg/9 hr, 30 mg/9 hr	Tablet, capsule, patch	PO, transdermal	Treatment of ADHD (C-II)

The treatment of bipolar disorder involves a combination of mood-stabilizing drugs (see Table 5-39) and psychotherapy. Several types of bipolar disorder exist. Treatment depends on the diagnosis as well as on the symptoms present. Schizophrenia is a complex brain disorder often resulting in an altered perception of reality. The selection of appropriate medications is based on the symptoms present. Symptoms are often categorized as positive (symptoms shown in excess, like hallucinations or delusions) or as negative (symptoms that are deficient, like social withdrawal or flat affect). Traditional antipsychotics are an older class of medications that are used to treat only positive symptoms. This class includes medications like fluphenazine and haloperidol, which have a potential to cause tardive dyskinesia (involuntary, repetitive body movements) and extrapyramidal side effects (antipsychotic drug side effects resulting in parkinsonism and abnormal involuntary movement, often referred to as acute dyskinesia). Atypical antipsychotics are used to treat both positive and negative symptoms. Agents in this class include olanzapine and risperidone. These agents cause less extrapyramidal side effects and are generally used more often than traditional agents.

Table 5-39. Bipolar Disorder and Schizophrenia

Generic Name	Brand Name	Common Strengths/Dosages	Dosage Forms	Route	Indication
lithium	Lithobid	150 mg, 300 mg, 450 mg, 600 mg, 300 mg/5 mL	Tablet, capsule, oral solution	PO	Treatment of bipolar disorder
aripiprazole	Abilify	2 mg, 5 mg, 10 mg, 15 mg, 20 mg, 30 mg, 300 mg, 400 mg	Tablet, parenteral	PO, IM	Treatment of schizophrenia
chlorpromazine	Thorazine	10 mg, 25 mg, 50 mg, 100 mg, 200 mg, 25 mg/mL	Tablet, parenteral	PO, IV, IM	Treatment of schizophrenia
clozapine	Clozaril	25 mg, 50 mg, 100 mg, 150 mg, 200 mg	Tablet	PO	Treatment of schizophrenia
fluphenazine	Prolixin	1 mg, 2.5 mg, 5 mg, 10 mg, 25 mg/mL	Tablet, parenteral	PO, IM	Treatment of schizophrenia
haloperidol	Haldol	0.5 mg, 1 mg, 2 mg, 5 mg, 10 mg, 20 mg, 5 mg/mL	Tablet, parenteral	PO, IM	Treatment of schizophrenia
lurasidone	Latuda	20 mg, 40 mg, 60 mg	Tablet	PO	Treatment of schizophrenia
olanzapine	Zyprexa	2.5 mg, 5 mg, 7.5 mg, 10 mg, 15 mg, 20 mg	Tablet, parenteral	PO, IM	Treatment of schizophrenia
paliperidone	Invega	1.5 mg, 3 mg, 6 mg	Tablet	PO	Treatment of schizophrenia
quetiapine	Seroquel	25 mg, 100 mg, 200 mg, 300 mg	Tablet	PO	Treatment of schizophrenia
risperidone	Risperdal	0.25 mg, 0.5 mg, 1 mg, 2 mg, 3 mg, 4 mg, 1 mg/mL	Tablet, oral solution	PO	Treatment of schizophrenia
thiothixene	Navane	1 mg, 2 mg, 5 mg, 10 mg, 20 mg	Capsule	PO	Treatment of schizophrenia
ziprasidone	Geodon	20 mg, 40 mg, 60 mg, 80 mg	Capsule	PO	Treatment of schizophrenia

Gout, which is the focus of Table 5-40, is a form of arthritis caused by an excess of uric acid in the blood. Too much uric acid can cause the formation of crystals in joints, often presenting as pain, stiffness, and swelling. Medications in this category aim at reducing uric acid levels. Uricosuric agents, like probenecid, increase the elimination of uric acid by the kidneys. These agents are contraindicated in patients with uric acid kidney stones and hypersensitivities. The xanthine oxidase inhibitor allopurinol exerts its action by inhibiting the conversion of hypoxanthine to uric acid. Patients should be monitored for the presence of an allergic reaction and the potential for hepatotoxicity. Uricosuric agents and xanthine oxidase inhibitors are used long term to reduce uric acid levels. Colchicine is indicated for acute flare-ups and may cause gastrointestinal upset.

Table 5-40. Gout

Generic Name	Brand Name	Common Strengths/Dosages	Dosage Forms	Route
allopurinol	Zyloprim	100 mg, 300 mg	Tablet	PO
colchicine	Colcrys	0.6 mg	Tablet, capsule	PO
febuxostat	Uloric	40 mg	Tablet	PO
probenecid*		0.5 g	Tablet	PO

*No brand name formulation is currently available.

The most common class of medications used to treat migraines, as shown in Table 5-41, is the 5-HT1 receptor agonists, often referred to as the "triptans" because they end in the USAN stem "triptan." These agents constrict blood vessels and reduce inflammation by targeting serotonin at the 5-HT1 receptor. These medications are used at the onset of symptoms and may cause asthenia (abnormal weakness), dizziness, and somnolence.

Table 5-41. Migraines

Generic Name	Brand Name	Common Strengths/Dosages	Dosage Forms	Route
acetaminophen, aspirin, caffeine	Excedrin Migraine *Available OTC	250 mg/250 mg/ 65 mg	Tablet, caplet	PO
almotriptan	Axert	6.25 mg, 12.5 mg	Tablet	PO
eletriptan	Relpax	20 mg, 40 mg	Tablet	PO
frovatriptan	Frova	2.5 mg	Tablet	PO
naratriptan	Amerge	1 mg, 2.5 mg	Tablet	PO
rizatriptan	Maxalt	5 mg, 10 mg	Tablet	PO
sumatriptan	Imitrex	5 mg, 20 mg, 25 mg, 50 mg, 100 mg, 6 mg/0.5 mL, 12 mg/mL	Tablet, spray, parenteral	PO, intranasal, SQ

Smoking cessation agents, as discussed in Table 5-42, are aimed at helping patients quit using tobacco. Buproprion exerts its primary effect by inhibiting dopamine reuptake by neuronal cells. The main side effects include insomnia and dry mouth. Buproprion may lower the seizure threshold and should be taken cautiously with other agents that may have similar effects. Varenicline is a nicotine agonist that prevents nicotine stimulation. Neuropsychiatric symptoms, such as depression and suicidal ideations, have been reported. A potential for nausea, seizures, and hypersensitivity is also possible while taking varenicline. Many nicotine replacement products are available over-the-counter. These agents are used to give the body nicotine, thus, reducing withdrawal symptoms. Side effects are usually mild and cease upon cessation of therapy. Pregnant patients and those with a history of cardiovascular disease should consult their physician before initiating therapy.

Table 5-42. Smoking Cessation

Generic Name	Brand Name	Common Strengths/Dosages	Dosage Forms	Route
buproprion	Zyban	75 mg, 100 mg, 150 mg, 200 mg, 300 mg	Tablet	PO
nicotine	Nicoderm CQ, Nicotrol, Nicotrol NS, Nicorette *OTC formulation available	7 mg, 14 mg, 21 mg, 10 mg/mL	Gum, patch, nasal spray	PO, nasal, transdermal
varenicline	Chantix	0.5 mg, 1 mg	Tablet	PO

SUMMARY

☐ Having an understanding of pharmacology is a fundamental component of pharmacy practice.

☐ Drug interactions can occur for a variety of reasons, including as a result of changes in metabolism, absorption, and excretion.

☐ Pharmacy technicians should be able to identify commonly prescribed medications, including the drug class, indication, common strengths, side effects, and duration of therapy.

☐ Drug endings may have similarities within a classification. Memorizing specific prefixes and suffixes may help you remember a drug class or an indication and is a great way to remember medications.

PHARMACOLOGY FOR TECHNICIANS PRACTICE QUESTIONS

1. Which of the following medications is a beta blocker used for the treatment of hypertension?

   (A) candesartan
   (B) diltiazem
   (C) lisinopril
   (D) metoprolol

2. Azithromycin is classified as a bacteriostatic anti-infective agent. Which of the following drugs also has bacteriostatic properties?

   (A) cephalexin
   (B) erythromycin
   (C) levofloxacin
   (D) penicillin

3. Medications ending in the USAN approved suffix "-afil" are used to treat

   _____.

   (A) gout
   (B) hyperlipidemia
   (C) impotence
   (D) osteoporosis

4. A suppository is a solid formulation used for what type of administration?

   (A) intravenous
   (B) oral
   (C) rectal
   (D) topical

5. A branch of pharmacology referring to the biological and physical effects of the drug on the body is referred to as _____.

   (A) pharmacodynamics
   (B) pharmacokinetics
   (C) pharmacotherapeutics
   (D) pharmacophysiology

6. Which of the following medications does NOT have a formulation that is available over-the-counter?

   (A) acyclovir
   (B) fluticasone
   (C) loperamide
   (D) omeprazole

7. The Controlled Substances Act places medications into one of five schedules based on the drug's medical use, abuse potential, and likelihood to cause dependence. Which of the following medications is classified as a controlled substance under this federal act?

   (A) omeprazole
   (B) ondansetron
   (C) oxazepam
   (D) oxybutynin

8. *Helicobacter pylori* is a type of bacteria associated with the formation and/or exacerbation of which of the following disease states?

   (A) acne vulgaris
   (B) peptic ulcer disease
   (C) oral thrush
   (D) otitis media

9. Which of the following medications is indicated in the treatment of epilepsy?

   (A) lansoprazole
   (B) levetiracetam
   (C) levofloxacin
   (D) lovastatin

10. Antibiotics may have a duration of therapy lasting _____ days.

    (A) 30
    (B) 21
    (C) 15
    (D) 10

ANSWERS EXPLAINED

1. **(D)** Metoprolol is a beta blocker, which is indicated by the suffix "-olol." Candesartan is an angiotensin receptor blocker (ARB). Diltiazem is a calcium channel blocker (CCB). Lisinopril is an angiotensin-converting enzyme (ACE) inhibitor.

2. **(B)** Erythromycin is a macrolide antibiotic with bacteriostatic activity. Cephalexin is a cephalosporin antibiotic containing bactericidal activity. Levofloxacin is a quinolone antibiotic with bactericidal activity. Penicillin is a bactericidal-type antibiotic in the penicillin class of antibiotics.

3. **(C)** Medications ending in the suffix "-afil" include the phosphodiesterese (PDE) inhibitors and are used to treat male impotence. Medications treating gout, hyperlipidemia, and osteoporosis do not end in the suffix "-afil."

4. **(C)** A suppository is used for either rectal or vaginal administration. Suppositories may not be injected intravenously, taken orally, or placed topically onto the skin.

5. **(A)** Pharmacodynamics refers to the biological and physical effects of the drug on the body. Pharmacokinetics is a branch of pharmacology referring to the rate of drug absorption, distribution, metabolism, and excretion. Pharmacotherapeutics is a branch of pharmacology that studies the therapeutic uses and effects of drugs. Pharmacophysiology is a branch of pharmacology that studies the actions of drugs upon living organisms.

6. **(A)** Acyclovir is an antiviral agent with no current over-the-counter formulation available. Fluticasone is available OTC as a nasal spray (Flonase). Loperamide has several oral formulations available OTC as Imodium. Omeprazole is available OTC as Prilosec in a tablet or capsule.

7. **(C)** Oxazepam (Serax) is a Schedule IV substance (in accordance with the Controlled Substances Act) used to treat anxiety. Omeprazole (Prilosec), ondansetron (Zofran), and oxybutynin (Ditropan XL) are not scheduled drugs under the Controlled Substances Act.

8. **(B)** *Helicobacter pylori* is associated with the formation and/or exacerbation of peptic ulcer disease. *H. pylori* is not associated with the formation of acne vulgaris, oral thrush, or otitis media.

9. **(B)** Epilepsy can be treated using levetiracetam (Keppra). Lansoprazole (Prevacid) is indicated for the treatment of gastroesophageal reflux disease (GERD). Levofloxacin (Levaquin) is an anti-infective quinolone-type antibiotic. Lovastatin (Mevacor) is indicated for the treatment of hypercholesterolemia.

10. **(D)** Typical antibiotic therapy lasts 7–10 days.

Pharmacy Law and Regulations

6

KNOWLEDGE DOMAIN 2.0

Pharmacy Law and Regulations   **12.50%**

→ Knowledge Area 2.1: Storage, handling, and disposal of hazardous substances and wastes (e.g., MSDS)

→ Knowledge Area 2.2: Hazardous substances exposure, prevention, and treatment (e.g., eyewash, spill kit, MSDS)

→ Knowledge Area 2.3: Controlled substance transfer regulations (DEA)

→ Knowledge Area 2.4: Controlled substance documentation requirements for receiving, ordering, returning, loss/theft, destruction (DEA)

→ Knowledge Area 2.5: Formula to verify the validity of a prescriber's DEA number (DEA)

→ Knowledge Area 2.6: Record keeping, documentation, and record retention (e.g., length of time prescriptions are maintained on file)

→ Knowledge Area 2.7: Restricted drug programs and related prescription-processing requirements (e.g., thalidomide, isotretinoin, clozapine)

→ Knowledge Area 2.8: Professional standards related to data integrity, security, and confidentiality (e.g., HIPAA, backing up and archiving)

→ Knowledge Area 2.9: Requirement for consultation (e.g., OBRA '90)

→ Knowledge Area 2.10: FDA's recall classification

→ Knowledge Area 2.11: Infection control standards (e.g., laminar air flow, cleanroom, hand washing, cleaning counting trays, countertop, and equipment) (OSHA, *USP* 795 and 797)

→ Knowledge Area 2.12: Record keeping for repackaged and recalled products and supplies (TJC, BOP)

→ Knowledge Area 2.13: Professional standards regarding the roles and responsibilities of pharmacists, pharmacy technicians, and other pharmacy employees (TJC, BOP)

→ Knowledge Area 2.14: Reconciliation between state and federal laws and regulations

→ Knowledge Area 2.15: Facility, equipment, and supply requirements (e.g., space requirements, prescription file storage, cleanliness, reference materials) (TJC, USP, BOP)

- ☐ Identify federal laws and regulations affecting pharmacy practice.
- ☐ Examine laws that govern controlled substances.
- ☐ Describe labeling requirements for both prescription and over-the-counter substances.
- ☐ Explain procedures relating to the ordering, receiving, and documentation of medications.
- ☐ Describe restrictions placed on the sales of products containing pseudoephedrine and ephedrine.
- ☐ Understand restrictions placed on the refill and transfer of prescriptions.
- ☐ Understand restrictions placed on the return, destruction, and theft of medications.
- ☐ Discuss federal laws that govern patient privacy.
- ☐ Understand infection control techniques and strategies.
- ☐ Explain facility, equipment, and supply requirements.

PHARMACY LAW

The PTCE certification exam follows federal guidelines and regulations. Federal laws take precedence unless the state law is stricter, in which case the state law governs. Pharmacy technicians should check with their State Board of Pharmacy for additional laws that may apply.

Federal laws and regulations have impacted pharmacy practice by protecting patients' well-being and maintaining efforts to ensure the safety and health of all patients. Many of these laws originated from crisis events, which brought attention to the issues of safety and security. These crisis events led to the creation of legislation that would not only provide these safety measures but would also shape reform in pharmacy practice.

Pure Food and Drug Act of 1906

- This act prohibited interstate commerce of misbranded and adulterated drugs, foods, and drinks.
- The focus was on purity, not safety.
- This act did not protect false therapeutic claims.
- Legislation did not require manufacturer labels to list active ingredients, directions for use or warnings, and safety concerns.

Federal Food, Drug, and Cosmetic Act (FFDCA) of 1938

- This act was produced in response to shortfalls of the Pure Food and Drug Act of 1906.
- Enactment of this legislation was hastened in 1937 due to the deaths of over 100 individuals who had consumed a sulfa-based elixir containing diethylene glycol, a chemical similar to ethylene glycol used in antifreeze.
- This act required drug labeling to include directions for use, warnings, and safety concerns.
- It provided mandates for premarketing approval of all drugs.

- This act ensured that the FDA oversees all provisions and classifies offenses as either misbranded or adulterated. A product may be labeled **misbranded** if it meets any of the following criteria:

1. The product is misrepresented, which is often seen in labeling (e.g., the omission of important information on the label).
2. The product does not comply with color additive provisions as established by the FFDCA.
3. The product is dangerous when used "in the dosage or manner or with the frequency or duration prescribed, recommended, or suggested in the labeling" as per the U.S. Food and Drug Administration, 2015.
4. The label fails to include the "name and place of business of the manufacturer, packer, or distributor and an accurate statement of the quantity of the contents in terms of weight, measure, or numerical count" as per the U.S. Food and Drug Administration, 2015.
5. "Any required wording is not prominently displayed as compared with other wording on the device or is not clearly stated" as per the U.S. Food and Drug Administration, 2015.

A product may be labeled **adulterated** if the drug "fails to conform to compendial standards of quality, strength, or purity" as per the U.S. Food and Drug Administration, 1980.

Tables 6-1 and 6-2 list the current drug labeling requirements for prescription and over-the-counter drugs (OTC), respectively. Figure 6-1 shows an example of an over-the-counter label.

Table 6-1. Prescription Drug Labeling Requirements*

- Highlights
- Limitations statement
- Product name and initial FDA approval date
- Boxed warning
- Recent major changes
- Indications and usage
- Dosage and administration
- Dosage form and strength
- Contraindications
- Warnings and precautions
- Adverse reactions
- Drug interactions
- Use in specialized populations
- Patient counseling information

*From the *American Journal of Health-System Pharmacy*, 2007

Table 6-2. OTC Drug Labeling Requirements*

- Active drug
- Uses
- Warnings
- Inactive ingredients
- Purpose
- Directions
- Other information, such as storage requirements
- Expiration date
- Batch or NDC number
- Name and address of the manufacturer, packer, or distributor
- Quantity of the product in the package
- Instructions in case of an overdose

*From the U.S. Food and Drug Administration, 2014

Drug Facts

Active ingredient (in each tablet) | **Purpose**
Chlorpheniramine maleate 2 mg...Antihistamine

Uses temporarily relieves these symptoms due to hay fever or other upper respiratory allergies: ■ sneezing ■ runny nose ■ itchy, watery eyes ■ itchy throat

Warnings
Ask a doctor before use if you have
■ glaucoma ■ a breathing problem such as emphysema or chronic bronchitis
■ trouble urinating due to an enlarged prostate gland

Ask a doctor or pharmacist before use if you are taking tranquilizers or sedatives

When using this product
■ drowsiness may occur ■ avoid alcoholic drinks
■ alcohol, sedatives, and tranquilizers may increase drowsiness
■ be careful when driving a motor vehicle or operating machinery
■ excitability may occur, especially in children

If pregnant or breast-feeding, ask a health professional before use.
Keep out of reach of children. In case of overdose, get medical help or contact a Poison Control Center right away.

Directions

adults and children 12 years and over	take 2 tablets every 4 to 6 hours; not more than 12 tablets in 24 hours
children 6 years to under 12 years	take 1 tablet every 4 to 6 hours; not more than 6 tablets in 24 hours
children under 6 years	ask a doctor

Drug Facts (continued)

Other Information ■ store at 20-25° C (68-77°F) ■ protect from excessive moisture

Inactive Ingredients D&C yellow no. 10, lactose, magnesium stearate, microcrystalline cellulose, pregelatinized starch

Image courtesy of the U.S. Food and Drug Administration

Figure 6-1. Over-the-counter (OTC) label example

The Comprehensive Drug Abuse Prevention and Control Act of 1970

- It is more commonly known as the Controlled Substances Act.
- This law requires registration, record keeping, and rules regarding dispensing of controlled drugs.
- Substances are placed into one of five categories called schedules. Table 6-3 lists these different schedules and what types of substances are placed into each.

Table 6-3. Controlled Substances Schedules

Schedule	Description	Example
Schedule I	- High potential for abuse - No legally accepted medical use in the U.S.	- heroin - LSD - peyote - methaqualone
Schedule II	- High potential for abuse - Substances may lead to severe psycholoigcal or physical dependence - Legally accepted medical use in the U.S.	- codeine - hydromorphone - methadone - meperidine - oxycodone - fentanyl - amphetamine - methylphenidate - hydrocodone (no more than 15 mg per dosage unit)
Schedule III	- Potential for abuse is less than Schedule II drugs - Substances may lead to moderate or low physical dependence and/or high psychological dependence	- buprenorphine - codeine (when used in combination products with no more than 90 mg of codeine per dosage unit) - ketamine - anabolic steroids
Schedule IV	- Potential for abuse is less than Schedule III drugs	- alprazolam - diazepam - carisoprodol - midazolam - temazepam
Schedule V	- Potential for abuse is less than Schedule IV drugs - Contains limited quantities of narcotics	- cough medications with no more than 200 mg of codeine per 100 mL or per 100 g - Robitussin AC - diphenoxylate

REGISTRATION

New pharmacies must first obtain a state license. Facilities that dispense controlled substances register with the DEA by using a **DEA 224 form**. The form can be obtained online or a written form can be requested by contacting the DEA. The certificate of registration should be maintained at the registered location and kept in an accessible place for inspections. Registration is valid for 3 years and can be renewed using a **DEA 224a form** available online. This form can be completed 60 days prior to the expiration date. In the event that the pharmacy needed a duplicate Certificate of Registration form (**DEA 223 form**), the pharmacy can request a copy online, via phone, or via email.

ORDERING, RECEIVING, AND DOCUMENTING REQUIREMENTS

Pharmacies must maintain complete and accurate inventories for all controlled substances, including those purchased, received, dispensed, or otherwise disposed of.

- Schedule II medications are ordered using a **DEA 222 form**, which is a triplicate form that must be handwritten or typed and then signed by the individual registered with the DEA.
- A maximum of 10 items may be ordered per form. The number of items should match the quantity marked on the bottom of the form. Copy 1 (top copy) is retained by the supplier. Copy 2 (middle copy) is forwarded to the DEA. Copy 3 (bottom copy) is received by the purchaser.
- The DEA 222 form is valid for only 60 days.

Upon receipt, the purchaser must record the number of items received and the date that they were received. All DEA 222 forms, including those that are incomplete or illegible, should not be thrown away. Instead, they must be maintained in the pharmacy for a minimum of 2 years.

- Schedule II prescriptions should be maintained for a period of two years, and they should be filed separately from Schedule III, IV, and V prescriptions.
- Schedule III, IV, and V prescriptions should be maintained for a period of 2 years.
- Schedule III, IV, and V prescriptions may be ordered online, over the phone, or via fax. All invoices should be maintained by the pharmacy, signed, dated, and stamped with a red "C." Invoices must be maintained for a minimum of 2 years.

Prescriptions containing controlled substances, and stock bottles containing controlled substances, may also have a red "C" stamp to visually note the presence of a controlled medication.

INVENTORY REQUIREMENTS

All controlled substances should be inventoried upon the very first day that the pharmacy opens (the first day of business). Federal law requires a biennial inventory of controlled substances. The inventory record must be kept in a retrievable location and maintained for 2 years.

- Inventory counts of Schedule II drugs should be kept separate in a separate file from inventory counts of Schedule III, IV, and V drugs.
- Schedule II drugs must be physically counted; Schedule III, IV, and V drugs can be estimated.

PRESCRIPTION RESTRICTIONS

Schedule II prescriptions may be either written or computer generated, but they must be presented in person at the pharmacy. The prescription is to be signed in ink or should contain a digital signature by the prescribing authority. It must also contain a valid DEA number. Institutions are granted an institutional DEA number. Prescribers from that hospital are given an identifier number to be used with the institutional DEA number. DEA numbers are required on all controlled prescriptions.

- DEA numbers consist of 2 letters and 7 numbers.
- The first letter of the DEA number will often be an A, B, F, or M, and it is used to identify the type of registrant.
- The second letter is the first letter of the prescribing individual's last name.
- Verification of a DEA number is determined by the following:

  ○ First add the 1st, 3rd, and 5th numbers.
  ○ Then add the 2nd, 4th, and 6th numbers. Multiply that sum by 2.
  ○ Finally, add together the sums of both of these numbers.
  ○ The digit in the ones place is referred to as the "check digit" number, and it should match the last digit in the DEA number.
  ○ Example: AB1234563

    STEP 1 $1 + 3 + 5 = 9$
    STEP 2 $2 + 4 + 6 = 12$
    $12 \times 2 = 24$
    STEP 3 $9 + 24 = \underline{33}$

The 3 in the ones place matches the last digit of the DEA number. Therefore, the DEA number is valid.

Schedule III or IV prescriptions may be handwritten or computer generated, but they must be signed by the prescriber in ink or must contain a digital signature. They may also be sent electronically. Depending upon state law, they may also be faxed or phoned into the pharmacy.

The use of DEA numbers on non-controlled prescriptions is strongly opposed by the DEA. In 2007, all covered health care providers were required to obtain a unique 10-digit identifier, known as a National Provider Identifier or NPI. Covered health care providers and health plans must use the NPI on all administrative and financial transactions, as mandated by HIPAA. NPI numbers are used to process pharmacy claims and are often found on the prescription or prescriber profile.

REFILL RESTRICTIONS

Prescriptions for Schedule II drugs may not be refilled. Schedule III and IV drugs may be refilled up to 5 times within 6 months after the date of issue. Partial fills for Schedule III and IV drugs are irrelevant as long as the total quantity dispensed meets the total quantity prescribed within the 6 month time frame. Each partial fill is recorded in the same manner as a refill. Partial fills (emergency fills) for Schedule II drugs may be dispensed if the pharmacist cannot supply the full quantity for a written or an emergency oral prescription. The pharmacist must note the quantity supplied on the front of the prescription. The remaining quantity must be supplied within 72 hours of the partial dispensing date. A new prescription must be presented for the remaining quantity to be dispensed. The prescribing physician should be notified of any prescriptions not picked up within 72 hours. Prescriptions for Schedule V and non-controlled prescriptions may be refilled as authorized by the prescriber.

TRANSFER RESTRICTIONS

The original prescription for Schedule III, IV, and V drugs may be transferred one time between pharmacies. Pharmacies that share an online database may transfer a Schedule III, IV, or V prescription up to the maximum number of refills as stated on the original prescription.

- All transferred prescriptions must be communicated between pharmacists.
- The transferring pharmacist must write "void" on the front of the prescription and include the name, address, and DEA number of the receiving pharmacy on the back.
- The receiving pharmacist's name should also be noted on the back of the prescription.
- The receiving pharmacist should write "transfer" on the front of the prescription and record the following:

  - The original date of issuance for the prescription
  - The number of refills
  - The original dispensing date
  - The number of refills remaining
  - The name, address, and DEA number of the transferring pharmacy
  - The name of the pharmacist who is receiving the transferred prescription
  - The name, address, and DEA number of the pharmacy where the prescription was originally filled (including the original prescription number)

- Both the original and transferred prescription should be filed and maintained for a period of 2 years.

RETURN, DESTRUCTION, AND THEFT REGULATIONS

Controlled substances may be returned between DEA registrants using a DEA 222 form. Outdated or damaged controlled substances may be destroyed using a DEA 41 form. The registrant destroying the medication must provide the following:

- His/her DEA registration number, name, and address on the DEA registration, as well as a valid telephone number
- An inventory of the controlled substances that are to be destroyed, including NDC numbers, names, strengths, forms, and quantities
- The date, location, and method of destruction
- The signatures of two witnesses who are authorized employees

Upon theft of a medication, the pharmacy must notify both the nearest DEA diversion office and the local police department and then fill out a **DEA 106 form**. The original form is sent to the DEA, and a copy of the form is retained by the pharmacy.

Poison Prevention Packaging Act (PPPA) of 1970

This act was passed in response to a growing number of accidental poisonings involving children. The Poison Prevention Packaging Act approved the Consumer Product Safety Commission's (CPSC) authority to identify household products and drugs that require child-resistant containers. Tests were performed, and a childproof container was deemed to be acceptable if no more than 20% of children could open the container. Exceptions for child-proof containers were determined for certain products as outlined in Table 6-4.

Table 6-4. Childproof Container Exemptions*

- OTC products available in a single-sized package with the label "This Package for Households Without Young Children" or "Package Not Child-Resistant"
- Powdered, unflavored aspirin and effervescent aspirin
- Sublingual nitroglycerin
- Inhalation aerosols
- Hormone replacement therapy
- Oral contraceptives in the original manufacturer's dispensing package
- Isosorbide dinitrate in dosage strengths of 10 milligrams or less
- Erythromycin ethylsuccinate containing no more than 8 grams or the equivalent of erythromycin
- Erythromycin ethylsuccinate tablets in packages containing no more than the equivalent of 16 grams of erythromycin
- Anhydrous cholestyramine in powder form
- Potassium supplements in unit dose forms, including individually wrapped effervescent tablets, unit dose vials of liquid potassium, and powdered potassium in unit dose packets, containing no more than 50 milliequivalents per unit dose
- Sodium fluoride drug preparations, including liquid and tablet forms, containing no more than 264 milligrams of sodium fluoride per package
- Betamethasone tablets packaged in the manufacturers' dispenser packages containing no more than 12.6 milligrams of betamethasone.
- Mebendazole in tablet form in packages containing no more than 600 milligrams of the drug
- Ethylprednisolone in tablet form in packages containing no more than 84 milligrams of the drug
- Colestipol in powder form in packages containing no more than 5 grams of the drug
- Pancrelipase preparations in tablet, capsule, or powder form
- Prednisone in tablet form when dispensed in packages containing no more than 105 milligrams of the drug

*As per the U.S. Consumer Product Safety Commission, 2005

Omnibus Budget Reconciliation Act (OBRA) of 1990

This act places expectations on the pharmacist by imposing counseling obligations, prospective drug utilization review (ProDUR) requirements, and record-keeping mandates. Pharmacists must provide a prospective drug utilization review for all Medicaid prescriptions under this act; this drug utilization may be done with or without the assistance of computers. The following areas are to be screened as part of the ProDUR process: therapeutic duplication, drug-disease contraindications, drug-drug interactions, incorrect drug dosage, incorrect duration of treatment, drug-allergy interactions, and clinical abuse/misuse of medication. An offer of counseling to discuss the patient's unique therapeutic drug regimens must also be made. OBRA '90 requires that this information includes:

- Drug name and description
- Intended use and action of the drug
- Route, dosage form, dose, and duration of drug therapy
- Common side effects, adverse effects, interactions, and therapeutic contraindications of the drug

- Techniques for self-monitoring of the drug
- Proper storage
- Drug-drug interactions or drug-disease interactions
- Prescription refill information
- Action to be taken in the event of a missed dose

Although federal requirements of OBRA '90 targeted Medicaid patients, state requirements established counseling regulations for both Medicaid and non-Medicaid patients. This state-level initiative resulted in all patients receiving the same patient counseling standards.

Health Insurance Portability and Accountability Act (HIPAA) of 1996

This provision profoundly affected the field of pharmacy by instituting privacy safeguards for all protected health information (PHI). Protected health information is defined as "individually identifiable health information . . . transmitted or maintained in any other form or medium." Pharmacies must do this by:

- Taking steps to limit the use of, disclosure of, and requests for PHI, including implementing policies and procedures on how PHI will be used. Pharmacies are also required to post the entire notice of privacy practice in a prominent location.
- Notifying individuals of the privacy practices by offering them to individuals upon first service and obtaining written authorization of receipt upon notice.
- Identifying a compliance officer.
- Offering training on regulations to all pharmacy individuals including pharmacists, pharmacy technicians, and other individuals who may work in the pharmacy.
- Disclosing PHI to "business associates" as warranted by HIPAA. Disclosures must also be made to all business associates who provide functions relating to data processing, billing, or claims processing.

RESTRICTED DRUG PROGRAMS AND PROVISIONS

Isotretinoin Safety and Risk Management Act of 2004

- This legislation was initiated due to the serious adverse effects, including spontaneous abortions and fetal abnormalities, resulting from the use of isotretinoin (Accutane).
- All practitioners, pharmacists, and patients must be included in the iPLEDGE registry.
- Patients must also complete a consent form outlining the potential consequences of taking the drug, obtain counseling about the potential risks and requirements for safe use, and comply with all required pregnancy testing.
- Prescriptions must be written for 30-day allotments. Prescriptions cannot be faxed, sent electronically, or phoned in.
- Prescriptions must be filled and picked up within a 7-day window, counting the date of the pregnancy test as day 1.
- This act requires blood testing before and 30 days after treatment.
- Treatment centers must be evaluated yearly to ensure program compliance.
- This act requires mandatory quarterly reporting of all isotretinoin adverse side effects and mandatory reporting of all isotretinoin deaths within 15 days of the incident.

Combat Methamphetamine Epidemic Act (CMEA) of 2005

Ephedrine, pseudoephedrine, and phenylpropanolamine are listed as "scheduled listed chemical products" under the Controlled Substances Act. This act places restrictions on products containing ephedrine, pseudoephedrine, and phenylpropanolamine.

- **SALES RESTRICTIONS:** There is a maximum limit of 3.6 g/day and 9 g/month of base product.
- **STORAGE REQUIREMENTS:** Products must be maintained behind the pharmacy.
- **RECORD-KEEPING REQUIREMENTS:** A written or an electronic logbook must be maintained with information pertaining to the product name, quantities sold, patient identifying information (name and address of the purchaser), date, and time of the sale.

Risk Evaluation and Mitigation Strategies (REMS) Program

This program provides limited access to medications as a joint effort between the drug manufacturer and the FDA. The REMS programs encourage safe and effective medication use. Medications are selected based on adverse effects, teratogenicity, abuse potential, and the necessity for appropriate dosing to minimize patient risks. The FDA may require manufacturers to submit a REMS program upon drug approval. Programs vary and may include the use of medication guides, communication plans, elements to assure safe use (ETASU), an implementation system, and a timetable for submission of assessments. Selected medications include buprenorphine, clozapine, darbapoetin, epoetin, fentanyl, hydromorphone, isotretinoin, naltrexone ER, oxycodone, rosiglitazone, thalidomide, and vigabtrin. Medications may also be part of a limited distribution program, which generally provides access to specialty medications, insurance assistance, and patient counseling services.

INFECTION CONTROL AND HAZARDOUS CHEMICAL STANDARDS

Infection control is a process used to prevent nosocomial, or health care–associated, infections. Increasing antimicrobial resistance and the emergence of new pathogens prompted concern for new standards of infection control. Hazardous materials and drugs produce adverse effects for the preparer.

The Occupational Safety and Health Administration (OSHA) requires employees to be protected from hazardous chemicals through hand washing and the use of **personal protective equipment**, including gowns, gloves, goggles, feet and hair covers, and masks. Glove selection depends on the type of preparation being compounded and the presence of allergies that may adversely affect the employee or patient. Nonpowdered gloves may be used when handling hazardous drugs, waste, or contaminants. Nonlatex gloves may be used by preparers and/or patients allergic to latex.

Facilities are expected to implement infection prevention and control processes. Hands should be appropriately washed and decontaminated before and after patient interactions, prior to the production of aseptic procedures, and upon contact with blood or other infectious materials. The use of appropriate personal protective equipment (PPE) must be based on the risk of contamination and the type of compounded preparation. All equipment should be cleaned and disinfected before and after the preparation of medications. Counting trays and spatulas must be disinfected using 70% isopropyl alcohol. Additional caution should be given to the preparation of antibiotics, including penicillins and sulfonamides that have allergy potential. The use of a designated counting tray and a spatula for these types of medications is appropriate and should be labeled as such. Laminar flow hoods should be cleaned before and after batch preparations and maintained as required by law. Counters should be clutter free and clean of any debris. Non-sterile compounding areas and sterile compounding areas should be cleaned and maintained as described in *USP* <795> and *USP* <797>.

Material safety data sheets (MSDS) are written communications provided by the manufacturer. They provide information about hazardous chemicals, including the associated hazards, proper handling and cleanup procedures, and proper selection of PPE. The MSDS should be consulted in case of accidental exposures. Eyewashes can be used for exposures to the eye. An initial incident report (IIR) may be used by the facility to document the exposure.

RECALLS

The Food and Drug Administration defines a drug recall as either an involuntary or a voluntary effort to remove a product from the market. The recall may be conducted by the drug manufacturer, by request of the FDA, or by a regulatory agency authorized by the FDA.

Recalls are classified by severity into three groups as shown in Table 6-5.

Table 6-5. Recall Classifications

Recall Category	Description	Example
Class I Recall	Involves violative products that are likely to cause serious adverse health consequences or death	– Label mix-up on a life-saving medication – For example, in 2008, heparin was recalled due to heparin contamination with oversulfated chondroitin sulfate.
Class II Recall	Involves violative products that may cause temporary health issues or where the probability of serious adverse health consequences is remote	– The presence of particles in a medication container – For example, in 2010, Ketorolac was recalled due to the presence of small particles in the medication vial.
Class III Recall	Involves violative products that are not likely to cause adverse health consequences	– Packaging issues or defective delivery devices – For example, in 2008, many fentanyl 75 mcg pain patches were recalled because the patch was leaking active drug.

The FDA may take other actions including an FDA market withdrawal or an FDA medical device safety alert. In an FDA market withdrawal, a withdrawal is issued for a product that has a minor violation that would not warrant legal action. For example, a product is withdrawn due to tampering without proof of manufacturing or distribution problems. In contrast, an FDA medical device safety alert is when a recall is issued for a medical device that may present an unreasonable risk of substantial harm.

PROFESSIONAL STANDARDS

Pharmacists, pharmacy technicians, interns, and other pharmacy personnel are expected to uphold a standard of conduct reflecting their commitment, honesty, integrity, and discipline to the health care field. These standards reflect their personal commitment and dedication to the patients they serve. Professional standards include the following:

- Ensuring the health and safety of the patient
- Promoting honesty and integrity in the profession
- Maintaining competency in his/her field of study
- Promoting the right to privacy for all patients
- Respecting and valuing the abilities of other technicians, pharmacists, and health care professionals
- Refusing to dispense, promote, or distribute products and services that do not meet standards as required by law
- Refusing to engage in activities that could discredit the profession
- Engaging in and supporting organizations that support the pharmacy profession

FACILITY EQUIPMENT AND SUPPLY REQUIREMENTS

The types of equipment and facilities vary depending on the pharmacy and services offered. State Boards of Pharmacy (BOP) provide guidelines on the amount of space and the types of equipment needed.

Pharmacies are required to have a monitored security system that transmits warnings of intrusions via an audible, electronic or visual signal. An auxiliary source of power must be equipped to provide continuous power in the event of a power failure or if the system is tampered with or disabled. The use of video surveillance technology may be used by pharmacies, to capture any activity where medications are stored, counted or dispensed, at all exit locations. Other security features may include physical barriers like steel doors or curtains, sensors used to detect movement, and alarmed doors and windows.

Pharmacies must have access to clean hot and cold water, the ability to lock Schedule II substances in a safe or other lockable device, and access to counters and medication-specific refrigerators and freezers. Pharmacies that provide compounded sterile preparations need to have a distinct compounding area complete with a laminar hood. The pharmacy should be neat and organized, uncluttered, well ventilated, and equipped with proper lighting.

Most pharmacies have electronic and written resources that can be accessed when questions arise. These resources support therapeutic decision making and improve patient outcomes. Electronic sources are usually incorporated into the pharmacy computer system and are accessed from any pharmacy computer.

Written pharmacy resources are outlined in Table 6-6.

Table 6-6. Pharmacy Resources and Their Features

Pharmacy Resources	Features
American Drug Index	- Dictionary format with alphabetical listings - Drug container and storage requirements - Charts and comparative tables to display information - Information on composition, strength, dosage form, schedule, and usage - Information on laboratory values, vaccine and immunological information, and manufacturers and distributors
Drug Facts and Comparisons	- Frequently updated - Comprehensive information on 22,000 Rx and 6,000 OTC products - Drugs are divided by therapeutic or by pharmaco-logical groups - Treatment guidelines - Manufacturer and distributor information - Canadian trade name index
FDA's *Approved Drug Products with Therapeutic Equivalence Evaluations (Orange Book)*	- Identifies the FDA's approved drug products on the basis of safety and efficacy - Contains therapeutic equivalency evaluations for prescription products
Handbook on Injectable Drugs	- A collection of monographs on commercially avail-able parenteral drugs - Information on preparation, stability, storage, administration, and compatibility
Physicians' Desk Reference®	- Compilation of medication package inserts providing information on drug mechanisms, drug interactions, contraindications, side effects, and warnings - Updated annually - Tablet identifier catalog
Remington's *The Science and Practice of Pharmacy*	- Covers 8 distinct topics, including orientation, pharmaceutics, pharmaceutical chemistry, testing/analysis/control, pharmacokinetics and pharmacody-namics, pharmaceutical and medicinal agents, phar-maceutical manufacturing, and pharmacy practice
United States Pharmacopeia Drug Information Volume 1 (USP-DI Vol. 1): Drug Information for the Health Care Professional	- Label and off-label uses for more than 11,000 drugs - Drug monographs with information, including indication, dosing, dosage form, pharmacology/pharmacokinetics, adverse effects, and patient counseling tips
United States Pharmacopeia Drug Information Volume 2 (USP-DI Vol. 2): Advice for the Patient	- Presented in layman terms for easy reading - Simplified drug monographs with information on proper drug use, precautions, side effects, and special considerations
United States Pharmacopeia-National Formulary (USP-NF)	- The official compendium of drug information from the United States Pharmacopeial Convention - Presents official monographs of information about drug substances and dosage forms, pharmaceutical ingredients, and drug standards and specifications

SUMMARY

☐ Pharmacy legislation helped shape pharmacy practice and pharmacy operations by providing many of the regulations currently used in practice.

☐ Restrictions on the use of medications vary. Pharmacy personnel should check their pharmacy policies and procedures, MSDS, and REMS for information about the proper usage and distribution of these medications.

☐ Pharmacies supply medications for different populations. The equipment and supplies pharmacies use vary based on the population they serve.

PHARMACY LAW AND REGULATIONS PRACTICE QUESTIONS

1. Which copy of the triplicate DEA 222 form does the purchaser retain?

   (A) copy 1 (top copy)
   (B) copy 2 (middle copy)
   (C) copy 3 (bottom copy)
   (D) All copies are forwarded to the DEA.

2. Which of the following statements is true regarding prescription refills?

   (A) Schedule II prescriptions can be refilled up to 5 times in 6 months.
   (B) Schedule III prescriptions can be refilled up to 5 times in 6 months.
   (C) Schedule II prescriptions can be refilled for up to 1 year.
   (D) Schedule III prescriptions can be refilled for up to 1 year.

3. According to federal law, how long must Schedule III, IV, and V invoices be maintained in the pharmacy?

   (A) 1 year
   (B) 2 years
   (C) 3 years
   (D) 4 years

4. Which of the following is an example of a misbranded drug?

   (A) The OTC product label is missing potential drug warnings.
   (B) The drug was manufactured in an unsanitary facility.
   (C) The drug leaves the pharmacy and is then redispensed.
   (D) The bottle contents are outdated.

5. Oxycodone is an example of a drug in what control schedule?

   (A) Schedule I
   (B) Schedule II
   (C) Schedule III
   (D) Schedule IV

6. Which regulation was prompted, in part, due to the death of over 100 individuals because of the addition of diethylene glycol to a sulfa-based elixir?

(A) Federal Food Drug and Cosmetic Act of 1938
(B) Health Insurance Portability and Accountability Act of 1996
(C) Comprehensive Drug Abuse Prevention and Control Act of 1970
(D) Poison Prevention Packaging Act of 1970

7. Which DEA form should be filled out in the event of a theft of a Schedule II substance?

(A) DEA 222
(B) DEA 41
(C) DEA 106
(D) No form is needed.

8. What are the maximum daily and monthly limits placed on the purchase of any pseudoephedrine-containing products?

(A) 1.2 g/day of base drug; 5 g/month of base drug
(B) 2 g/day of base drug; 6 g/month of base drug
(C) 2.8 g/day of base drug; 7.5 g/month of base drug
(D) 3.6 g/day of base drug; 9 g/month of base drug

9. What does REMS stand for?

(A) Risk Evaluation and Mitigation Strategies
(B) Risk Effort and Medical Strategies
(C) Return Effect and Manipulation Systems
(D) Recovery Evaluation and Master Strategies

10. Which of the following reference books provides information directed toward the patient?

(A) *USP-DI Volume I*
(B) *USP-DI Volume 2*
(C) *USP-NF*
(D) *Drug Facts and Comparisons*

ANSWERS EXPLAINED

1. **(C)** Copy 3 (bottom copy) is retained by the purchaser. The only copy forwarded to the DEA is copy 2.

2. **(B)** Schedule III prescriptions may be refilled up to 5 times in 6 months. Schedule II prescriptions cannot be refilled.

3. **(B)** Federal law mandates that Schedule III, IV, and V invoices be maintained in the pharmacy for a minimum of 2 years.

4. **(A)** The omission of potential drug warnings is an example of misbranding. The production of a drug in unsanitary conditions is an example of adulteration. Drugs that are redispensed after leaving the pharmacy or are outdated are considered adulterated.

5. **(B)** Oxycodone is classified as a Schedule II drug as defined by the Controlled Substances Act. Schedule I drugs do not have any legal medical use in the United States.

6. **(A)** The Federal Food Drug and Cosmetic Act of 1938 was prompted, in part, by the deaths of over 100 individuals who took a sulfa-based elixir containing diethylene glycol, an ingredient found in antifreeze. The Health Insurance Portability and Accountability Act of 1996 was enacted to place privacy safeguards on all protected health information (PHI). The Comprehensive Drug Abuse Prevention and Control Act of 1970 placed controlled substances into one of five schedules based on each substance's abuse potential and legal status. The Poison Prevention Packaging Act of 1970 was enacted in response to a growing number of accidental poisonings in children.

7. **(C)** A DEA 106 form must be filled out in the event of a theft of a Schedule II substance. Schedule II substances are controlled. Therefore, the DEA must be alerted using a DEA 106 form. A DEA 222 form is used to purchase or transfer Schedule II medications. A DEA 41 form is filled out for any outdated or damaged controlled substances.

8. **(D)** The maximum daily limit for pseudoephedrine-containing products is 3.6 g of the base drug. The maximum monthly limit for pseudoephedrine-containing products is 9 g of the base drug.

9. **(A)** REMS is the abbreviation for Risk Evaluation and Mitigation Strategies.

10. **(B)** *USP-DI Volume 2* provides information geared toward the patient. *USP-DI Volume 1* provides information geared toward the health care professional. *USP-NF* provides drug monographs and information about the purity and quality of drugs. *Drug Facts and Comparisons* provides comprehensive medication information.

Sterile and Non-Sterile Compounding

7

KNOWLEDGE DOMAIN 3.0

Sterile and Non-Sterile Compounding   **8.75%**

→ Knowledge Area 3.1: Infection control (e.g., hand washing, PPE)
→ Knowledge Area 3.2: Handling and disposal requirements (e.g., receptacles, waste streams)
→ Knowledge Area 3.3: Documentation (e.g., batch preparation, compounding record)
→ Knowledge Area 3.4: Determine product stability (e.g., beyond use dating, signs of incompatibility)
→ Knowledge Area 3.5: Selection and use of equipment and supplies
→ Knowledge Area 3.6: Sterile compounding processes
→ Knowledge Area 3.7: Non-sterile compounding processes

LEARNING OBJECTIVES

☐ Define extemporaneous compounding, including both sterile and non-sterile compounding.
☐ Understand the role of the United States Pharmacopeia, and identify the chapters essential to compounding procedures.
☐ Describe safety procedures, including infection control standards, handling, and disposal requirements.
☐ Understand the documentation process, including the types of records used.
☐ Differentiate between the three risk levels given to sterile compounding procedures.
☐ Identify ingredients used in compounding processes.
☐ Describe equipment commonly used in compounding.
☐ Perform sterile and non-sterile compounding calculations.

Manufacturers supply dosage forms to meet the needs of a majority of their patients. Sometimes a dosage form is unavailable, is not currently on the market for that drug, or is not carried by the pharmacy. In these cases, the pharmacist uses his or her chemistry background and knowledge of medications in order to make a special preparation. This process of mixing and preparing drug components to meet a patient's need is called **extemporaneous compounding**. Technicians may be called upon to assist the pharmacist with these preparations. Compounded preparations can be made to adjust a dose, flavor a medication, reformulate the drug to remove an ingredient that a patient is allergic to (such as gluten), or even change a dosage form to one more suitable for the patient (e.g., tablet to a suspension).

> **Compounding vs. Manufacturing:** Compounding is the formulation of an individual compound made specifically to meet a patient's need. It is not commercially available, and it is not available to be resold by the patient or the prescriber. Manufacturing involves batch compounding of FDA-approved compounds that are then sold to pharmacies or health care practitioners.

Extemporaneous compounding can be broken down into two categories: sterile compounding and non-sterile compounding. Sterile compounding is used for intravenous solutions, parenteral nutrition, and ophthalmic formulations. Non-sterile compounding is used for tablets, capsules, creams, ointments, suspensions, suppositories, transdermal applications, and troches.

The United States Pharmacopeial Convention (USP) is the leading authority in setting standards for product safety and purity. This nonprofit organization publishes a compendium called the *USP-NF* (*National Formulary*) with standards for chemical substances, compounded products, dosage forms, medical supplies, and dietary supplements. *USP <797>* (**Chapter 797**) provides specific procedures and methods used for compounding sterile preparations. *USP <795>* (**Chapter 795**) describes compounding practices and procedures for non-sterile preparations.

STERILE COMPOUNDING PROCESSES

Sterile compounding is a process reserved for injectable products, as well as for medications to be instilled into the eye. These products require special precautions and additional safety measures to ensure product sterility.

Compounding prescriptions is an integral component of pharmacy practice. The pharmacy can acquire commercially made parenteral products and diluents. These products can be used as is, or they can be formulated to meet a patient's needs. Although these products are used often in pharmacy practice, non-commercially available formulations may still need to be compounded. Compounding specific formulations is necessary because patients with allergies to preservatives or diluents may require non-commercially available compounds prepared in the pharmacy. In addition, medication strengths for certain populations (i.e., pediatric or geriatric) may not be available and therefore must be prepared by the pharmacy. Other reasons include stability issues or combination therapies that are not commercially available.

Safety

Sterile preparations must be formulated according to purported norms, ensuring that the product meets identity, potency, quality, and purity standards. A failure to ensure that these norms are met may result in an adulterated or a misbranded product.

In order to meet safety standards, all sterile preparations must be formulated in a designated sterile compounding area. This area has to be distinct and separate, and it may not be used for non-sterile compounding procedures. This area is referred to as a controlled area or a buffer area. The laminar flow workbench must be located in this area. The pharmacy also contains an area called an anteroom, which is separate and distinct from the buffer area. The anteroom is used to decontaminate supplies and equipment. Personnel must also use this area to perform hand washing and gowning procedures. All unpacking and opening of boxes should be confined to the anteroom in order to reduce the number of particles in the buffer area.

Compounding pharmacists and technicians must abide by all federal and state laws. In addition, proper infection control procedures must be maintained to prevent harm as a result of:

- Non-sterility due to microbial contaminants
- The presence of bacterial endotoxins
- The incorrect strength of intended ingredients in excess of monograph limits
- Physical and chemical contaminants
- Poor-quality ingredients used in compounding

Infection control quality standards are based on the best sterile compounding processes and scientific documentation. Any individual involved in formulating compounded sterile preparations (CSPs) must be trained, skilled, and evaluated on proper compounding techniques and procedures. These techniques and procedures include:

- Hand washing and disinfection of sterile equipment
- Selection of appropriate personal protective equipment (PPE)
- Formulation of CSPs in ISO Class 5 devices (see the section on sterile compounding equipment later in this chapter)
- Identification of products and weighing of ingredients
- Performing calculations as needed
- Maintaining sterility while performing aseptic procedures
- Performing quality control measures
- Labeling and inspecting CSPs

CSPs can be subdivided into three distinct categories. These categories are determined based on the potential for microbial growth during compounding procedures. Sources of contamination may include non-sterile components used in compounding procedures, the contamination of a compound due to inappropriate conditions within the compounding environment, and spillage of solid or liquid matter during compounding. Table 7-1 lists the CSP risk levels.

Table 7-1. Compounded Sterile Preparation Risk Levels*

Risk Level	Description
Low risk	- Compounded using aseptic manipulations in an ISO Class 5 environment - Compounding involves no more than three commercially available products and no more than two entries into any sterile container or bag - Manipulations must follow aseptic guidelines when using ampules, syringes, or needles and during the transfer of formulations
Medium risk	- Pooling multiple vials or containers to prepare a CSP for one or more patients - Compounding involves more than one vial transfer - A long compounding process is required (i.e., dissolution or preparation of a homogenous mixture) - An example of a medium-risk CSP is the preparation of the total parenteral nutrition formulations using an automated device
High risk	- Using non-sterile formulations to prepare CSPs (including those intended for oral administration) - Sterile components, antimicrobial-free CSPs, and sterile surfaces exposed to air quality worse than an ISO Class 5 - Compounding personnel not garbed or inappropriately garbed - Measuring or mixing sterile ingredients in non-sterile devices

*The information in this table is currently being reviewed for potential structural changes by the United States Pharmacopeia. The proposed revisions would collapse the three levels of CSP contamination risk into two categories based on the conditions under which these preparations are made and the time to be used. At the time of this publication, those proposed revisions are still only under consideration and have not yet been adapted.

Compatibility issues are also an area of concern. Compatibility may occur between one or more drugs or even between a drug and an IV solution. Incompatibility issues can be due to many factors, including visible changes or chemical changes. Examples of visible changes include a color change, a cloudy appearance, or a change in viscosity. Examples of chemical changes include the formation of a gas or the formation of a precipitate. Calcium phosphate is an example of a precipitate formed through a chemical incompatibility when sodium phosphate or potassium phosphate are combined with calcium gluconate. The formation of a calcium phosphate precipitate can be avoided by adding the phosphate component first and then flushing out the line before adding any of the potentially incompatible components.

Handling and Disposal

Disposal of pharmaceutical waste must meet all state and federal guidelines according to the U.S. Environmental Protection Agency (EPA). Hazardous waste can either be categorized into one of four categories (P, U, K, or F)—as listed in the Resource Conservation and Recovery Act—or be categorized as meeting a hazardous waste characteristic. These characteristics include toxicity, corrosiveness, ignitability, and reactivity. The P and U lists are discarded commercial chemical products specific to pharmaceutical hazardous wastes. They include drugs such as chemotherapeutic agents, warfarin, and nicotine.

Pharmacies that prepare hazardous drugs must have a separate negative pressure room to house engineering controls. These controls are to be used for hazardous preparations and are separate from controls used for nonhazardous preparations. Hazardous waste should be clearly labeled as "hazardous drug waste." This waste is placed into leak-proof trash bags that are similarly labeled. Hazardous waste receptacles should also be labeled as such and placed near areas where hazardous drugs are prepared. Stored hazardous waste should be kept separate from nonhazardous waste until it is picked up and transferred to a treatment facility.

Red sharps containers are used to dispose of used needles and syringes and other breakable items.

Agents Used in Formulation

CSPs are made using various components, including those listed in Table 7-2.

Table 7-2. Agents Used When Preparing CSPs

Component	Definition	Example
Antimicrobial preservatives	Used for bacteriostatic preparations to prevent bacteria from growing	- IV solutions: benzyl alcohol - Ophthalmics: benzalkonium chloride 0.01%
Antioxidants	Prevent oxidation of the component drug	- metabisulfite (used for low pH values) - bisulfite (used for intermediate pH values) - sulfite (used for high pH values)
Chelating agents	Reduce toxic effects of metals by binding to form complexes that can be removed	- edetate sodium
Emulsifiers	Used to create a uniformed concentration of an active drug in solution	- sodium lauryl sulfate
pH buffers	Help stabilize a solution against degradation	- phosphate - citrate
Solute	A substance dissolved in a solvent (dissolving substance)	- Active drug - Inactive drug used to increase stability
Tonicity agents	Help adjust formulation to an appropriate isotonic range	- sodium chloride
Vehicle	Serve as solvents with little to no therapeutic activity or toxicity	- sterile water for injection - normal saline (0.9% sodium chloride injection)
Water-miscible solvents	A solution used to dissolve drugs with low water solubility	- polyethylene glycol

Sterile preparations require the use of containers used to hold the formulation. Containers include those used before, during, and after aseptic preparation. They should be free of microbial pathogens. In addition, these containers should not interact with the formulation, resulting in a change to the strength, quality, or purity of the preparation. Examples of containers include: single- and multiple-dose containers, and glass containers. Single-use containers (i.e., vials and ampules) do not contain antimicrobial preservatives and should be used immediately. Vials should be used no more than 6 hours after the initial needle puncture (*USP* <797>). Open ampules should not be stored.

Multiple-dose containers have antimicrobial preservatives, allowing for the withdrawal of contents over a period of time. There is a beyond use date (BUD) of 28 days unless otherwise specified by the manufacturer (see Table 7-7).

Glass containers are preferred in sterile preparations. Borosilicate glass is the most commonly used glass material. Plastic containers are not commonly used and pose problems, including leaching, difficult inspection due to clarity issues, and sorption of drug molecules through plastic. Additionally, container closures are sterile, usually made of rubber, and free from pyrogens and particles. Closures are also subject to coring and require proper inspection.

Sterile Preparation Equipment

Sterile preparations are prepared in ISO Class 5 (International Organization for Standardization) environments. ISO guidelines classify cleanrooms by the size and number of airborne particles per cubic meter of air. An ISO Class 5 environment may also be referred to as a Class 100 environment, based on a previous guideline set by the U.S. Federal Standard that denoted the cleanroom based on the number of particles per cubic foot of air. Both standards are still used interchangeably today. Class 5 environments cannot contain more than 100 particles (0.5 microns) per cubic foot. The most common equipment used to achieve these conditions is the **laminar flow hood**.

The laminar flow hood provides an ultraclean environment by using a high-efficiency particulate air (HEPA) filter. Two types of laminar flow hoods are used in compounding. Horizontal laminar flow hoods take room air in from the top. The air is then processed by the HEPA filter, filtered, and blown out horizontally over the work surface toward the operator (from the back to the front). Vertical laminar flow hoods also receive room air from the top. The air is then processed by the HEPA filter, filtered, and blown down vertically across the work surface and toward the operator (top to bottom). Horizontal laminar flow hoods are used for a majority of CSPs, while vertical laminar flow hoods are reserved for chemotherapeutic agents. See Figure 7-1.

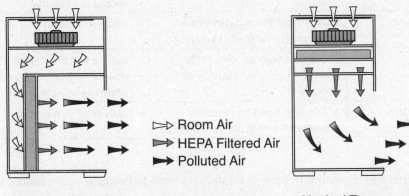

Room Air
HEPA Filtered Air
Polluted Air

Horizontal Type   Vertical Type

Figure 7-1. Laminar flow hood airflow

Laminar flow hoods can be used to prepare IV admixtures, ophthalmic solutions, and sterile products. They are also used when reconstituting powdered drugs and preparing unit-dose syringes. The laminar flow hood should be running continuously. If the hood is turned off, run the hood for 30 minutes before using the work surface. Inspection and recertification of the hood should be completed every six months.

Cleaning a laminar flow hood should be done before and after any manipulations within the hood. First, sterile water is used to remove large pieces of dirt on the interior surfaces of the hood. Then sterile isopropyl alcohol (70% isopropyl alcohol) is used to disinfect interior surfaces. In order to clean the inside of the hood properly, the operator should use a lint-free cloth to wipe from top to bottom and from back to front with the isopropyl alcohol. The alcohol should be allowed to air dry before compounding is resumed.

The operator should work at least 6 inches into the hood to avoid contamination. The outer edges of the hood should also be avoided when compounding preparations. All plastic covers and paper should be removed before supplies are placed into the hood. Extreme effort should be made not to block airflow while processing compounds. Skill and practice are needed to learn proper finger placement. The area between the HEPA filter and the sterile object is known as the "critical area." When there is an interruption or blockage of airflow to this area, turbulence can form. The area of turbulence could extend outside of the hood, in turn, allowing contaminants to enter the sterile workplace.

Biological safety cabinets are reserved for hazardous substances, including chemotherapeutic agents. Air is taken from the top, passed through the HEPA filter (taking up the entire ceiling of the hood), and moved down toward the work surface area. As air approaches the work surface, it is pulled through vents located on the sides, front, and back of the cabinet, where it is recirculated back into the cabinet.

Needles and syringes are also used to prepare admixtures. Figure 7-2 contains a picture depicting the parts of a syringe and a needle.

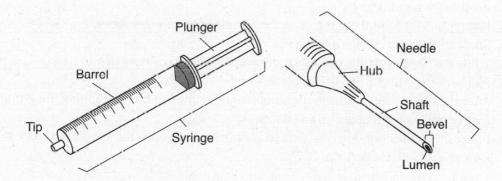

Figure 7-2. Parts of a syringe and a needle

A **needle** has two parts: the shaft and the hub. The shaft is the stem and has a bevel (diagonal point) on one end. The hub is the other end of the needle and attaches to the syringe. Also note that the shaft contains a hollow bore referred to as the lumen. Needles are referred to by their size. Needle lengths vary from $\frac{3}{8}$ inch to $3\frac{1}{2}$ inches. Another way to designate size is by referring to the needle's gauge. This refers to the size of the lumen, measured inversely, with sizes measuring from 13 (largest-size lumen) to 32 (smallest-size lumen). Some needles come attached to the syringe, while others are available in individual packaging. Selecting the appropriate needle is determined by the viscosity of the solution and the vial in which it is to be administered. Used needles should be discarded into a sharps container. Some needles contain a safety cap that automatically locks to protect the user from finger pricks. **Filter needles** are specialized needles that contain a filter used to catch any particles that may be present in an ampule. The filter needle is used to withdraw solution from the ampule. Then a nonfiltered needle can be attached to add the medication to the bag of solution.

Syringes have two main components: the barrel and the plunger. The barrel is a hollow tube with an open end on one side. Within the barrel is a plunger, which is a piston-type rod that moves within the plunger and is used both to draw and to release fluid. The tip of the syringe contains a point of attachment that is used to attach a needle. Some syringes contain a tapered tip allowing the needle to be held on by friction. Other needles have a locking device that allows the needle to be secured by turning and locking the needle in place. Graduation lines indicate the volume of solution. Capacity varies with syringes and ranges in size from 1 to 60 mL. Syringes are also disposable and should not be reused.

Vials are glass containers that supply a majority of the injectable medications used in compounding procedures. They contain a flip-top cover that should be removed before proceeding. Once revealed, this exposes a rubber stopper that must be sterilized with 70% isopropyl alcohol swabs before needle entry. Needles may cause coring of the rubber stopper, resulting in pieces of the rubber entering the solution. To avoid this, the operator should practice penetrating the rubber stopper with the tip and bevel at the same point. This is done by first penetrating the stopper with the bevel side up at a 45-degree angle and then inserting the needle straight in.

When using a vial, remember to follow these aseptic technique steps:

TIP

The following areas should be avoided during preparation: needle shaft, inner core of the needle hub, syringe plunger, syringe barrel tip and vial, and the IV bag rubber entry points.

1. Remove the cover of the vial, and disinfect the rubber stopper using 70% isopropyl alcohol.
2. Withdraw a volume of air into the syringe that is equivalent to the volume of the drug intended to be withdrawn.
3. Uncap the needle, and insert it using the technique mentioned above.
4. Inject air from the syringe into the vial.
5. While the needle is in the vial, invert the vial and hold it with one hand.
6. Pull back the plunger, and draw out the liquid.
7. After the medication has been drawn out, remove any bubbles by tapping the syringe and/or pulling the plunger up and down.
8. Inject the medication into the desired container, or remove the needle and lock the syringe using a Luer Lock tip.
9. Dispose of the needle in a sharps container in accordance with pharmacy policies and procedures and with Joint Commission patient care and safety standards.

Ampules are single-use containers made of glass. Once opened, they must be used and discarded. Ampules contain a top portion called the head, a middle neck portion, and a bottom portion called the body. Solution should be directed toward the body of the ampule before opening. This can be done by tapping the tip (head) of the ampule or by swirling the ampule.

You should know the proper technique to open an ampule and withdraw medication. Proper technique involves the following steps:

1. Clean the head and neck of the ampule with 70% isopropyl alcohol.
2. Place the alcohol swab around the neck of the ampule. This will help reduce the chance of glass fragments cutting your fingers.
3. Hold the head of the ampule with one hand using your thumb and index fingers. With your other hand, grab the body of the ampule using your thumb and index fingers.
4. Using pressure and a swift motion, snap the ampule neck by moving your hands away and out.
5. Tilt the ampule, and insert a filter needle into the ampule with the bevel side up. Pull back the plunger, and draw out the medication.
6. Remove the filter needle, replace it with a regular needle, and inject it into the desired product.

Plastic **intravenous (IV) bags** are used for diluting and administering medications to patients. IV bags are available in various sizes: 50, 100, 250, 500, and 1,000 mL. Parenteral nutrition bags are also found in 2,000 mL and 3,000 mL sizes. Bags that are 100 mL or smaller are referred to as small-volume parenteral (SVP) bags and are infused intermittently. Bags larger than 100 mL are referred to as large-volume parenteral (LVP) bags and are infused continuously. Although plastic IV bags are more commonly used, PVC (polyvinyl chloride) bags are also available. PVC bags are reserved for drugs that can adhere to the plastic (e.g., Taxol). The top has a looped plastic extension piece with a center hole used to hang the IV bag during administration. The bottom of the bag contains two ports. One port is a sterile administration port. The port usually has a cover that needs to be removed prior to being used. In order to use the port, it has to be punctured. Administration sets contain a spike that will puncture the administration port and allow for medication to drip through. The second port is the medication port, which needs to be sterilized with isopropyl alcohol before use. IV bags are available in a variety of solutions. Common IV solutions are listed in Table 7-3.

Table 7-3. Common IV Solutions

IV Solution	Description
NS	0.9% NaCl in water
$\frac{1}{2}$ NS	0.45% NaCl in water
D5W	Dextrose 5% in water
LR (lactated Ringer's)	Normal saline with electrolytes and buffer
D5NS	5% dextrose in 0.9% normal saline
$\frac{1}{4}$ NS	0.225% normal saline
D5 $\frac{1}{2}$ NS	5% dextrose in 0.45% normal saline
D5 $\frac{1}{4}$ NS	5% dextrose in 0.225% normal saline
D10W	10% dextrose in water

Common injectable routes of administration are listed in Table 7-4.

Table 7-4. Common Injectable Routes of Administration

Injectable Route	Description
Subcutaneous (SC, SQ)	Injections made under the skin (e.g., insulin, vaccinations)
Intra-arterial (IA)	Injections made into an artery (usually reserved for situations when injection into a vein is not possible)
Intramuscular (IM)	Injections made into a muscle (typical muscles include deltoid and gluteal muscles)
Intravenous (IV)	Injections made into a vein (e.g., a large-volume parenteral, a small-volume parenteral)
Epidural	Medication is delivered through a catheter placed in the space outside of the spinal canal
Intradermal (ID)	Injections made into the dermal layer of the skin (e.g., tuburculin)
Intrathecal	Injections made into the spinal canal

Other sterile preparations include ophthalmic (eye) and inhalation (inhaled through mouth) solutions.

Intravenous therapy is the riskiest type of administration because it circumvents the body's natural barriers. The combination of parenteral dosage forms for administration via a unit product is called an IV admixture. Patients who receive IV therapy are typically the most vulnerable. IV admixtures must absolutely be free of contamination. Improper solutions can cause occlusions, infections, and even death. Intravenous piggyback (IVPB) is a term used when referring to a small-volume parenteral bag (SVP) that is hung alongside a large-volume parenteral (LVP) bag. These bags use the same IV tubing, with the SVP attached to the injection port.

TOTAL PARENTERAL NUTRITION (TPN) SOLUTIONS

TPNs provide patients with nutrition via intravenous administration. This process bypasses the typical process of digestion. TPNs may be used for patients with bowel obstructions, ulcerative colitis, pediatric GI disorders, or short-bowel disorder. These preparations are compounded using aseptic procedures. TPN compounders can be used to aid in the production of TPNs through the assistance of computer software and robotics. Reservoirs, referred to as channels, hold amino acids, dextrose, fats, and other additives that can then be pumped into TPN bags.

TPNs are administered in the right atrium of the heart using a central line. TPNs typically consist of 50% dextrose solution, 20% fat emulsion, and 10% amino acids. Administration through a peripheral IV access line is called peripheral parenteral nutrition (PPN). These preparations usually contain 25% dextrose solution, 10% amino acids, and 10% fat emulsion.

Solutions are available premixed by manufacturers, allowing pharmacies to add necessary vitamins, medications, and electrolytes as prescribed. Administration techniques vary. However, they may include 2-in-1 or 3-in-1 individualized admixtures. 2-in-1 admixtures infuse dextrose and amino acids first followed by the addition of the fat emulsion and any additives. 3-in-1 admixtures allow for the simultaneous infusion of amino acids, fats, and dextrose. Examples of additives include sodium chloride (NaCl), potassium chloride (KCl), multivitamins with iron (MVI), magnesium sulfate ($MgSO_4$), and calcium gluconate (Ca gluconate).

NON-STERILE COMPOUNDING PROCESSES

Many different prescriptions can be made using non-sterile techniques. The pharmacist will evaluate the appropriateness of the order and determine product selection. Ingredient selection should be based on National Formulary (NF) or USP guidelines and should meet safety and purity standards. Table 7-5 contains a list of commonly made compounds.

Table 7-5. Compounded Preparations

Compound	Description
Capsules	Active drug is contained in a cylinder-shaped shell made of gelatin or methylcellulose
Creams	Oil in water (o/w) emulsion
Emulsions	A mixture of two or more liquids that are immiscible
Gels	A suspension of a solid in a liquid medium
Lozenge/troche	A tablet that is designed to be dissolved in the mouth
Ointment	Water in oil (w/o) emulsion
Paste	Formed by mixing a solid with a small amount of a liquid levigating agent
Powder	A finely ground mixture of an active and/or an inactive drug
Solution	A liquid dosage form where the active ingredient is dissolved in the liquid vehicle
Suppository	A solid dosage form containing a base ingredient (e.g., cocoa butter) that is inserted into the vagina, rectum, or urethra
Suspension	A liquid dosage form where the active ingredient is dispersed in the liquid vehicle; must be shaken prior to use
Tablet	A solid dosage form made by compression or molding

Compounded preparations may include one, two, or multiple ingredients. Active ingredients produce a pharmacological response or change. Inactive ingredients are needed to fill prescriptions but do not produce a pharmacological response. A list of common inactive ingredients is displayed in Table 7-6.

Table 7-6. Commonly Used Inactive Ingredients

Inactive Ingredients	Description	Example
Acidifying agents	Provide acidic medium; bring stability to the formulation	citric acid
Alkalizing agents	Provide alkalizing medium; bring stability to the formulation	ammonia solution
Colorants	Provide color to preparations	FD&C red #3
Emulsifying agents	Maintain dispersion of fine particles of liquid in vehicles	benzalkonium chloride
Flavorants	Provide flavor or odor to a preparation	menthol
Gelling agents	Used to increase viscosity by thickening and stabilizing the preparation	Carbopol 940
Levigating agents	Help reduce particle size	mineral oil
Lubricants	Prevent ingredients from clumping	magnesium stearate
Preservatives	Protect formulation from microbial growth	methylparaben
Suspending agents	Increase viscosity to prevent sedimentation of powder in liquid	sodium lauryl sulfate
Sweeteners	Colorless, odorless agents that bring sweetness to a preparation	sorbitol
Wetting agents	Disperse air on the surface of drug molecules with liquid	betadex sulfobutyl ether sodium

Safety

Personnel performing non-sterile compounding procedures should wear a clean laboratory jacket. Hair bonnets, gloves, face masks, shoes, and aprons may also be worn. Clothing selection is based on personal protection and prevention of drug contamination.

Documentation

Proper records should be kept of all compounded preparations. *USP* <795> requires pharmacies to maintain master formulation records as well as compounding records for each preparation. Master formulation records are the official "recipes" prepared before a unique formulation is made. They are kept in the pharmacy and filed alphabetically. Pharmacists and technicians can use these records in order to duplicate a prescription. Master formulation records include the following:

- List of ingredients (including official names and amounts)
- List of equipment needed to compound the prescription
- Calculations used to prepare and verify each ingredient
- Instructions for preparing the compound, including the mixing order
- Labeling requirements (beyond use date, storage requirements, generic names, and quantities of each ingredient and prescription number)
- Compatibility and stability requirements

Any time a compound is made, the following should be recorded in the compounding record:

- Preparer (e.g., pharmacist, pharmacy intern, technician as allowed by state law)
- All product names, lot numbers, and quantities used (even those quantities that may have been tossed due to error)
- Master formulation record reference
- Mixing order
- Beyond use date
- Date of preparation and prescription number
- Storage requirements (e.g., refrigeration, protection from light, shake before use)
- Label (duplicate of master formulation)
- Description of final preparation (ointment, cream, etc.)

All documentation should be typed or written in a standard format to prevent errors and to allow for easy access and determination of the prepared compound. Preparations made according to a manufacturer's labeling instructions do not require additional documentation. All other preparations require both a master formulation record and a compounding record. Records must be maintained in accordance with state law and must be kept for the same amount of time as that required for prescriptions. In addition, all equipment maintenance records and purchase records should be retained by the pharmacy.

> Four sets of records pertaining to non-sterile compounding should be maintained by the pharmacy: master formulation records, compounding records (including batch records), equipment maintenance records, and purchase records.

Pharmacies must maintain standard operating procedures (SOPs), which ensure accountability, quality, standards, and safety for all compounded preparations. This includes SOPs for personnel, the pharmacy, equipment, documentation, preparations, and packaging. In addition, Material Safety Data Sheets (MSDS) must be readily available for personnel. MSDS contain information about hazards, including flammability of chemicals and procedural guidelines.

Stability and Beyond Use Dating

Stability refers to the ability of a substance to remain unchanged over time while maintaining its initial characteristics. Chemical compatibility concerns, as well as proper beyond use date labeling, are both vital to stability.

Chemical compatibility refers to stability, specifically the ability for the substance to remain stable when mixed with other substances. Chemical incompatibilities include visible as well as invisible changes. A change in color or the formation of a precipitate, such as calcium phosphate, are examples of visible changes. The formation of gases or of volatile chemicals, in contrast, are examples of invisible changes.

The **beyond use date** is defined by the *USP-NF*, General Chapter <795>, as "the date after which a compounded preparation should not to be used; determined from the date the preparation is compounded." Medications may include stability information in their package insert or labeling. In the absence of stability information, packaged, light-resistant, temperature-controlled non-sterile compounded medications may use the beyond use dates listed in Table 7-7.

Table 7-7. Maximum Non-Sterile Beyond Use Dates

Formulation	Beyond Use Date (BUD) Maximum
Nonaqueous solutions (i.e., capsule without water)	BUD no later than 6 months or BUD equal to earliest expiration date of any active pharmaceutical ingredient (API)
Oral solutions containing water (i.e., oral suspension)	BUD no later than 14 days from reconstitution date (must be kept at the controlled temperature as indicated on the package label)
Topical solutions and semisolid formulations containing water (i.e., ointment)	BUD no later than 30 days

Equipment and Supplies

Compounding equipment may vary, and it depends on the type of preparations made. Compounding equipment includes the following:

- Glass mortar and pestle, which provide smooth surfaces ideal for suspensions, oily agents, and chemotherapeutic agents
- Wedgewood or porcelain mortar and pestle, which provide a rough surface ideal for emulsions and blending powders
- Stainless steel, hard rubber, and plastic spatulas, which are used for mixing powders, ointments, and creams
- Weighing papers and cups
- Graduated cylinders

    ○ Used to measure liquids
    ○ Amount measured should be no less than 20% of the cylinder's capacity
    ○ Liquid measurements are measured at eye level by verifying the volume at the bottom of the meniscus; this is the curved surface, called the meniscus, that appears due to surface tension (see Figure 7-3)

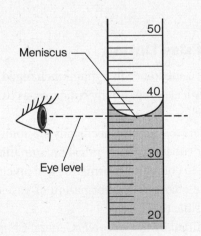

Figure 7-3. Reading a meniscus

- Ointment slab or ointment mixing paper, which are used for mixing ointments
- Suppository and troche molds

- Capsule preparation
  - The powder used to fill the capsules is mixed using geometric dilution and particle size is blended using trituration
  - The powder is then gathered together and compressed to form a block allowing for an easier punch method
  - Capsules are prepared using a punch method where the capsule components are separated, held vertically, and the open end is punched into the powder until filled
  - Each capsule is then weighed to ensure an appropriate fill
  - Capsule capacity can be determined by using a capacity table
  - Capsule sizes vary with the smallest size being 000 and the largest size being 5. The size of the capsule and approximate amount contained within are inversely proportionate. The smallest size, 000, will carry an approximate amount of 1,000 mg of powder, whereas the largest size, 5, will carry an approximate amount of 100 mg of powder

- Stir rods, funnels, and beakers, which are used to mix formulations
- Hot plate
- Refrigerator and freezer
  - Temperatures should be checked and logged in accordance with the law and pharmacy standards
  - Freezer temperatures may vary from –20°C to –10°C (–4°F to 14°F)
  - Refrigerator temperatures may vary from 2°C to 8°C (36°F to 46°F)

- Electronic balance
  - Used to determine the weight of material used in compounded prescriptions
  - Newer technology than the Class A prescription balance
  - Digital readout
  - Sensitivity reading of 0.1 mg

- Class A prescription balance with brass weight sets (see Figure 7-4)
  - Used to determine the weight of material being compounded
  - Must be calibrated; this process involves using a known weight and properly assessing the scale for accuracy
  - Can measure compounds ranging in weight from 120 mg to 120 g
  - Sensitivity reading of 6 mg, meaning that 6 mg of that substance will move the pointer of the balance one division off equilibrium
  - Weights are cylindrical and range in weight from 1 g to 50 g, with fractional weights ranging from 10 mg to 500 mg

- Prescription vials, ointment jars, capsule and suppository boxes or containers, and liquid bottles

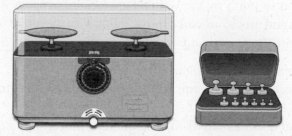

Figure 7-4. Class A prescription balance and brass weights

When weighing ingredients using the Class A Prescription Balance, the following steps should be used:

1. Lock the balance by turning and arresting the knob and by placing the weighing paper onto each pan.
2. Verify that the internal weights are set to zero.
3. Unlock the balance, level the weights, and then relock the balance.
4. Place the desired weight onto the right pan and the material to be weighed onto the left pan.
5. Unlock the weights, and observe the indicator arrow.
6. Lock the weights, and make any needed changes.
7. Write down the final measurement with the top down, and check your work.
8. Return the weights and supplies, and clean the balance.

Techniques Used to Prepare Prescriptions

The preparation of non-sterile prescriptions is customized according to industry and legal standards to maintain potency and purity. Compounding pharmacists will ensure that the final preparation is pure and accurate, properly labeled, and maintained. The following are techniques used to produce compounded preparations:

- **TRITURATION** reduces the particle size of an ingredient by grinding it into a powder (e.g., by using a mortar and pestle).
- **SPATULATION** uses a spatula to mix ingredients in a plastic bag, on ointment paper, or via another medium.
- **LEVIGATION** grinds a powder by incorporating a liquid.
- **PULVERIZATION** is the process of reducing particle size in a solid by using a substance in which the particle is soluble (e.g., camphor, alcohol).
- **GEOMETRIC DILUTION** is a technique used when mixing different quantities of two or more ingredients to achieve a homogenous mixture.

  ○ First the smaller-quantity ingredient is mixed with an equal part of diluent (base) until the ingredient is incorporated in the diluent.
  ○ The diluent is continually added in small amounts until all has been incorporated and a homogenous mixture has been formed.

Standards

Non-sterile compounding refers to any oral, transdermal, vaginal, or rectal medicinal preparations formulated using strict standards. These preparations must adhere to all rules as conveyed by *USP* <795>, the first set of enforceable standards guiding non-sterile aseptic technique preparation set forth by the United States Pharmacopeia. This publication provides both guidelines and procedures for compounding with the intent of protecting both the patient and pharmacist. These standards include:

- Ensuring pharmaceutical ingredient purity and potency
- Maintaining accuracy when mixing compounds in order to make customized medications
- Providing proper documentation on compounding procedures
- Maintaining and supplying proper packaging, storage, and labeling

- Keeping all work surfaces and equipment clean
- Using purified water when mixing compounds or when cleaning surfaces and equipment

Compounds can be prepared for specialty practices, including:

- Dermatology
- Home care
- Hormone replacement therapy
- Hospice
- Men's health
- Pediatrics
- Podiatry
- Veterinary medicine
- Women's health

A proper environment must be maintained with adequate space designated for compounding. Separate and distinguishable areas are needed for sterile and non-sterile compounding procedures. The order and arrangement of all supplies, equipment, containers, and labels must be kept to prevent any cross contamination. The compounding facility should have an abundant supply of both clean hot water and clean cold water. This supply should include purified water for washing equipment and supplies as well as for compounding prescriptions that require the addition of water. Controlled lighting and temperature are necessary to avoid contamination and decomposition.

Non-sterile compounding can be divided into three distinct categories. Table 7-8 provides information about each category.

Table 7-8. Non-Sterile Compounding Categories

Category	Description	Examples
Simple non-sterile compounding	Preparations made according to standard formulas or recipes	- alprazolam oral suspension - captopril oral solution
Moderate non-sterile compounding	Preparations made using ingredients that require special handling	- fentanyl patch - morphine sulfate suppository
Complex non-sterile compounding	Complex preparations requiring additional training and equipment	- extended-release tablets - transdermal dosage forms

Steps for Compounding Non-Sterile Formulations

Steps for compounding non-sterile formulations are as follows:

1. Obtain the prescription.
2. Calculate the quantity of ingredients needed to make the preparation.
3. Wash your hands.
4. Document the ingredients needed to fill the prescription.
5. Obtain the equipment, ingredients, and materials needed to fill the prescription.
6. Clean the compounding area and equipment.
7. Obtain verification of the ingredients used and the quantities calculated prior to compounding.

8. Compound the preparation using the calculated formula.
9. Label the preparation.
10. Document the preparation on the compounding log.
11. Clean and store all equipment and materials.

The pharmacist then performs another check, termed the final check, where he or she will verify the ingredients used, the calculations performed, the weight of the ingredients, the color, the odor (if present), and the pH (if needed). Auxiliary labels may be added as warranted. The pharmacist then signs off on the compound; this ensures consistency and accuracy.

Batch orders are prepared in anticipation of medication orders. These preparations may be determined based on need, and they should maintain similar standards. All batch orders should maintain consistency of ingredients. Labels for batch orders must contain a lot number, and extra labels should be tossed after a batch has been completed. Labeling requirements should be consistent with the formatting presented on the master formulation record.

Calculations

Making calculations is a critical component of compounding prescriptions. Pharmacy technicians must understand how to determine quantities of ingredients accurately. Having a working knowledge of the metric system as well as familiarity with percentages and proportions is crucial. Familiarity with roman numerals, system conversions, and metric and temperature conversions can be found in Appendix H.

PERCENTAGES AND STRENGTHS

Percentages refer to a quantity out of 100. Percentages can be considered to be a fraction. For example, the quantity 75% means $\frac{75}{100}$. Interpreting percentages can be tricky, especially when determining the units involved. Remember the following facts:

- Volume/volume percent (v/v%) is measured in mL/100 mL. This is used for liquids.
- Weight/weight percent (w/w%) is measured in g/100 g. This is used for ointments and creams.
- Weight/volume percent (w/v%) is measured in g/100 mL. This is used for drugs dissolved in solutions.

When converting a percentage to a fraction, the denominator is always 100. Let's look at the following examples.

> **TIP**
>
> **Make sure you are using the correct conversion factor and units when you set up proportions. Always double-check your answer!**

➡ Example 1 _____

20 mL of glycerin is dissolved in water to make 80 mL of final solution. What is the percent strength of glycerin?

Answer: Calculate the percent strength by dividing the amount of active ingredient by the total weight or volume of the product. Then multiply the result by 100 and add a percent sign (%).

The active ingredient is glycerin, and the final volume is 80 mL.

$$\frac{20 \text{ mL}}{80 \text{ mL}} \times 100 = x$$

$$0.25 \times 100 = x$$

$$25\% = x$$

➡ Example 2

A prescription is written for ibuprofen 15% cream. How much ibuprofen powder is needed to prepare 30 grams of the compound?

Answer: First set up your proportion. A proportion is a statement of equality between two ratios. Make sure to put what you want on the left side and what you need on the right side: WANT = NEED.

The prescription is written for 15% strength; this is what we want. 15% means $\frac{15 \text{ g}}{100 \text{ g}}$.

The problem also tells us that we need 30 g of the cream.

$$\frac{15 \text{ g}}{100 \text{ g}} = \frac{x}{30 \text{ g}}$$

We can now cross multiply and solve for x.

$$(15 \text{ g})(30 \text{ g}) = (x)(100 \text{ g})$$

$$450 \text{ g} = (x)(100 \text{ g})$$

$$x = \frac{450 \text{ g}}{100 \text{ g}}$$

$$x = 4.5 \text{ g}$$

This means that 4.5 g of ibuprofen powder is needed to prepare this prescription.

➡ Example 3

The prescription below is written for benzocaine gel 240 g:

benzocaine USP 2%

carbopol 940 NF 2%

alcohol USP 90%

distilled Water 6%

How much benzocaine and carbopol are needed to prepare this prescription?

Answer: To solve this problem, you must determine the amount of each individual ingredient needed to make this preparation. The question does not ask for the amount of alcohol or sterile water needed to formulate this preparation, so only calculate the amount of benzocaine and carbopol. Set up a proportion for each ingredient using 240 g as the total amount of the final preparation.

$$\text{benzocaine: } \frac{2 \text{ g}}{100 \text{ g}} = \frac{x}{240 \text{ g}}$$

$$100x = 480 \text{ g}$$
$$x = 4.8 \text{ g}$$

$$\text{Carbopol: } \frac{2 \text{ g}}{100 \text{ g}} = \frac{x}{240 \text{ g}}$$

$$100x = 480 \text{ g}$$
$$x = 4.8 \text{ g}$$

You will need 4.8 g of benzocaine and 4.8 g of carbopol to fill this prescription.

DILUTING STOCK SOLUTIONS

The concentration of a medication is the amount of drug (e.g., mg, g) given in a specified volume (e.g., mL). Concentrations may be expressed as a percent, fraction, or ratio. Stock solutions are concentrated solutions used to prepare less-concentrated solutions. These less-concentrated solutions (dilutions) are prepared by adding a diluent such as sterile water.

Remember the following formula when solving these sorts of problems.

$$C1 \times V1 = C2 \times V2$$

where C1 is the initial concentration, V1 is the initial volume, C2 is the final concentration, and V2 is the final volume.

➥ Example 1 _____

400 mL of a 40% solution is diluted to 500 mL. What is the percent strength of the resulting solution?

Answer: To solve this problem, determine which components are given in the problem. This problem gives us a final volume of 500 mL with an initial volume of 400 mL. We are also given an initial concentration of 40%. An equation must be set up to determine the final concentration.

$$40\% \times 400 \text{ mL} = x \times 500 \text{ mL}$$
$$16,000\% \text{ mL} = x \times 500 \text{ mL}$$

Divide both sides by 500 mL to solve for x. Make sure to cancel units.

$$\frac{16,000\% \text{ mL}}{500 \text{ mL}} = x$$

$$32\% = x$$

The resulting solution will have a percent strength of 32%.

This problem can also be solved using the ratio and proportion method.

First calculate the number of grams contained in 400 mL of the 40% solution.

$$\frac{40 \text{ g}}{100 \text{ mL}} = \frac{x}{400 \text{ mL}}$$

$$x = \frac{400 \text{ mL} \times 40 \text{ g}}{100 \text{ mL}}$$

$$x = 160 \text{ g}$$

This tells us that 160 g is diluted in 500 mL. Percent strength can be determined by calculating the number of grams in 100 mL.

$$\frac{160 \text{ g}}{500 \text{ mL}} = \frac{x}{100 \text{ mL}}$$

$$x = \frac{160 \text{ g} \times 100 \text{ mL}}{500 \text{ mL}}$$

$$x = 32 \text{ g} = 32\% \text{ (Remember that percent is g per 100 mL)}$$

ALLIGATIONS

Alligations are used to prepare a concentration of solution that is not commercially available. These solutions are made by mixing together two solutions where one solution contains a higher concentration and the other contains a weaker concentration. The solutions must be expressed in percentages with the desired solution strength lying between the stronger and weaker concentrations.

Alligations can be solved using a table that looks similar to a tic-tac-toe board. See Table 7-9 below.

Table 7-9. Setting Up an Alligation Problem

Higher % strength solution (H)		Number of parts in higher % strength solution (P − L)
	Desired (product) % strength solution (P)	
Lower % strength solution (L)		Number of parts in lower % strength solution (H − P)

➥ Example 1 _____

How many mL of a 50% solution and of a 25% solution are needed to prepare 2 liters of a 40% solution?

Answer: First set up a tic-tac-toe layout using the information provided, and solve for the number of parts of each solution.

Number of parts in higher % strength solution = (P – L)
Number of parts in lower % strength solution = (H – P)

50%		15 parts
	40%	
25%		10 parts

Next determine the total number of parts by adding them together.

15 + 10 = 25 total parts

Then set up a proportion using the parts of each concentration. Remember to convert liters to milliliters (1 L = 1,000 mL, so 2 L = 2,000 mL).

$$\frac{15}{25} \times 2,000 \text{ mL} = 1,200 \text{ mL of 50\% solution}$$

$$\frac{10}{25} \times 2,000 \text{ mL} = 800 \text{ mL of 25\% solution}$$

Check your work by adding the total amounts of each concentration and comparing your answer to the total volume of the preparation, which in this case is 2,000 mL.

1,200 mL + 800 mL = 2,000 mL

INFUSION RATES AND DRIP RATES

Orders written for the rate at which an IV is infused are called infusion rates. These rates are expressed in mL/min, mL/hour, or amount of drug/time.

Here are some examples.

➥ Example 1 _____

infuse at 80 mL/hr
infuse 1,000 mL over 8 hours
infuse 20 mg per minute
rate of infusion = $\dfrac{\text{volume of fluid}}{\text{time of infusion}}$

Based on this information, what is the rate of infusion in mL/hour of 1,000 mL of drug "X" to be infused over 8 hours?

Answer: Using the formula given:

$$\text{rate of infusion} = \frac{1{,}000 \text{ mL}}{8 \text{ hrs}}$$

$$\text{rate of infusion} = 125 \text{ mL/hr}$$

This equation can also be manipulated to solve for time.

➡ Example 2

$$\text{time of infusion} = \frac{\text{volume of fluid}}{\text{rate of infusion}}$$

The rate of infusion is 125 mL/hr, and the volume of infusion is 500 mL. How long will the IV bag last?

Answer: Using the formula above:

$$\text{time of infusion} = \frac{500 \text{ mL}}{125 \text{ mL/hr}}$$

$$\text{time of infusion} = 4 \text{ hours}$$

IV sets are used to deliver IVs to patients. These sets are calibrated for a specific number of drops per mL. Pharmacy technicians are expected to calculate the rate of infusion in drops per minute.

Common drop (gtts) factors are 10 gtts/mL (macro sets), 15 gtts/mL, and 60 gtts/mL (micro sets).

Use the following formula to solve for the infusion flow rate:

$$\text{infusion flow rate (gtts/min)} = \frac{\text{volume (mL)}}{\text{time (min)}} \times \text{drop factor (gtts/mL)}$$

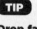

TIP

Drop factors can be found on the IV administration package.

➡ Example 3

What is the infusion rate of a 1 L lactated Ringer's solution with a flow rate of 125 mL/hr and a drop factor of 15 gtts/mL?

Answer: Recognize that 1 L = 1,000 mL.

$$\text{infusion flow rate (gtts/min)} = \frac{125 \text{ mL}}{60 \text{ min}} \times \frac{15 \text{ gtts}}{1 \text{ mL}}$$

$$\text{infusion flow rate (gtts/min)} = 31.25 \approx 31 \text{ gtts/min}$$

OTHER CALCULATIONS/DOSES BASED ON BODY WEIGHT AND BODY SURFACE AREA

Many pediatric, geriatric, oncology, corticosteroid, and antibiotic medications are dosed based on body weight (usually mg/kg). These problems require conversions from pounds to kilograms (1 kg = 2.2 lb).

➡ Example 1

The prescriber orders a drug to be dosed at 15 mg/kg/day. What is the daily dose for a 132 lb patient?

Answer:

$$132 \, \cancel{lbs} \times \frac{1 \, kg}{2.2 \, \cancel{lbs}} = 60 \, kg$$

Then set up a ratio and proportion using the given dosing regimen.

$$\frac{15 \, mg}{1 \, kg} = \frac{x}{60 \, kg}$$

$$(15 \, mg)(60 \, kg) = (1 \, kg)(x)$$

$$900 \, mg \text{ per day} = x$$

Doses based on body weight can be determined using a nomogram, which is a chart used to determine body surface area (BSA) based on the patient's height and weight. Nomograms may be used if the BSA is not given in the problem. The BSA is used to calculate doses for patients receiving chemotherapeutic agents and is measured in m^2.

➡ Example 2

A patient has a BSA of 1.54 m^2. Calculate the dose of fluorouracil, in mg, for the patient if the doctor has ordered 400 mg/m^2 daily.

Answer: Set up a proportion.

$$\frac{400 \, mg}{1 \, m^2} = \frac{x}{1.54 \, m^2}$$

$$(400 \, mg)(1.54 \, m^2) = (x)(1 \, m^2)$$

$$616 \, mg = x$$

SUMMARY

- [ ] Sterile compounding procedures are based on standards set by the United States Pharmacopeia per *USP* <797>. These procedures require sterile techniques, PPE, and proper hand-washing procedures.

- [ ] Personnel must demonstrate an understanding and knowledge of aseptic procedures, including infection control, prior to working on any medication orders. Demonstration of additional knowledge and training, including familiarity with calculations, is essential.

- [ ] Non-sterile compounding procedures are based on standards set by the United States Pharmacopeia (*USP* <795>).

- [ ] Pharmacy personnel prepare non-sterile compounded medications according to standards of quality in order to maintain product sterility and accuracy.

- [ ] Proper selection of materials for non-sterile and sterile compounding formulations is determined from the prescription, common practices, and current guidelines.

STERILE AND NON-STERILE COMPOUNDING PRACTICE QUESTIONS

1. Which of the following equipment is NOT used in non-sterile compounding procedures?

    (A) graduated cylinder
    (B) mortar and pestle
    (C) prescription vial
    (D) laminar flow hood

2. Pharmacy personnel use various techniques when compounding preparations. Which of the following statements best describes levigation?

    (A) the process of grinding a powder through the incorporation of a liquid
    (B) the process of reducing a particle's size by incorporating a substance in which that particle is soluble
    (C) the process of reducing the particle size of an ingredient by grinding it into a powder
    (D) the process of using a spatula to mix ingredients.

3. Compounded sterile preparations are categorized by risk levels. Which of the following does NOT describe a low-risk level?

    (A) compounded using aseptic manipulations in an ISO Class 5 environment
    (B) sterile components, antimicrobial-free CSPs, and sterile surfaces exposed to air quality worse than an ISO Class 5
    (C) compounding involving no more than three commercially available products and no more than two entries into any sterile container or bag
    (D) manipulations must follow aseptic guidelines when using ampules, syringes, and needles and during the transfer of formulations

4. Laminar flow hoods should be disinfected with what type of solution?

   (A) betadine solution
   (B) 70% isopropyl alcohol
   (C) antibacterial soap
   (D) 95% isopropyl alcohol

5. What is the appropriate beyond use date (BUD) for an oral suspension that does not have stability information on the product label?

   (A) BUD no later than 30 days
   (B) BUD no later than 6 months or equal to the earliest expiration date of any active pharmaceutical ingredient
   (C) BUD no later than 14 days from the reconstitution date
   (D) BUD no later than 1 year

6. Which of the following units are used when interpreting an expression of a percentage (e.g., 10%)?

   (A) mg/mL
   (B) mg/L
   (C) g/mL
   (D) g/L

7. Which way does air flow in a horizontal laminar flow hood?

   (A) from back to front
   (B) from top to bottom
   (C) from side to side
   (D) from bottom to top

8. Which of the following devices should be calibrated prior to use?

   (A) Class A prescription balance
   (B) graduated cylinder
   (C) laminar flow hood
   (D) mortar and pestle

9. What type of medication is dosed based on BSA?

   (A) antihistamines
   (B) corticosteroids
   (C) chemotherapeutic agents
   (D) antibiotics

10. 3-in-1 TPN admixtures allow for simultaneous infusion of what ingredients?

   (A) fats, multivitamins, and dextrose
   (B) dextrose, amino acids, and fats
   (C) protein, sugar, and fats
   (D) amino acids, dextrose, and lactated Ringer's

ANSWERS EXPLAINED

1. **(D)** Graduated cylinders, mortars and pestles, and prescription vials are all examples of equipment used in non-sterile compounding procedures. Laminar flow hoods are used in sterile compounding procedures.

2. **(A)** Levigation is the process of grinding a powder through the incorporation of a liquid. Pulverization is the process of reducing a particle's size by incorporating a substance in which that particle is soluble. Trituration is the process of reducing the particle size of an ingredient by grinding it into a powder. Spatulation is the process of using a spatula to mix ingredients.

3. **(B)** Sterile components, antimicrobial-free CSPs, and sterile surfaces exposed to air quality worse than an ISO Class 5 is an example of a high-risk level.

4. **(B)** Laminar flow hoods should be cleaned with sterile water and disinfected with 70% isopropyl alcohol (sterile isopropyl alcohol).

5. **(C)** The *USP* <795> lists beyond use date usage criteria for products that do not have stability information on package inserts or product labeling. Nonaqueous solutions have a BUD of no later than 6 months. Aqueous solutions (e.g., suspensions) have a BUD of no later than 14 days from the reconstitution date. Topical solutions have a beyond use date of no later than 30 days. *USP* <795> does not have a BUD of 1 year listed for any product formulations.

6. **(C)** Percentages may be expressed as g/mL, mL/mL, and g/g.

7. **(A)** Horizontal laminar flow hoods take room air in from behind the HEPA filter located at the back of the unit. The air is then processed by the HEPA filter, filtered, and blown out horizontally over the work surface toward the operator (from the back to the front).

8. **(A)** The Class A prescription balance must be calibrated prior to use. Graduated cylinders, as well as mortars and pestles, are supplies used in non-sterile compounding. Laminar flow hoods are used in the preparation of sterile compounded products.

9. **(C)** Chemotherapeutic agents are dosed based on body surface area (BSA). Antihistamines, corticosteroids, and antibiotics are based on weight.

10. **(B)** 3-in-1 TPN admixtures allow for the simultaneous infusion of dextrose, amino acids, and fats.

Medication Safety

8

KNOWLEDGE DOMAIN 4.0

Medication Safety   **12.50%**

→ Knowledge Area 4.1: Error prevention strategies for data entry (e.g., prescription or medication order to correct patient)
→ Knowledge Area 4.2: Patient package insert and medication guide requirements (e.g., special directions and precautions)
→ Knowledge Area 4.3: Identify issues that require pharmacist intervention (e.g., DUR, ADE, OTC recommendation, therapeutic substitution, misuse, missed dose)
→ Knowledge Area 4.4: Look-alike/sound-alike medications
→ Knowledge Area 4.5: High-alert/risk medications
→ Knowledge Area 4.6: Common safety strategies (e.g., tall man lettering, separating inventory, leading and trailing zeros, limit use of error prone abbreviations)

LEARNING OBJECTIVES

☐ Identify possible sources of medication errors, including the role of each party in reducing errors.
☐ Compare and contrast knowledge deficit vs. performance deficit.
☐ Identify common look-alike/sound-alike drug names.
☐ Identify common high-alert/high-risk medications.
☐ Be familiar with common safety strategies used to limit potential errors.

The Food and Drug Administration has received over 95,000 reports of medication errors since 2000. These reports were voluntarily made through an adverse event reporting system called MedWatch. Why do medication errors occur? Are they due to patient misuse, practitioner error, or even an error in the pharmacy? All of these can be true. In 2016, the National Coordinating Council for Medication Error Reporting and Prevention (NCCMERP) defined a medication error as "any preventable event that may cause or lead to inappropriate medication use or patient harm while the medication is in the control of the health care professional, patient, or consumer." (© 2016 National Coordinating Council for Medication Error Reporting and Prevention. All Rights Reserved.)

An awareness of the existence of medication errors is the first step in preventing these errors from happening in the future. Medication errors can occur anywhere and at any time. They must be taken seriously. Health care professionals, patients, and their families are all responsible for identifying and preventing errors when possible.

Potential errors may include:

- Wrong patient
- Wrong route
- Wrong drug
- Wrong dosage form
- Wrong strength
- Wrong rate of administration
- Wrong time
- Wrong technique
- Wrong doctor
- Wrong preparation of dose
- Skipped dose
- Patient is not informed that the prescription has been called in

CAUSES OF MEDICATION ERRORS

Medication error sources may include deficits in the following categories as outlined in Table 8-1.

Table 8-1. Knowledge Deficit vs. Performance Deficit

Knowledge Deficit	Performance Deficit
- Lack of knowledge or training - Employee may not have been given the information needed to perform the task	- Employee has the knowledge, but the knowledge is not applied to the situation - Lack of sleep or illness - Personal problems - Employee is not paying attention to his or her job and/or may be distracted by background noises, such as talking, radio, phone ringing, etc.

A thorough evaluation of a medication error will discover why an error occurred and work toward preventing similar errors in the future. Did the practitioner make a mistake when writing the prescription? Did he or she select the wrong drug when typing out the electronic script? What errors were made when the pharmacy technician entered the script? Did the pharmacist perform a drug utilization review when checking the script for errors?

ERROR PREVENTION STRATEGIES

In order to implement medication error prevention strategies, you must identify possible sources for medication errors. Errors do not just occur from one source. In fact, the causes of errors can be quite complex. Possible sources for medication errors include doctors, nurses, the pharmacy, and patients and their family members.

Tables 8-2, 8-3, 8-4, and 8-5 are categorized by the individual(s) responsible for the error. Each table lists potential causes of errors and their respective solutions.

Table 8-2. Causes of Errors and Solutions—Prescribers

Error	Solution
Illegible handwriting	Use a computer to type the prescription or write legibly.
Ambiguous orders	Write specific instructions. Do not use the phrase "as directed."
Incomplete orders	Write complete instructions indicating the drug name, route, strength, frequency, quantity, and directions for use.
Verbal orders	Repeat the order to the pharmacist. Use written or faxed orders.
Inappropriate use of decimal points	Always include a zero before a decimal point.
Unapproved abbreviations	Avoid using abbreviations.
Dosage calculations	Require an independent double check.

Table 8-3. Causes of Errors and Solutions—Nurses

Error	Solution
Poor labeling	Read the label 3 times.
Patient identifiers	Use the bar coding system to identify the patient and the medication.
Borrowing medications	Avoid borrowing medications.
Unit dose vs. floor stock	Use unit-dose medications when available.

Table 8-4. Causes of Errors and Solutions—The Pharmacy

Error	Solution
Labeling orders	Use standard format.
Misinterpretation	Avoid distractions. Verify patient information, including date of birth.
Calculations	Require an independent double check.
Sound-alike drugs	Require indications for all high-risk drugs.
Transcription	Repeat back all phone orders.

Table 8-5. Causes of Errors and Solutions—Patients and Family Members

Error	Solution
Patients bringing medications from home	Bring a list of medications, and leave the medications themselves at home.
Family members bringing medications from home	Bring a list of medications, and leave the medications themselves at home.
Family members pushing buttons on the PCA pump	Explain tolerance considerations to family members.

ISSUES THAT REQUIRE PHARMACIST INTERVENTION

Multiple situations require pharmacist intervention. **Drug utilization review (DUR)** is a structured, comprehensive review strategy employed by pharmacists to review a patient's prescriptions, health history, and medication data. Changes in drug therapy may be necessary based on results of the DUR. According to the Academy of Managed Care Pharmacy, these reviews are performed on every prescription, help maintain accuracy in drug therapy, and improve patient outcomes.

Adverse drug events (ADE) are checked during the DUR process. During a prospective DUR, the patient's therapy is checked for accuracy and optimal care. Part of this process includes verifying that drug-drug interactions are not present. Drug-drug interactions can occur between prescription drugs or even between prescription and over-the-counter medications. It is important to resolve any ADE because drug-drug interactions can result in a change in the effect of the drug, resulting in an adverse drug event.

Over-the-counter (OTC) recommendations Pharmacy technicians should never counsel a patient. Pharmacy personnel should take a thorough patient history at the in-window. This should include the patient's medication history as well as both prescription and over-the-counter medications that he or she is taking. All medications should be reviewed. The pharmacist on duty should handle any requests for over-the-counter medication recommendations. Pharmacists should select a proper medication and strength based on the patient's allergies and prescription drug profile.

Therapeutic interchanges allow for the substitution of a medication to an alternative, usually from a nonpreferred drug to one that is preferred. Many factors help determine the need for a therapeutic substitution, including cost. It is important to recognize that the patient needs to be informed of the therapeutic substitution.

Misuse of a medication is taking a medication for any reason other than the one for which it was prescribed. A misuse could be intentional or unintentional. Pharmacy personnel should be observant and proactive when dealing with patients exhibiting misuse or abuse tendencies. Misuse and abuse can be differentiated by looking at the patient's intentions and motivations. According to the Substance Abuse and Mental Health Administration Center for Behavioral Health Statistics and Quality, in 2011, drug misuse and abuse resulted in more than 1.4 million cases or emergency department (ED) visits. Figure 8-1 shows the spectrum of prescription drug abuse.

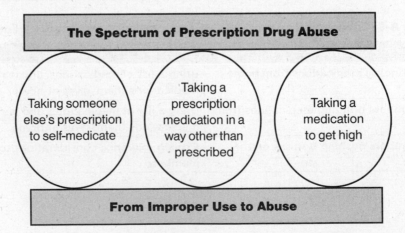

Figure 8-1. The spectrum of prescription drug abuse

With **intentional misuse,** the patient is dependent on the medication and requires a larger dose than prescribed.

- The patient may take his or her medication inappropriately, including taking the prescription medication more often than prescribed.
- The patient may be taking someone else's prescription, often to self-medicate.
- The patient may take the prescription medication after it's no longer needed.

With **unintentional misuse**, the patient may or may not be dependent on the medication.

- The patient may use his or her asthma inhaler all day long, even though it is meant for emergencies.
- The patient may take double the dose to relieve urgent pain. As time goes on, he or she becomes addicted to or reliant on increased doses due to tolerance issues.

Missed or skipped doses can occur for many reasons. The patient may have forgotten to take the dose or may have even run out of the medication. The caregiver could have failed to give the patient his or her medication on time, or the caregiver may have forgotten to give the patient the dose altogether. These situations require counseling from the pharmacist because patients should not assume that the missed dose can simply be taken with the next dose. Pharmacists can help identify and resolve situations that may be affecting optimal drug therapy. If a patient continues to miss doses, it can ultimately affect his or her health.

PATIENT INFORMATION

Manufacturers must provide medication guides and patient package inserts for drugs deemed to have serious and significant risks. These written guides and inserts must be given to patients. They inform patients about the risks and benefits of the prescription medications.

Patient package inserts, or PPIs, are written summaries of patient information about specific risks and benefits. PPIs are based on the FDA-approved package insert. This insert provides clinical information about the drug and is written in consumer friendly terminology. The FDA mandates that certain classes of medications, such as estrogen-containing medications and oral contraceptives, include PPIs. In 2006, the FDA made a revision stating that all PPIs must also include a table of contents and a summary section that highlights the benefits and risks.

Medication guides are another form of written patient information. Medication guides address issues specific to particular drugs and drug classes. They contain FDA-approved information that can help patients avoid serious adverse events.

HIGH-ALERT MEDICATIONS

The Institute for Safe Medication Practices (ISMP) defines high-alert medications as "drugs that can cause significant and considerable harm when used in error." Safeguards—including DUR reviews, pharmacist checks, and patient education—are all important steps in reducing errors and minimizing harm (see Figures 8-2 and 8-3).

Classes/Categories of Medications
adrenergic agonists, IV (e.g., **EPINEPH**rine, phenylephrine, norepinephrine)
adrenergic antagonists, IV (e.g., propranolol, metoprolol, labetalol)
anesthetic agents, general, inhaled and IV (e.g., propofol, ketamine)
antiarrhythmics, IV (e.g., lidocaine, amiodarone)
antithrombotic agents, including: ■ anticoagulants (e.g., warfarin, low molecular weight heparin, IV unfractionated heparin) ■ Factor Xa inhibitors (e.g., fondaparinux, apixaban, rivaroxaban) ■ direct thrombin inhibitors (e.g., argatroban, bivalirudin, dabigatran etexilate) ■ thrombolytics (e.g., alteplase, reteplase, tenecteplase) ■ glycoprotein IIb/IIIa inhibitors (e.g., eptifibatide)
cardioplegic solutions
chemotherapeutic agents, parenteral and oral
dextrose, hypertonic, 20% or greater
dialysis solutions, peritoneal and hemodialysis
epidural or intrathecal medications
hypoglycemics, oral
inotropic medications, IV (e.g., digoxin, milrinone)
insulin, subcutaneous and IV
liposomal forms of drugs (e.g., liposomal amphotericin B) and conventional counterparts (e.g., amphotericin B desoxycholate)
moderate sedation agents, IV (e.g., dexmedetomidine, midazolam)
moderate sedation agents, oral, for children (e.g., chloral hydrate)
narcotics/opioids ■ IV ■ transdermal ■ oral (including liquid concentrates, immediate and sustained-release formulations)
neuromuscular blocking agents (e.g., succinylcholine, rocuronium, vecuronium)
parenteral nutrition preparations
radiocontrast agents, IV
sterile water for injection, inhalation, and irrigation (excluding pour bottles) in containers of 100 mL or more
sodium chloride for injection, hypertonic, greater than 0.9% concentration

Specific Medications
EPINEPHrine, subcutaneous
epoprostenol (Flolan), IV
insulin U-500 (special emphasis)*
magnesium sulfate injection
methotrexate, oral, non-oncologic use
opium tincture
oxytocin, IV
nitroprusside sodium for injection
potassium chloride for injection concentrate
potassium phosphates injection
promethazine, IV
vasopressin, IV or intraosseous

*All forms of insulin, subcutaneous and IV, are considered a class of high-alert medications. Insulin U-500 has been singled out for special emphasis to bring attention to the need for distinct strategies to prevent the types of errors that occur with this concentrated form of insulin.

*Copyright 2014 Institute for Safe Medication Practices (ISMP)

Figure 8-2. ISMP list of high-alert medications in acute care settings

Classes/Categories of Medications	Specific Medications
antiretroviral agents (e.g., efavirenz, lami**VUD**ine, raltegravir, ritonavir, combination antiretroviral products)	carBAMazepine
chemotherapeutic agents, oral (excluding hormonal agents) (e.g., cyclophosphamide, mercaptopurine, temozolomide)	chloral hydrate liquid, for sedation of children
hypoglycemic agents, oral	heparin, including unfractionated and low molecular weight heparin
immunosuppressant agents (e.g., aza**THIO**prine, cyclo**SPORINE**, tacrolimus)	met**FORMIN**
insulin, all formulations	methotrexate, non-oncologic use
opioids, all formulations	midazolam liquid, for sedation of children
pediatric liquid medications that require measurement	propylthiouracil
pregnancy category X drugs (e.g., bosentan, **ISO**tretinoin)	warfarin

*Copyright 2011 Institute for Safe Medication Practices (ISMP)

Figure 8-3. ISMP list of high-alert medications in community/ambulatory health care

LOOK-ALIKE/SOUND-ALIKE MEDICATIONS

These medications tend to sound the same when spoken and/or may look similar when written. Ultimately, these medications require pharmacists and pharmacy technicians to take extra precautions. The Institute for Safe Medication Practices (ISMP) maintains a list of common look-alike/sound-alike drugs.

In order to avoid errors, these drugs should be separated on the shelf. Other strategies include the use of tall man lettering. This tactic requires the use of capital letters to designate areas of words that are dissimilar. For example, the insulin drugs Novolog and Novolin may look or sound the same. The use of tall man lettering highlights the differences between the drug names: NovoLOG and NovoLIN.

REDUCING ERRORS USING SAFETY STRATEGIES

Errors can occur anywhere and at any time. Pharmacies take many measures to eliminate errors, including separating inventory, using tall man lettering, educating their staff on the use of leading or trailing zeros, and limiting the use of error-prone abbreviations.

Separating inventory is an important step in eliminating errors. Medications with similar names should be separated on the shelf. High-risk medications should be stored separately from regular stock medications. Other examples include placing similar medication formulations together (e.g., liquid medications together, IV medications together, and ointments and creams together). This strategy allows the medication seeker to look only in the specific area of the formulation needed, resulting in less chance of an error.

Tall man lettering highlights areas of similar-sounding or similar-looking words to emphasize the dissimilarities. In addition to being used as a technique to limit errors when identifying look-alike/sound-alike drug names, manufacturers have even adapted this technique and often use it on the medication bottle to bring attention to the drug name. The technician must consult with the pharmacist on any look-alike/sound-alike medications.

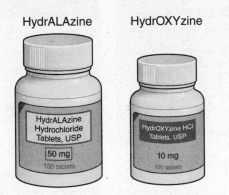

Figure 8-4. HydrALAzine/HydrOXYzine tall man lettering

Another way to eliminate medication errors is to avoid the use of error-prone abbreviations. Many abbreviations may be misinterpreted. Abbreviations like QID may be misinterpreted for QD. D/C may be interpreted as either discharge or discontinue depending on the circumstance. A complete list of abbreviations can be found in Appendix G of this book.

Mathematics and calculations are an imperative part of the pharmacy. Errors can occur when pharmacy personnel do not follow the same techniques when writing numbers with decimal points. Writing decimals incorrectly can lead to medication errors. Two common errors are trailing zeros and naked decimal points. To avoid trailing zeros, write 5 instead of 5.0. To avoid naked decimal points, write 0.5 instead of .5.

Can you read the prescription shown in Figure 8-5?

TIP

Remember, periods are sometimes difficult to see. This can lead to a 10-fold error. Be sure to be as clear as possible!

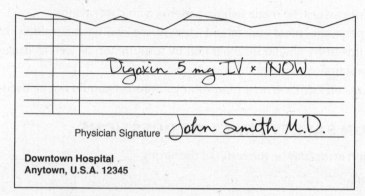

Figure 8-5. Sample Digoxin medication order

This prescription should read "Digoxin 0.5 mg." A dose of 5 mg would have resulted in the patient receiving 10× the prescribed dose.

How about Figure 8-6? Can you read it?

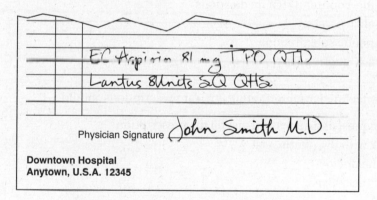

Figure 8-6. Sample insulin medication order

Lantus is long-acting insulin. In this particular prescription, the amount of Lantus may be misread and interpreted as 80 units instead of 8 units.

SUMMARY

☐ Errors may occur due to prescribers, administrators, pharmacy personnel, or even patients or their family members.

☐ It is important to determine the source of the error and then come up with a plan to resolve the situation and eliminate future errors.

☐ The pharmacist should always review look-alike/sound-alike and high-risk drugs before having the technician fill a prescription.

☐ Pharmacists should perform a drug utilization review (DUR) for each prescription to determine if any potential changes need to be made.

☐ Prescriptions should be screened for potential adverse drug events (ADE). Therapeutic substitutions can also be made to help patients with cost savings.

☐ Pharmacy personnel must understand when to use leading and trailing zeros.

☐ Pharmacy inventory should be separated by formulation as well as usage. Medications with similar names should be separated on shelves.

☐ Abbreviations on ISMP's error-prone abbreviations list should not be used.

MEDICATION SAFETY PRACTICE QUESTIONS

1. A medication error may be the result of the wrong _____.

   (A) prescriber
   (B) dosage form
   (C) day's supply
   (D) All of the above.

2. The drugs Zyrtec 10 mg and Zoloft 10 mg are examples of _____.

   (A) over-the-counter (OTC) medications
   (B) look-alike names
   (C) therapeutic substitutions
   (D) tall man lettering

3. Pharmacy technicians interpreting unclear prescriptions should _____.

   (A) not request assistance and just fill the prescription
   (B) check with the pharmacist
   (C) call the doctor
   (D) All of the above.

4. "AlprazOLam" is an example of a medication with _____.

   (A) tall man lettering
   (B) a look-alike/sound-alike name
   (C) a drug utilization review
   (D) HIPAA

5. Which of the following is an example of a knowledge deficit?

   (A) Personnel are distracted by noise.
   (B) An employee comes into work with a fever and a cough.
   (C) The employee lacks training.
   (D) The employee is going through a difficult time in his/her personal life.

6. Which of the following is an example of an error caused by the prescriber?

   (A) illegible handwriting
   (B) family members bringing in medications for the patient without staff approval
   (C) borrowing medications from another patient
   (D) labeling error

7. True or False: Abuse and/or misuse of medications may be unintentional or intentional.

8. Error prevention strategies in the pharmacy setting include _____.

   (A) separating the inventory of medications with similar names
   (B) avoiding the use of error-prone abbreviations
   (C) organizing mediations by formulation
   (D) All of the above.

9. True or False: Medication guides contain FDA-approved information that can help patients avoid serious adverse effects.

10. Medication errors can occur for many reasons. Which of the following is a reason why a patient may miss or skip a dose?

   (A) The patient forgot to take the medication.
   (B) The patient's caregiver did not give the medication to the patient.
   (C) The patient ran out of the medication.
   (D) All of the above.

ANSWERS EXPLAINED

1. **(D)** A medication error can occur due to any, or all, of these reasons.

2. **(B)** These drugs are among many on ISMP's common look-alike/sound-alike drug name list.

3. **(B)** Pharmacy technicians should check with the pharmacist before proceeding to fill the prescription.

4. **(A)** Tall man lettering is used to distinguish dissimilarities and differentiate similar-looking drug names.

5. **(C)** The other choices are examples of performance deficits.

6. **(A)** Choice (B) is an error due to family members. Choice (C) is an error due to the pharmacy. Choice (D) is an error due to a nurse.

7. **True** Abuse and/or misuse may be unintentional or intentional. Pharmacy personnel should be cautious and examine a patient's medical history to evaluate for any potential dependency or abuse issues.

8. **(D)** Error prevention strategies include all of these choices.

9. **True** Medication guides address medication issues, adverse effects, or warnings for groups of medications. The patient can read the information in the medication guide to avoid serious adverse effects.

10. **(D)** A patient may skip or miss a dose due to any, or all, of these reasons.

Pharmacy Quality Assurance

9

KNOWLEDGE DOMAIN 5.0

Pharmacy Quality Assurance   **7.50%**

→ Knowledge Area 5.1: Quality assurance practices for medication and inventory control systems (e.g., matching National Drug Code (NDC) number, bar code, data entry)

→ Knowledge Area 5.2: Infection control procedures and documentation (e.g., personal protective equipment [PPE], needle recapping)

→ Knowledge Area 5.3: Risk management guidelines and regulations (e.g., error prevention strategies)

→ Knowledge Area 5.4: Communication channels necessary to ensure appropriate follow-up and problem resolution (e.g., product recalls, shortages)

→ Knowledge Area 5.5: Productivity, efficiency, and customer satisfaction measures

LEARNING OBJECTIVES

☐ Describe the continuous quality improvement process.

☐ Understand continuous quality improvement procedures, including prevention strategies.

☐ Define quality control and quality assurance.

☐ Identify quality-related events and understand document procedures related to these events.

☐ Identify organizations and their roles in quality assurance procedures, including medication-reporting methods.

☐ Explain infection control procedures, including proper hand washing.

☐ Know the importance of communication among pharmacy members, patients, and health care providers.

CONTINUOUS QUALITY IMPROVEMENT (CQI)

Pharmacies have an obligation to uphold high standards of quality, safety, and efficacy in order to avoid medication errors and provide superior health care. Quality is an implication of worth, a standard of excellence. While the pharmacist oversees the prevention and management of medication errors, it is the responsibility of all pharmacy team members to ensure safety in the health system. Many pharmacies have implemented **continuous quality improvement (CQI)** programs to ensure that these standards are met. CQI programs can improve outcomes and customer satisfaction while decreasing costs and liability. The basic outline for this process is "detect and document-evaluate-report-prevent."

Pharmacy CQI plans should include the following:

- An evaluation of the medication use process
- A process for identifying and tracking medication errors
- Definitions of medication error categories
- An increase in awareness and reporting of medication errors by involving health care professionals, patients, and caregivers
- Systems to detect errors and the development of interventions to correct the deficiency
- A focus on improvements rather than on punitive aspects of medication error reporting
- A respect for the confidentiality of all parties involved in the medication error

Continuous quality improvement methods institute a process of review, assessment, and implementation. The American Society of Clinical Pharmacists has indicated that assessments include an evaluation of the cause(s) of error(s) as well as a review of data to determine potential trends, frequency, significance, and outcomes of medication errors. **Prevention strategies** should include interventions for reducing errors. These may include the following:

- **Fail-safes** and **constraints** that include a change in the system itself or in the individual's interaction with the system may be implemented. An example of this is the integration of the register with the computer system to block a prescription from being rung up unless it was verified by the pharmacist.
- The use of **forcing functions**, often referred to as a "lock and key," provide a stop in the system, requiring important information to be provided before proceeding. Medications must be scanned using a bar code that will match the NDC of the selected drug to the profiled medication. Pharmacies commonly use this function to insert a notation before overriding a high-alert medication.
- Pharmacies are implementing **automation and computerization** through medication use processes that are designed to assist in filling prescriptions and can lessen the fallibility of human memory reliance. Common examples of this include using electronic processing software with clinical decision support systems, the use of e-prescribing or CPOE to avoid transcription or misinterpreting errors, the assistance of robots and dispensing technology to count or fill prescriptions, and the use of warnings, alerts, and flags in computer systems.
- **Standardization** is also integrated to provide a uniform approach to avoid variation or complexity. This is accomplished through the use of preprinted prescription blanks containing commonly used protocols (e.g., corticosteroid tapering) or frequently prescribed medications to reduce the potential for confusing or missing directions or even for illegible handwriting.
- **Redundancies**, **reminders**, and **checklists** are also used as an intervention strategy by incorporating duplicate checks, audits, or verifications to provide information in an accessible format. This includes having more than one person verify the prescription, using independent double checks for high-alert medications, using the brand and generic names of medications when communicating about a prescription, counseling patients about medications, using auxiliary labels to provide warnings and alerts, and using preprinted prescription blanks with prompts for pertinent information like allergies, indication, or date of birth.

- **Education standards** and **information technology** are used to convey a level of knowledge and understanding in pharmacy practice. Pharmacy personnel may be required to complete continuing education (CE) hours or certification in advanced areas of practice. Proper training procedures, including infection control procedures, may also need to be renewed as required by law.
- **Pharmacy policies** and **procedures** should be maintained and followed, and protocols must be in place for the recording and transcription of prescriptions. CQI initiatives should incorporate goals and measurable standards. Any interventions should be analyzed and assessed frequently, allowing for changes to be made as needed; management of these initiatives requires the understanding of two key terms:
  - **Quality control**: identifying areas that require change due to inconsistency
  - **Quality assurance**: implementing a systematic review of quality-related events (QRE) to uphold the quality of care standards and their review over time.

QUALITY-RELATED EVENTS

A **quality-related event** is the inappropriate dispensing or administration of a prescribed medication. These events include, but are not limited to, variations or the failure to identify or manage:

- Clinical abuse/misuse
- Drug-allergy interactions
- Drug-disease contraindications
- Drug-drug interactions
- Inadequate or incorrect packaging, labeling, or directions
- Incorrect dosage or duration of treatment
- Incorrect drug
- Incorrect drug strength
- Incorrect patient
- Overutilization or underutilization
- Therapeutic duplication

The occurrence of a QRE should be documented and maintained as required by the corresponding State Board of Pharmacy (see Figure 9-1). Documentation must be completed the same day as the incident's occurrence. Documentation must include a description and an analysis of the event and the actions taken.

Quality-Related Event Documentation

I. QRE Prescription Data   Prescription No.: _____

Attach copy of: ☐ prescription   ☐ label   ☐ photo copy of vial (mark all available)

II. QRE Data

QRE Type: (select all that apply)

A. Prescription processing error:

☐ (1) Incorrect drug
☐ (2) Incorrect strength
☐ (3) Incorrect dosage form
☐ (4) Incorrect patient
☐ (5) Inaccurate or incorrect packaging, labeling, or directions
☐ (6) Other: _____

B. A failure to identify and manage

☐ (1) Over/under utilization
☐ (2) Therapeutic duplication
☐ (3) Drug-disease contraindication
☐ (4) Drug-drug interactions
☐ (5) Incorrect duration of treatment
☐ (6) Incorrect dosage
☐ (7) Drug-allergy interaction
☐ (8) Clinical abuse/misuse

Prescription was received by the pharmacy via: ☐ telephone   ☐ written   ☐ computer   ☐ fax

Prescription was: ☐ new   ☐ refill

III. QRE Contributing Factors

Day of the week and time of QRE: _____

# of new prescriptions: _____   # of refill prescriptions: _____   RPh to tech ratio: _____

RPh staff status: ☐ regular staff   ☐ occasional/substitute staff

# of hours RPh on duty: _____   Average # of prescriptions filled per hour: _____

# of other RPhs on duty: _____   # of support staff on duty: _____

Describe preliminary root contributors:

_____

_____

_____

_____

Describe remedial action taken:

_____

_____

_____

Name and title of preparer of this report: _____

Date: _____

Figure 9-1. Sample Quality-Related Event (QRE) Documentation

ORGANIZATIONS

Specific organizations oversee the quality of care by setting minimum standards for adherence. These organizations and their roles in quality assurance are outlined in Table 9-1.

Table 9-1. Organizations and their Roles in Quality Assurance

Organizations	Roles in Quality Assurance
Institute for Safe Medication Practices	- Nonprofit national organization dedicated to medication error prevention and safe medication practices - Operates a voluntary practitioner error-reporting program called the National Medication Errors Reporting Program (MERP) - Reviews all medication errors reported to the Patient Safety Authority in Pennsylvania - Publishes resources for health professionals and consumers - Medication safety tools include lists of look-alike/sound-alike drugs and potentially dangerous abbreviations
State Board of Pharmacy	- Ensures that pharmacists and technicians (as allowed by their state) meet certain standards for licensure and/or registration - Regulates pharmacies and other entities that manufacture or distribute medications - May require medication error reporting
The Joint Commission	- Evaluates and accredits health care organizations, including hospitals, laboratories, and nursing homes - Provides certification programs and/or services in disease specific care, integrative care, palliative care, perinatal care, health care staffing, and primary care - Accreditation is a symbol of quality, indicating that the health care organization is committed to meeting specific performance standards - Provides national safety goals and considerations, including infection control and medication errors
United States Pharmacopeia	- Established standards for medication identity, purity, quality, and strength, as well as standards for food ingredients and dietary supplements - Publishes and oversees the United States Pharmacopeia and National Formulary (*USP-NF*), which contains standards for biological and chemical drug substances, compounds, medical devices, dosage forms, excipients, and dietary supplements - Provides labeling requirements for single-dose and multi-dose medications - *USP-NF* maintains standards on compounding practices, including *USP* <797> on sterile compounding practices and *USP* <795> on non-sterile compounding practices

INFECTION CONTROL PROCEDURES

Training should include infection control procedures to prevent the spread of nosocomial or health care–associated infections. This includes procedures on hand washing, the use of personal protective equipment (PPE), and needle recapping. Preparers of compounded sterile preparations should wear PPE, including a gown, shoe and hair covers, masks (including face shields when necessary), and sterile gloves.

USP <797> requires that proper hand-washing procedures are used. It also specifies the order in which PPE should be put on. That order is as follows:

1. Remove outer garments, along with any cosmetics and visible jewelry, before entering the cleanroom or sterile environment.
2. Remove artificial nails, which are prohibited.
3. The order of putting on garb is directed from dirtiest to cleanest. It begins with putting on approved shoes or shoe covers. Shoe covers are to be worn once and then removed after exiting the cleanroom.
4. Don a head cover and a facial hair cover (if applicable).
5. Don a face mask and an eye shield. The eye shield is mandatory during the disinfection and preparation of hazardous drugs.
6. Clean your hands. Proper hand-washing procedures can be completed by using the following steps. First remove debris from under your fingernails using nail cleaner and water. Then wash your hands vigorously, making sure to include the forearm up to the elbow for a minimum of 30 seconds using antimicrobial soap and water. The use of scrubbing brushes should not be used on the skin as they can damage the skin or cause shedding. Last, completely dry the skin using lint-free wipes or an electronic hand dryer.
7. Don a nonshedding gown that fits snuggly around your wrists and your neck enclosure.
8. Enter the cleanroom or compounding area.
9. Use a waterless, alcohol-based hand scrub to cleanse your hands further.
10. Don sterile, powder-free gloves. Hazardous compounding procedures also require the use of chemotherapy gloves and eye shields.

QUALITY ASSURANCE GUIDELINES

Additional quality assurance guidelines involve needle recapping, recalls, shortages, and communication. Needles should never be recapped because of the potential for needle sticks. The use of Luer Lock needles is preferred for hazardous preparations. Needles should remain attached to the syringe and be placed into a red sharps container following the preparation of nonhazardous formulations. Needles should never be bent, manipulated, or directed toward the body.

Computer processing systems and automated inventory control systems are used to assist in quality assurance measures involving recalls and shortages. These systems detect potential shortages and adjust order quantities accordingly. Manual inventory systems rely on the continual assessment of inventory; initial levels of inventory, as well as minimum and maximum par levels, need to be established. Supply or manufacturing shortages do not require an explanation by the manufacturer. Instead, the pharmacy should attempt to find an alternative source. Pharmacies can check with distributors and manufacturers for alternative lists.

Medication recalls are established by the FDA and are classified according to severity. Once a drug is recalled, the pharmacy must determine if it has that drug in stock. Patients are notified and advised to stop taking the medication. The medication can then be returned to the pharmacy for substitution or credit. The pharmacy returns recalled medication to the manufacturer for credit. Any medication that was recalled and pulled from shelves should be supplemented, and new medications should be ordered.

Effective communication among the pharmacist, the pharmacy technician, the patient, and the health care provider is necessary to facilitate safe and productive medication delivery. Lines of communication among all parties should be clear to facilitate exchanges of information. The intake process serves as a time for the pharmacy technician to gather information. This information is used to screen for interactions and contraindications. The pharmacy uses other methods to provide patients with information. Prescriptions may have auxiliary labels, package inserts, or medication drug guides. Pharmacists also offer counseling, which serves as another point of interaction and a point of verification. Recalls, shortages, refill requests, prior authorizations, and insurance issues should always be conveyed to the patient. This can be done over the phone or face to face. Patients with complaints should be dealt with in a positive manner. The acronym HEAT is often used when handling patient complaints (**H**ear the patient out, **E**mpathize with the patient, **A**pologize, and **T**ake action).

SUMMARY

- ☐ Continuous quality improvement plans are an essential component of pharmacy practice. Pharmacy teams can improve pharmacy services by implementing procedures that allow for continual monitoring and improvement.

- ☐ Prevention strategy plans are used to reduce errors, including quality-related event errors, and should be included in CQI plans.

- ☐ Many organizations have roles in quality assurance and have instituted minimum standards for quality of care. Their role in pharmacy practice varies. However, their commitment to the field and patient care is evident in the programs and publications they have developed.

- ☐ Standards of quality are also seen in compounding procedures, where personnel must adhere to guidelines to maintain sterility when preparing sterile preparations.

- ☐ Pharmacy personnel have a responsibility to provide quality service and maintain great customer satisfaction. Effective communication is critical. Pharmacy-patient interactions should remain positive, even in difficult situations.

PHARMACY QUALITY ASSURANCE PRACTICE QUESTIONS

1. Which of the following is NOT a preventative strategy used to reduce medication errors?

   (A) providing a notation before overriding a high-alert medication
   (B) the use of auxiliary labels to provide warnings and alerts
   (C) inadequate or incorrect packaging, labeling, or directions
   (D) the use of e-prescribing or CPOE to avoid transcription or misinterpretation errors

2. Which organization oversees the National Medication Errors Reporting Program (MERP)?

   (A) ISMP
   (B) TJC
   (C) State Board of Pharmacy
   (D) USP

3. Proper hand-washing technique requires washing the hand from the forearm to the _____.

   (A) elbow
   (B) shoulder
   (C) neck
   (D) face

4. Which of the following is NOT a process used in continuous quality improvement programs?

   (A) detect and document
   (B) evaluate
   (C) report
   (D) pursue

5. What should the preparer do with his or her needle and syringe following the compounding of a nonhazardous, sterile prescription?

   (A) Recap it, and toss it into the sharps container.
   (B) Do not recap it; toss it in the sharps container.
   (C) Remove the needle, and toss it into the sharps container.
   (D) Use the Luer Lock, and toss it into the waste receptacle.

6. A recall was issued by the FDA for medication "X." Who should contact the patient to let him know that his medication has been recalled?

   (A) FDA
   (B) pharmacy
   (C) manufacturer
   (D) prescriber

7. What should be removed before entering the cleanroom or sterile compounding area?

    (A) outer garments
    (B) cosmetics
    (C) jewelry
    (D) All of the above.

8. The identification of errors that require change due to inconsistencies is called
   _____.

    (A) continuous quality improvement
    (B) quality assurance
    (C) quality control
    (D) quality

9. What is the minimum amount of time that your hands should be washed before you participate in preparing sterile compounding procedures?

    (A) 30 seconds
    (B) 45 seconds
    (C) 60 seconds
    (D) 120 seconds

10. What items should be placed into a sharps container?

    (A) syringes and needles
    (B) vials
    (C) hazardous waste
    (D) gloves

ANSWERS EXPLAINED

1. **(C)** This is an example of a quality-related event that can lead to inappropriate dispensing.

2. **(A)** The Institute for Safe Medication Practices (ISMP) established a voluntary medication error-reporting system called the National Medication Errors Reporting Program (MERP). The Joint Commission (TJC) accredits and offers certification to health care organizations. State Boards of Pharmacy are responsible for licensure, registration, and regulation procedures of pharmacists, pharmacy technicians, pharmacy interns, manufacturers, and distributors. The United States Pharmacopeia (USP) provides purity, identity, quality, and strength standards for medications and other compounds.

3. **(A)** *USP* <797> provides procedures for infection control, including proper hand-washing techniques. It states that hands should be cleaned from the forearm to the elbow.

4. **(D)** The basic outline for any continuous quality improvement (CQI) program is "detect and document-evaluate-report-prevent." CQI programs should look at errors and determine ways to prevent future errors from occurring.

5. **(B)** Used needles should never be removed from the syringe or recapped because of the potential to cause accidental needle sticks. Luer Lock fixings are used to attach the needle to the syringe and are reserved for the preparation of hazardous compounds.

6. **(B)** Either the FDA or the manufacturer can issue a recall. When the pharmacy is alerted of the recall, it must pull any of that drug it may have on its shelves. The pharmacy must then alert those patients who may be on that drug. The pharmacy can also alert the prescriber and request that a prescription be written for an alternative.

7. **(D)** Before entering the cleanroom or sterile compounding area, personnel should remove all outer garments, cosmetics, and jewelry.

8. **(C)** Quality control is the process of reviewing areas for inconsistencies and making changes as needed. This differs from quality assurance, which is the review of QRE to evaluate for quality and systematic changes over time. Continuous quality improvement is a process to detect and document, evaluate, report, prevent, and review a plan to increase patient outcomes and customer satisfaction. Quality is a term that refers to a standard, or degree, of excellence.

9. **(A)** According to the *USP* <797>, the minimum amount of time that should be spent on hand washing is 30 seconds.

10. **(A)** Syringes and needles are placed into red sharps containers. Vials, hazardous waste, and gloves should be disposed of according to the directions in the policy and procedure manual.

Medication Order Entry and Fill Process

10

KNOWLEDGE DOMAIN 6.0

Medication Order Entry and Fill Process   **17.50%**

→ Knowledge Area 6.1: Order entry process
→ Knowledge Area 6.2: Intake, interpretation, and data entry
→ Knowledge Area 6.3: Calculate doses required
→ Knowledge Area 6.4: Fill process (e.g., select appropriate product, apply special handling requirements, measure, and prepare product for final check)
→ Knowledge Area 6.5: Labeling requirements (e.g., auxiliary and warning labels, expiration date, patient specific information)
→ Knowledge Area 6.6: Packaging requirements (e.g., type of bags, syringes, glass, pvc, child resistant, light resistant)
→ Knowledge Area 6.7: Dispensing process (e.g., validation, documentation, and distribution)

LEARNING OBJECTIVES

☐ Learn the order entry process.
☐ Understand the intake process, including prescription interpretation and data entry.
☐ Calculate doses required in order to process prescriptions, including a day's supply
☐ Understand the fill process, including proper product selection, measurements, and preparation for the pharmacist's final check.
☐ Be familiar with packaging requirements.
☐ Understand the prescription-dispensing process.

INTRODUCTION

Pharmacy technicians are responsible for processing many of the prescriptions that come into the pharmacy. The process of filling a prescription can be broken down into 5 steps:

1. Receiving the prescription
2. Translating the prescription
3. Entering the prescription into the computer system
4. Filling the prescription
5. Verifying the prescription and providing patient consultation

The pharmacy technician may complete only the first four steps. Verification of prescriptions and patient consultations requires additional education and training. Therefore, the last step may be completed only by the pharmacist.

This process utilizes a computerized prescription system. Pharmacy computer systems can vary, and training is provided to technicians upon hiring. Pharmacy technicians must be able to understand the computer system and learn how to process prescriptions efficiently and accurately.

> **Note:** Laws vary from one state to another, and some states may allow pharmacy interns to consult with patients. As a rule of thumb, remember that pharmacy technicians may *not* provide any patient consultations.

RECEIVING THE PRESCRIPTION

Prescriptions may arrive to the pharmacy in various formats. A traditional written prescription pad may be used. In addition, prescriptions may also be faxed, sent electronically as an e-script to the pharmacy's computer system, called into the pharmacist who will then transcribe the prescription to a telephone prescription pad, or sent using a computerized prescriber order entry (CPOE) system in an institutionalized setting. Table 10-1 provides more information about these various methods.

Table 10-1. Prescription Transmission Methods

Type of Prescription	Notes
Written prescription	**Community pharmacy:** – Usually delivered to the pharmacy by the patient. – May be difficult to read or interpret. – The pharmacy must be aware of potential fraudulent prescriptions, and must be able to identify fraudulent activity. **Hospital pharmacy:** – Inpatient medication orders can be hand delivered by the hospital staff, sent via pneumatic tube systems, or submitted by the patient in an outpatient pharmacy setting.
Faxed prescription	**May be used in hospital or community pharmacies:** – Faxed prescriptions should include the physician's office letterhead and the manual signature of the practitioner. Some states may require a statement of validity to be sent with the faxed prescription. – C-II prescriptions may be accepted by the pharmacy (in accordance with state law) if the original, written, signed prescription is presented to the pharmacist prior to dispensing.
Called-in prescription	**May be used in hospital or community pharmacies:** – The prescription is called in by a prescribing individual and transcribed by the pharmacist on a pharmacy-approved prescription pad. – The pharmacist writes down the prescription information and repeats the prescription order to the prescriber to ensure accuracy. – State laws vary, and some states may allow pharmacy interns to perform this step under the supervision of a pharmacist.

Type of Prescription	Notes
e-script prescription	**Community pharmacy:** – Increasingly popular method used by physicians and other prescribing health professionals in an effort to focus on error prevention. – Prescribing individuals can use computers or other approved handheld devices to enter prescription information. – The prescription information is sent electronically through a secured system to the patient's preferred pharmacy, where it can be filled. – Laws currently regulate whether controlled substances can be sent via e-script, and those laws vary by state. States that recognize these scripts require the physician's digital signature to be saved on file.
CPOE prescription	**Hospital pharmacy:** – Used by practitioners to order medications for patients under their care. – This is becoming the standard for prescription entry in an institutionalized setting. – Prescriptions are ordered on a 24-hour basis. – The practitioner can select priority of fill (STAT or as ordered). – In some institutionalized settings, this eliminates the need for the pharmacy technicians to interpret the medication order, allowing pharmacists to complete this step. This method allows the technician to fill orders, thus, speeding up the process.

PATIENT INFORMATION IN A COMMUNITY SETTING

It is very important to retrieve all of the necessary information from the patient before he or she leaves your intake window. The pharmacy computer system includes patient profiles that contain patient-sensitive information, including the patient's name, address, allergies, and medication history, as well as the prescriber's name and the insurer's name. The computer system can also identify and flag drug interactions.

The technician should always ask the patient a series of questions when receiving a prescription. The technician must know if a patient has previously filled a prescription at the pharmacy. If the person has, the technician can ask the patient for identifying information, including the person's name and date of birth to locate the patient profile. Some pharmacies may require patient identification for controlled prescriptions. For new patients, it is imperative to collect the following information for the patient profile:

- Full name of the patient
- Current address
- Date of birth
- Telephone number (preferably cell phone number)
- Allergies to any medications
- Other medications (including over-the-counter, vitamins, and herbs)
- Medical conditions
- Insurance information
- Service preference, including childproof caps or easy-open caps
- Whether the patient will wait for the prescription or when he/she will return to pick it up
- HIPAA compliance handout and/or signature

The pharmacy may use a patient intake form like the one in Figure 10-1. Alternatively, the pharmacy may simply enter the information directly into the computer. After you have verified all of the information, ask the patient if he or she would like to wait for the prescription or if the person plans on returning at a later point. Prescriptions are prioritized based on waiting time. Some pharmacies may even offer delivery services for patients.

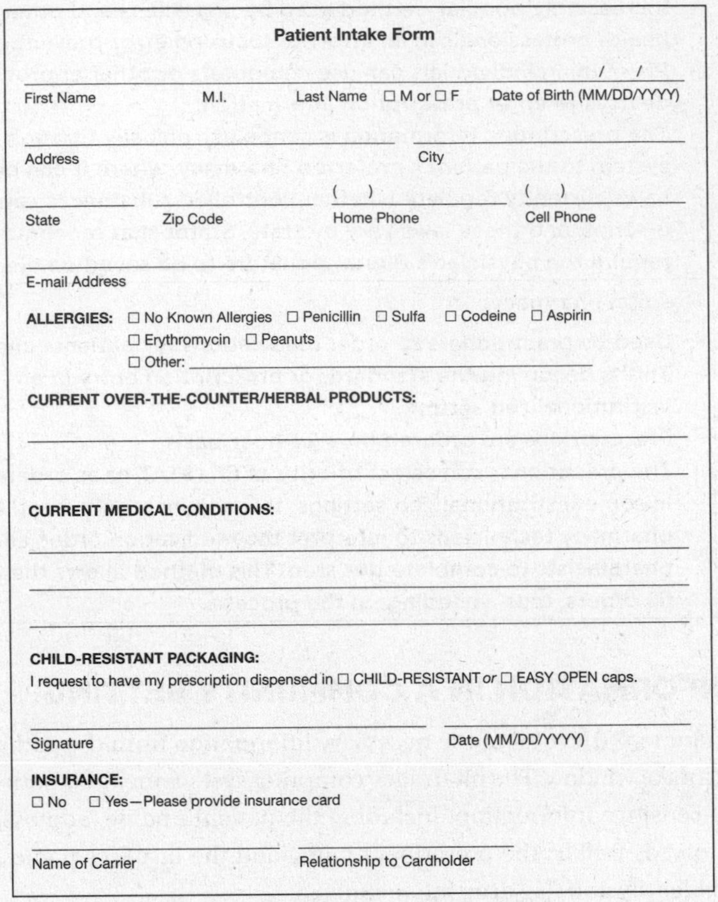
Patient Intake Form

First Name M.I. Last Name ☐ M or ☐ F Date of Birth (MM/DD/YYYY)

Address City

State Zip Code Home Phone ( ) Cell Phone ( )

E-mail Address

ALLERGIES: ☐ No Known Allergies ☐ Penicillin ☐ Sulfa ☐ Codeine ☐ Aspirin ☐ Erythromycin ☐ Peanuts ☐ Other:

CURRENT OVER-THE-COUNTER/HERBAL PRODUCTS:

CURRENT MEDICAL CONDITIONS:

CHILD-RESISTANT PACKAGING:
I request to have my prescription dispensed in ☐ CHILD-RESISTANT *or* ☐ EASY OPEN caps.

Signature Date (MM/DD/YYYY)

INSURANCE:
☐ No ☐ Yes—Please provide insurance card

Name of Carrier Relationship to Cardholder

Figure 10-1. Patient intake form

PATIENT INFORMATION IN A HOSPITAL SETTING

Prescriptions in institutionalized settings are referred to as medication orders. They may be written in a patient's chart, sent as a CPOE order, or even written on a standardized hospital medication order form. Patient information is generally gathered by other hospital professionals in this setting, and it should include the following information:

- Patient number and identification number (medical record number)
- Room number
- Date of birth
- Height and weight (may be needed for dosage calculations)
- Laboratory values (may be needed for dosage calculations)
- Diagnosis, if available

This information is typically found on the medication order or by accessing the patient's information via the hospital computer system. Hospitals place security restrictions on the type of information that health professionals may access. Pharmacy technicians may be restricted from accessing specific patient information and can ask the pharmacist for help if they are unsure about what information is needed.

TRANSLATING THE PRESCRIPTION

Prescriptions provide important information for filling, compounding, dispensing, and administering a medication. Once a prescription is signed, it is considered a legal document. You must verify the patient's name before entering prescription information. Patients may have common last names or even similar birth dates. Some patients may be a second- or third-generation family member. New prescriptions are scanned into the computer, and information is entered into the appropriate patient profile fields. The parts of a prescription are displayed in Figure 10-2.

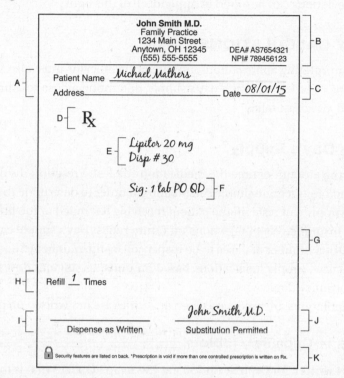

A. Patient information, such as name, address, date of birth, age, height, weight, and allergy information
B. Prescriber information, including name, DEA number (required for controlled prescriptions), and other contact information
C. Date of prescription, which is typically good for a year from the date the prescription is written for noncontrolled prescriptions; controlled prescription laws vary from state to state
D. Superscription, which is the Rx symbol indicating how to take the prescription and is translated to mean "take thus"
E. Inscription, which includes the medication and quantities to be dispensed
F. Transcription or signa, which are directions for patient use
G. Subscription, which are additional directions to the pharmacist for preparing the prescription (can be used for preparations or labeling)
H. Number of authorized refills
I. Dispense as written (DAW) code or signature line indicating that a brand or a generic product is being dispensed
J. Prescriber's signature
K. Security markings used to authenticate the prescription

Figure 10-2. Sample written prescription

Note: Prescription styles vary, but they should include similar standard information. Some states may not mandate the presence of DEA numbers on noncontrolled prescription orders.

It is now time for the technician to translate the prescription. This step is vital, and it is done by deciphering the prescription abbreviations. Prescription abbreviations include those used to indicate route, dosage form, quantity, and measurement. A list of commonly used pharmacy abbreviations can be found in Appendix F of this book.

PHARMACY CALCULATIONS

In addition to interpreting abbreviations, pharmacy technicians must also know how to perform calculations in order to input a day's supply, determine a dose to administer based on the dose at hand, or adjust refills.

Calculating Day's Supply

Day's supply is the amount of time the medication will last. Prescriptions do not always last 30 or 90 days and often require simple calculations in order to determine the day's supply. An incorrect day's supply can result in the patient receiving too much or too little of the medication, as well as insurance claim rejections on future refills. Day's supply can be determined by dividing the total number of doses to be dispensed by the number of doses taken per day. Hospital pharmacies supply medications based on units, or singular doses, and provide an additional supply once depleted.

Note that calculations are necessary when quantities are not written on prescriptions.

 Example 1—Capsules/Tablets

A prescription is written for Cephalexin 250 mg #30 1 cap PO TID. What is the day's supply?

Answer:

$$\frac{1 \text{ day}}{3 \text{ caps}} = \frac{x \text{ days}}{30 \text{ caps}}$$

Cross multiply and solve for x.

$$x = 10 \text{ days}$$

The next example is a bit trickier and requires some investigation. In order to calculate day's supply, you will need to know how many "puffs" are in one inhaler. This information can be found by looking at the inhaler package.

TIP

When calculating day's supply, make sure to convert both the prescribed dose and the total amount of the drug in the container to the same unit.

➡ Example 2—Inhalers

A prescription is written for ProAir inhaler 2 puffs QID. A ProAir inhaler has 200 puffs. What is the day's supply?

Answer: First determine the amount of puffs in one day. 2 puffs QID is the same as 2 puffs, 4 times a day, or 8 puffs a day. Then move on to calculating the day's supply.

$$\frac{8 \text{ puffs}}{1 \text{ day}} = \frac{200 \text{ puffs}}{x \text{ days}}$$

Cross multiply and solve for x.

$$x = 25 \text{ days}$$

Example 3 deals with oral liquids. Oral liquids are generally not dispensed in the original container unless the amount to be dispensed is equivalent to the stock bottle amount or if the prescription is written for a complete bottle to be dispensed. Calculations are needed in order to determine the total amount, in mL, to be dispensed.

> **Note:** In order to determine what size bottle is needed for the volume of medication prescribed, take the total volume in mL (if not already given in oz) and divide by 30. For example, a 120 mL prescription would be dispensed in a 4 oz bottle.

➡ Example 3—Oral Liquids

A prescription is written for Dilantin 125 mg/5 mL # 8 oz, 1 tsp PO BID. What is the day's supply?

Answer: First convert oz to mL.

$$\frac{x \text{ mL}}{8 \text{ oz}} = \frac{30 \text{ mL}}{1 \text{ oz}}$$

Cross multiply and solve for x.

$$x = 240 \text{ mL}$$

Now look at the total quantity to be taken in one day.

$$5 \text{ mL} \times 2 = 10 \text{ mL/day}$$

Finally, determine day's supply.

$$\frac{x \text{ days}}{240 \text{ mL}} = \frac{1 \text{ day}}{10 \text{ mL}}$$

Cross multiply and solve for x.

$$x = 24 \text{ days}$$

Many times, the prescription will specify an amount of time that the patient should take the medication. It is best to determine the appropriate day's supply based on the amount of drops the patient will use daily. The pharmacy technician should check the amount of mL contained in one bottle and select the appropriate size that will maintain the course of therapy as prescribed. In addition, it is customary to assume a conversion factor of 20 drops/mL (typically used for ophthalmic and otic solutions) when determining the total amount of drops per bottle. Some pharmacies may be conservative and use a conversion factor of 15 drops/mL (typically reserved for ophthalmic and otic suspensions). Third-party payers may also require a conversion factor of 16 drops/mL when determining day's supply. Check with the pharmacist before proceeding.

➡ Example 4—Eyedrops and Eardrops

A prescription is written for Cipro HC Otic suspension, 4 gtts ad BID × 7 days # 10 mL. What is the day's supply?

Answer: Calculate the actual day's supply based on a conversion factor of 15 drops/mL. First determine the amount of drops contained in the bottle.

$$x \text{ drops/bottle} = 10 \text{ mL} \times 15 \text{ drops/mL}$$
$$x = 150 \text{ drops/bottle}$$

Next determine the volume of drops a patient will use per day, and calculate the number of days this prescription will last. The script states: 4 gtts ad BID. This means that the patient will use 4 drops in the right ear twice a day for a total of 8 drops a day.

$$\frac{1 \text{ day}}{8 \text{ drops}} = \frac{x \text{ days}}{150 \text{ drops}}$$

Cross multiply and solve for x.

$$x = 18.75 \text{ days} \approx 18 \text{ days}$$

This answer is rounded down because the medication will not last the patient until the end of his or her course of treatment on the 19th day.

Insulin prescriptions are written in units. Day's supply calculations are determined based on 1 mL = 100 units. Insulin may also be referred to as U-100, meaning that each mL contains 100 units. Typical sizing for insulin includes both 10 mL vials (1,000 units) and 3 mL syringes (available as a quantity of 5 syringes for a total quantity of 15 mL or 1,500 units).

➡ Example 5—Insulin

A prescription is written for Humulin-N U-100 Insulin 10 mL vial, 35 U SC QD. What is the day's supply?

Answer: There are 100 units/mL. First determine the total number of units in the 10 mL vial of insulin.

$$\frac{100 \text{ U}}{1 \text{ mL}} = \frac{x \text{ U}}{10 \text{ mL}}$$

Cross multiply and solve for x.

$$x = 1{,}000 \text{ U}$$

Then solve for the total day's supply of this prescription.

$$\frac{35 \text{ U}}{1 \text{ day}} = \frac{1{,}000 \text{ U}}{x}$$

Cross multiply and solve for x.

$$x = 28.57 \text{ days} \approx 28 \text{ days}$$

Do not round up because the patient will not have enough to last until the next day.

Day's supply calculations for ointment/cream prescriptions are not as concrete and require some additional information. It is important to note that ointments/creams vary in size. The day's supply depends on how often the patient will use the medication and how large of an area the patient will use the ointment or cream on. If an amount is not specified, err on the side of caution and use 1 g/dose to calculate day's supply.

➡ Example 6—Ointments/Creams

A prescription is written for hydrocortisone cream 2.5% cream, 30 g tube, apply once daily to affected area. What is the day's supply?

Answer: For this example, we will use 1 g/dose to calculate the day's supply. First determine the total number of doses available in a 30 g tube.

$$\frac{1 \text{ gram}}{1 \text{ dose}} = \frac{30 \text{ g}}{x \text{ doses}}$$

Cross multiply and solve for x.

$$x = 30 \text{ doses}$$

Now solve for the total day's supply for this prescription.

$$\frac{1 \text{ dose}}{1 \text{ day}} = \frac{30 \text{ doses}}{x \text{ days}}$$

Cross multiply and solve for x.

$$x = 30 \text{ days}$$

TIP

Labels for inhaler, liquid, and insulin preparations should include a beyond use date when appropriate.

Now practice day's supply using the following community and hospital pharmacy prescriptions.

➡ Prescription 1 _____

> **John Smith M.D.**
> Family Practice
> 1234 Main Street
> Anytown, OH 12345   DEA# AS7654321
> (555) 555-5555   NPI# 789456123
>
> Patient Name _Ava Thomas_____
> Address_____ Date _08/01/15_
>
> **Rx**
>   _Robitussin #120_
>
>   _Sig: 1 tsp PO q4-6H PRN_
>
>
>
>
> Refill _0_ Times
>
>   _John Smith M.D._
> _____   _____
> Dispense as Written   Substitution Permitted
>
> 🔒 Security features are listed on back. *Prescription is void if more than one controlled prescription is written on Rx.

1. What is the total quantity of this medication to be dispensed to the patient?

2. What is the minimum day's supply for this prescription?

3. How many refills are on this prescription?

Answers:

1. The total is 120 mL. This can also be interpreted as 4 oz.

2. The minimum day's supply is 4 days.

   1 teaspoonful by mouth every 4–6 hours as needed.

$$5 \text{ mL} \times 6 \text{ doses/day} = 30 \text{ mL/day}$$

$$\frac{30 \text{ mL}}{1 \text{ day}} = \frac{120 \text{ mL}}{x \text{ days}}$$

   Cross multiply and solve for x.

$$x = 4 \text{ days}$$

3. There are no refills on this prescription.

TIP

Remember, one teaspoonful is equivalent to 5 mL.

➡ Prescription 2 _____

```
                      John Smith M.D.
                      Family Practice
                      1234 Main Street
                    Anytown, OH 12345        DEA# AS7654321
                      (555) 555-5555         NPI# 789456123
   _____
   Patient Name  Philip Johns
   Address_____  Date 08/01/15

      Rx
                 Xalatan #2.5

                 Sig: 1 gtt OU QD




   Refill  2  Times


   _____          John Smith M.D.
      Dispense as Written          Substitution Permitted

   🔒 Security features are listed on back. *Prescription is void if more than one controlled prescription is written on Rx.
```

1. Translate the sig code into plain English.

2. Is this prescription written for an eardrop or an eyedrop?

3. What is the day's supply?

Answers:

1. Instill 1 drop in each eye every day.

2. This prescription is written for an eyedrop.

3. The day's supply is 25 days.

$$2.5 \text{ mL} \times 15 \text{ gtts/mL} = 37.5 \text{ gtts}$$

$$\frac{2 \text{ gtts}}{1 \text{ eye}} = \frac{37.5 \text{ gtts}}{x}$$

Cross multiply and solve for x.

$$x = 18.75 \text{ days} \approx 18 \text{ days}$$

This answer is rounded down because the medication will not last the patient until the end of the course of treatment on the 19th day.

Other Calculations: Calculations for Dispensing Fees, Co-Pays, and Cash Register Calculations

Dispensing fees are costs associated with filling the prescription. They are determined by a contractual agreement between a third party and the pharmacy. Dispensing fees for prescriptions include the cost of labor, equipment, medications, and rent.

Co-pays are determined by a contractual agreement between a third party and the patient. They are fixed dollar amounts that may reflect a percentage of the medication cost.

Cash register calculations require the technician to give the correct change to the patient. In addition, patients who pay cash for their prescriptions are charged a **usual and customary price** (U&C). These prices reflect the medication's cost (average wholesale price or AWP) and a professional fee. Some pharmacies also provide discounts to patients without insurance coverage.

➡ Example 1

What is the co-pay for a prescription of prednisone 20 mg # 10 if the co-pay is 20% of the U&C price of the prescription? The U&C price for prednisone 20 mg #10 is $4.76.

Answer: 20% is the same as saying $\frac{20}{100}$ or 0.2. To determine the co-pay, multiply the percentage by the U&C price.

$$0.2 \times \$4.76 = \$0.95$$

The co-pay for this prescription is $0.95.

➡ Example 2

A third-party contract allows for pharmacy reimbursement of prescription "X" based on the following formula: 80% of AWP + $1.65 dispensing fee. The AWP for prescription "X" is $34.20. Determine the pharmacy reimbursement for prescription "X."

Answer: 80% is the same as saying $\frac{80}{100}$ or 0.8. Pharmacy reimbursement can be determined by multiplying the AWP by 0.8 and adding the dispensing fee.

(0.8	×	$34.20)	+	$1.65	=	$29.01
percentage	×	AWP	+	dispensing fee	=	pharmacy reimbursement

The pharmacy's reimbursement is $29.01.

➡ Example 3

A patient's prescription costs $75.25, and a patient gives you $80.00. How much change should the patient receive?

Answer: There are multiple ways of counting out change, and the currency you provide to the patient can vary based on how you count out change. Here is one method you can use. Start counting out the currency using the smallest denomination of money that will get you to the next coin or bill size. Start with the purchase price of $75.25, and count to the amount given to you, $80.00.

3 quarters (75¢) will make $76.00

4 dollars ($4.00) will make $80.00

The patient should receive $4.75 in change.

➡ Example 4

A patient qualifies for a pharmacy discount of 5% on her prescription costs. What is the cost that the patient will pay if the retail price of her prescription is $6.15?

Answer: 5% is the same as saying $\frac{5}{100}$ or 0.05. To determine the amount the patient will pay, multiply the percentage by the prescription cost.

$$0.05 \times \$6.15 = \$0.31$$

This is the discount that the patient will receive. Subtract this amount from the prescription cost to determine the discounted amount to be paid by the patient.

$$\$6.15 - \$0.31 = \$5.84$$

The patient will pay a discounted amount of $5.84.

PRESCRIPTION ENTRY INTO THE COMPUTER SYSTEM

Community Pharmacy

When processing prescriptions, each prescription is automatically assigned a prescription number by the pharmacy computer system. Refills of the prescription will carry the same prescription number. Patients can use this number to refill their prescriptions. When processing a refill request, the technician should verify that refills are available. If no refills are available, alert the pharmacist to contact the physician for a new prescription. Your pharmacy may also choose to send refill requests electronically to the prescriber; this process can be completed by the pharmacy technician. If a refill request is processed too early, the third-party payer may choose to reject the claim. Refills for controlled substances should not be filled too early because of the potential for abuse. A DAW code may also be required by your computer in order to process a prescription. Examples of DAW codes include:

- 0 = no product selection indicated
- 1 = substitution not allowed by provider
- 2 = substitution allowed; patient requested product
- 3 = substitution allowed; pharmacist selected product
- 4 = substitution allowed; generic medication is not in stock
- 5 = substitution allowed; brand name drug dispensed as generic
- 6 = override
- 7 = substitution not allowed; brand name drug mandated by law
- 8 = substitution allowed; brand name drug not available
- 9 = other

TIP

You may have to figure out why a claim has been rejected. A good place to start is by checking all person codes, group codes, and patient-identifying information.

Before a label can be printed, the system must send a claim to the patient's insurance company or other third-party payer. The third party will then respond online within a few moments stating if the claim has been paid or rejected. This is called **adjudication**.

Once the patient and prescription information have been correctly entered into the computer system, the computer will generate a prescription label (see Figure 10-3). The prescription label contains the following:

1. Pharmacy's name and address
2. Number used by the pharmacy to identify this drug for refills
3. Person for whom the drug is prescribed
4. Instructions about how often and when to take the drug
5. Name of the drug and the strength of the drug
6. Number of refills before a certain date
7. Doctor's name
8. Drugstore's phone number
9. Prescription fill date
10. Warning: Do not use this drug after this date _____

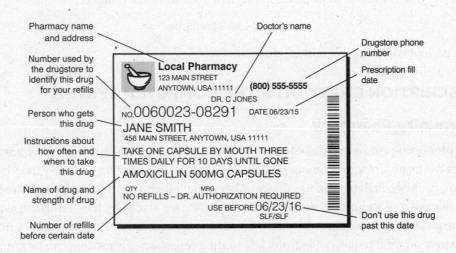

Figure 10-3. Prescription label

The FDA requests, but does not require, the label to include the medication's **National Drug Code** number, also known as the NDC number, as shown in Figure 10-4. This is a 10-digit number unique not only to the drug but also to the strength and form of the drug product. This number is used to confirm proper selection of the product. NDC placement on the prescription label varies; check with your State Board of Pharmacy for more information.

Labeler		Drug		Package
12345	–	101	–	50
XYZ Company		Sunscreen		50 mL Tube

Figure 10-4. National Drug Code number

The medication's expiration date is based on information supplied by the manufacturer. The expiration date can be expressed as a month and a year. Alternatively, it can be listed as a day, month, and year. If just the month and year are indicated, the drug can be used or dispensed until the last day of that month. For example, if the expiration date is written as 2/17, the drug does not actually expire until 2/28/2017.

INSURANCE INFORMATION

Modern computer systems allow pharmacies to bill insurance companies in real time. This means that pharmacies can bill the insurance company and receive a response within moments stating either that the claim has been paid or that it has been rejected. Pharmacy technicians should be familiar with common private, federal, and state-administered prescription plans and services. When entering plan information, the following information must be gathered:

- Name of the plan
- Patient ID number
- Group number—this identifies the patient's employer or association
- Pharmacy BIN number, which is a 6-digit bank identification number necessary to route online claims for payment correctly
- Person code—this indicates if the patient is the primary cardholder (00 or 01), the spouse (01 or 02), or a dependent child (02 or 03)
- Provider service's phone number, which is the insurance company's (or other provider's) phone number

The pharmacy technician will scan the insurance card into the computer. This process allows a visual of the card to be retained in the patient's profile. Figure 10-5 shows a sample insurance card.

WELLS INSURANCE

MEMBER NAME: JANE DOE EFFECTIVE DATE: 12/15/2016

IDENTIFICATION #: SUFFIX:
999999999 01

GROUP #: 1234567
RX GROUP #: INSGROUP01
BIN #: 555555

RETAIL RX: $10/$25/$45
MAIL ORDER RX: $25/$45/$60

MEMBER SERVICES: 1-800-987-1234
CLAIMS / INQUIRIES: 1-800-123-6789

Figure 10-5. Insurance card

Some insurance companies require a co-payment by the patient. If one is required, the amount will be indicated on the insurance card. Any rejections by the insurance company will state a general message regarding why the claim has been rejected. Some issues can be easily resolved, including an incorrect plan or group number. Other issues may require a call to the insurer to get the claim paid.

Many computer software systems notify the user of any drug-drug interactions or allergy concerns by flagging issues in the prescription. The pharmacist should be alerted, and an evaluation of the concern should be completed by the pharmacist. New computer systems have built-in barriers that prevent technicians from moving forward in the fill process until concerns have been evaluated.

Hospital Setting

Prescriptions in a hospital setting are referred to as medication orders. They are received via one of the methods mentioned in Table 10-1. Once the medication order has been verified, it can be filled. Insurance claims are handled by the hospital business office. They are not verified by the pharmacy department.

PREPARING THE PRESCRIPTION

Once the label has been generated, the pharmacy technician can begin to prepare the prescription. The pharmacy technician will locate the product, verify its NDC, and count the appropriate number of tablets or measure the appropriate quantity of liquid as stated on the prescription.

Community pharmacies use amber-colored vials in which to place tablets and capsules. These vials are available in a variety of sizes. The technician should choose an appropriate vial size that will fit the quantity of pills needed for the prescription. Unless otherwise stated, all prescription vials, bottles, and other products should be dispensed with a child-resistant cap. Figure 10-6 shows a variety of vials and child-resistant caps. If a patient chooses not to have a child-resistant cap, the appropriate field in his or her patient profile should be marked for future filling purposes.

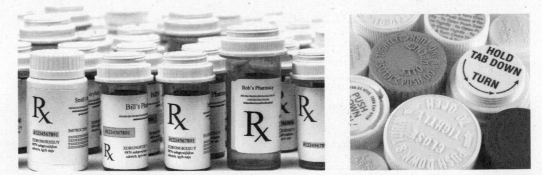

Figure 10-6. Prescription vials and child-resistant caps

Pharmacy technicians may use automated filling and dispensing machines that fill and label bottles with correct quantities of ordered drugs. They may also use a counting tray, as shown in Figure 10-7. It is a tray designed for counting tablets from a stock bottle into a prescription. A counting tray contains a side container area that allows for tablets to slide into the prescription bottle after being counted. Tablets are typically counted in groups of 5 to maintain consistency and ease when filling medication orders.

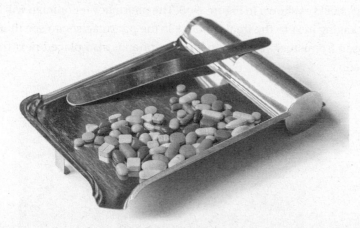

Figure 10-7. Counting tray

Some retail pharmacies and hospital pharmacies employ the use of automated robots to assist in filling prescriptions. Hospitals that have a horizontal and vertical rail system can use automated arms to assist in locating medications and filling patient carts. Automated packaging systems are also available. Medications can be poured into a reservoir after medication-identifying information is entered to generate a unit package label. The automated packaging machine dispenses and packages one dose of medication at a time.

Once the desired pill or product is put into an appropriate container, the finished prescription label is placed onto the container along with any auxiliary labels that may be necessary. Auxiliary labels are labels alerting patients about specific warnings, foods, or medications to avoid, about potential side effects, and about other cautionary interactions. Common examples include "take with food" and "medication should be taken with plenty of water."

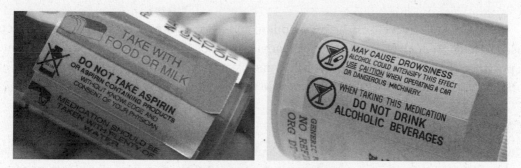

Figure 10-8. Auxiliary labels

Prescriptions for controlled substances must contain the following warning on the prescription label: "Caution: Federal law prohibits the transfer of this drug to any person other than the patient for whom it was prescribed."

Some medications may also be prepackaged, such as inhalers, eyedrops, eardrops, oral contraceptives, insulin vials, creams, ointments, and gels. With these products, the prescription label is affixed directly onto the package or container. Other medications may need to stay in their original packaging. One example of this is nitroglycerin, which is available in an airtight, amber-colored glass vial to protect the contents from degradation.

The final step of the preparation process is to organize the completed product for the pharmacist's final check, as shown in Figure 10-9. The pharmacy technician will leave stock bottles or other packaging next to the final product so the pharmacist can see that the correct product was chosen from stock. The original prescription is also placed next to the final product for comparison.

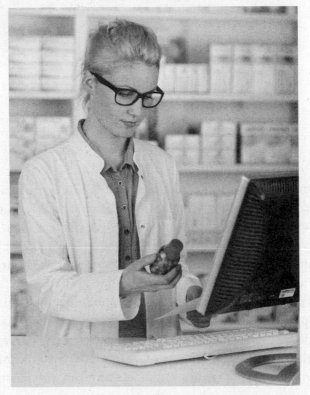

Figure 10-9. Checking a prescription

The pharmacist will check the prescription, and the technician will return any products used to their proper place. The technician or pharmacist will then place the prescription into a prescription bag with the receipt attached and place it into the will-call area for pickup. The original prescription will be filed and stored in the pharmacy.

CUSTOMER PICKUP

Completed prescriptions are usually filed alphabetically by the patient's last name, either in bins or another storage area as shown in Figure 10-10. They may be placed into paper or plastic bags depending on the pharmacy. Pharmacy personnel must be sensitive to the confidential nature of prescription information, and they must be sure to follow HIPAA privacy regulations.

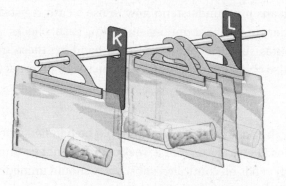

Figure 10-10. Prescriptions for customer pickup

Patients picking up prescriptions will approach the will-call area. Most pharmacies have a waiting area for patients as well as a placeholder in line where patients can wait until the pharmacy technician is ready to have them approach the counter. This placeholder is necessary to maintain HIPAA privacy regulations.

The pharmacy technician obtains the prescription from the storage area and verifies the patient's personal information, including his or her name, date of birth, address, and the number of prescriptions he or she is picking up. The technician should find only requested prescriptions. Some states also require patients to show identification to pick up scheduled substances and substances containing pseudoephedrine. The technician then scans the prescription into the point of sale (POS) system to let the computer know that the patient has picked up his or her prescription. The POS system can also advise the technician if other prescriptions are ready. The patient is asked if he or she has any questions for the pharmacist. A signature log is used to document both the prescription being picked up and the acceptance or denial of counseling by the pharmacist (see Figure 10-11).

Technicians may also be responsible for handling cash registers. Most pharmacy cash registers have integration systems and automatically communicate with the pharmacy's computer system. The bar code on the prescription label not only allows the cash register and the pharmacy computer system to know that the prescription has been picked up, but it also sends co-pay information to the cash register. The technician requests the co-pay from the patient at the time of pickup. After receiving the co-pay and providing change, if needed, the patient is given the prescription.

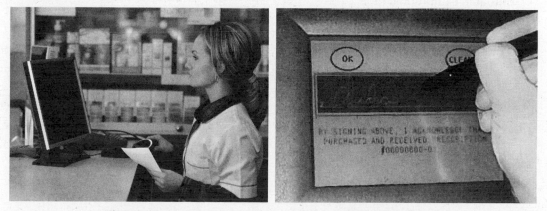

Figure 10-11. Scanning and signing for a filled prescription

Pharmacy technicians must understand how to use a cash register. Patients pay for prescriptions with a variety of payment options, including cash, checks, and credit cards. Store policies and procedures should be followed when handling these transactions. Pharmacy technicians should also check identification as instructed by pharmacy and store personnel.

SUMMARY

- [ ] Retail pharmacy third-party billing issues should be handled before filling the prescription. Prescriptions filled a few days or a week early may not go through insurance.
- [ ] Requests for early refills on controlled substances should immediately involve the pharmacist to avoid disputes and potential abuse issues.
- [ ] A new-patient profile must be added for new patients. All patient information, including billing information, must be taken at the time of prescription entry.
- [ ] Hospital pharmacies do not deal with insurance. Insurance is processed through the hospital business office.
- [ ] Medications are unit dosed and based on a 24-hour time frame or on an as-needed basis.
- [ ] The pharmacist must review any prescription flags that occur during processing before continuing to prepare the prescription.
- [ ] All drug products should be verified by the NDC number available on the medication stock bottle or product. Verification of the correct product is essential. Any discrepancies should be reviewed before continuing prescription preparation.
- [ ] Child-resistant caps must be used unless otherwise stated by the patient and documented in the patient profile.
- [ ] Appropriate auxiliary labels should be placed onto the prescription vial to identify pertinent warnings, cautions, or concerns.
- [ ] Technicians should always be courteous and provide patients with timely service.
- [ ] Signature logs are required. Pharmacy technicians should be aware of all prescriptions that require signatures, including any OTC pseudoephedrine products.
- [ ] Pharmacy technicians are responsible for reordering stock when needed. This process may include electronic ordering through a wholesaler, applying stickers to products as needed, putting items onto shelves, and filling invoices. Orders must also be unpacked and checked.
- [ ] Pharmacy technicians are also responsible for keeping the pharmacy neat and clean. This includes rearranging stock bottles so that labels face forward and checking bottles for outdated expiration dates.

MEDICATION ORDER ENTRY AND FILL PROCESS PRACTICE QUESTIONS

1. _____ requires community pharmacists to offer counseling to Medicaid patients regarding medications.

    (A) OBRA
    (B) The FDA
    (C) The DEA
    (D) HIPAA

2. An NDC number is _____ digits long and is _____ for all drugs.

    (A) 8; different
    (B) 8; the same
    (C) 10; different
    (D) 10; the same

3. Patient information that must be entered into the computer includes the patient's _____.

    (A) name and date of birth
    (B) telephone number and address
    (C) medication allergies and medication safety cap preference
    (D) All of the above.

4. A signature log is used in a pharmacy _____.

    (A) to log medications that need to be ordered
    (B) for patients to sign for prescriptions received
    (C) to document patient signatures for their patient profile
    (D) by pharmacists to document prescriptions filled

5. A PRN order is an order for a medication that is used on a(n) _____ basis in a hospital.

    (A) twice a day
    (B) daily
    (C) as needed
    (D) immediate

6. In the NDC number 0415-5258-26, the last two numbers indicate the _____.

    (A) dosage form
    (B) manufacturer
    (C) package size
    (D) drug strength

7. How many tablets should be dispensed, given the following order?

    amoxicillin 250 mg tabs; sig 1 tab BID × 10 days

    (A) 10
    (B) 20
    (C) 30
    (D) 40

8. A drug container has the expiration date of 07/2018. On which of the following days does this bottle actually expire?

    (A) 6/30/2018
    (B) 7/01/2018
    (C) 7/31/2018
    (D) 8/01/2018

9. Which of the following pieces of information is NOT located on the prescription label?

    (A) pharmacy name
    (B) prescriber's name
    (C) medication strength
    (D) prescriber's address

10. Which of the following is NOT a valid method for presenting a prescription for a noncontrolled medication?

    (A) via mail to a retail pharmacy
    (B) submitted to a pharmacy as an e-script
    (C) presented to a pharmacy in person
    (D) faxed to a pharmacy

ANSWERS EXPLAINED

1. **(A)** The 1990 Omnibus Budget and Reconciliation Act (OBRA) calls for this requirement.

2. **(C)** An NDC number is a 10-digit number that is not only unique to the drug but also to the strength and form of the drug product.

3. **(D)** All of this data should be entered into the patient information screen.

4. **(B)** A signature log is a book or an electronic signing tool used to document prescriptions received by the patient.

5. **(C)** PRN is an abbreviation used to indicate an as needed basis. Twice a day, choice (A), is reflective of a BID, which is an abbreviation used to indicate taking a medication twice daily. Daily, choice (B), is reflective of a QD, which is an abbreviation used to indicate taking a medication daily. Immediate, choice (D), is reflective of STAT, which is an abbreviation used to indicate an immediate need.

6. **(C)** The last two numbers of a product's National Drug Code indicate the package size of the product.

7. **(B)** 1 tablet × twice a day = 2 tablets a day × 10 days = 20 total tablets dispensed.

8. **(C)** Unless a product has a clear expiration date (month, day, year), it is assumed that an expiration date with a month and year format does not expire until the last day of the month.

9. **(D)** The prescriber's address is not indicated on the prescription label. However, the prescription label does indicate the prescriber's name.

10. **(A)** Retail pharmacies do not accept prescriptions sent via the mail. Instead, prescriptions may be presented in person, faxed, phoned in, or sent as an e-script.

Pharmacy Inventory Management

11

KNOWLEDGE DOMAIN 7.0

Pharmacy Inventory Management   **8.75%**

→ Knowledge Area 7.1: Function and application of NDC, lot numbers, and expiration dates
→ Knowledge Area 7.2: Formulary or approved/preferred product list
→ Knowledge Area 7.3: Ordering and receiving processes (e.g., maintain par levels, rotate stock)
→ Knowledge Area 7.4: Storage requirements (e.g., refrigeration, freezer, warmer)
→ Knowledge Area 7.5: Removal (e.g., recalls, returns, outdates, reverse distribution)

LEARNING OBJECTIVES

- [ ] Identify specific pharmacy technician roles in inventory management.
- [ ] Describe the importance of a formulary, including the differences between an open and a closed formulary.
- [ ] Explain the function and application of a National Drug Code (NDC) as well as lot numbers and expiration dates.
- [ ] Understand ordering and receiving processes, including how to maintain par levels and rotate stock.
- [ ] Identify specific storage requirements.
- [ ] Explain situations that can result in medications being removed from the pharmacy.

The pharmacy technician's role in inventory management is a significant part of his or her daily role. Inventory management may include returning prescriptions to stock, introducing new products to shelves, new generic product transitions, recalls, maintaining par levels, and completing cycle counts.

Each hospital maintains a specific formulary. A formulary is a continually updated list of medications stocked in the pharmacy. It is based on therapeutic implications, necessity, and cost. A hospital's Pharmacy and Therapeutics (P & T) Committee is composed of medical professionals who develop and maintain the formulary.

Formularies can be open or closed. Open formularies have no limitations to medication access; closed formularies have a concrete list of medications. Some institutions also have restrictions on their formularies, limiting institutional drug uses.

MEDICATION-SPECIFIC NUMBERS

The **National Drug Code**, most commonly referred to as the **NDC**, is a 10-digit, 3-segment number identifying the labeler (manufacturer), product, and package.

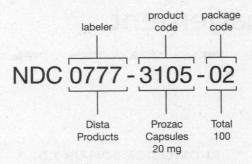

Figure 11-1. National Drug Code

The NCD consists of three segments:

- **FIRST SEGMENT:** This sequence of four or five numbers identifies the labeler (manufacturer or distributor). The Food and Drug Administration (FDA) assigns this segment.
- **SECOND SEGMENT:** These three or four middle digits refer to the package strength, dosage form, and formulation.
- **THIRD SEGMENT:** The final one or two digits identify the package form and size.

The NDC is used to verify product selections when filling a prescription. Pharmacy technicians can also scan the NDC bar code when ordering or to verify counts.

Medications contain a second set of numbers called a **lot number**. This is a unique number issued by the manufacturer. It is assigned to a batch of medications during production. This number helps to identify and, in the event of a problem, isolate any medications with potential problems that occurred during production. It is usually stamped on the side of the packaging. Recalls will always state the lot number(s) involved for consumer verification. When a pharmacy receives a recall notice, they will pull the medication from shelves, med-carts, and storage areas to return it to the manufacturer.

The third set of numbers that is found on medications is the **product expiration date**. This set of numbers can be found on over-the-counter (OTC) medications as well as on prescription medications. OTC medications and stock prescription medications receive an expiration date as determined by the manufacturer. Prescription medications that are repackaged and placed into vials for patient use also receive a beyond use date. Typically, the expiration dates for a prescription medication are set for one year from the date the medication is repackaged unless the manufacturer's expiration date comes before that. Medications that are reconstituted (e.g., children's antibiotics) and intravenous (IV) medications also have a beyond use date.

Expired medications may be returned to the distributor for reimbursement. Each distributor determines its own return policy and may require authorization before returns are accepted and reimbursement is granted. Pharmacy technicians must check for expired drugs. Some strategies used to decrease the amount of expired drugs in the pharmacy include using colored stickers to designate the month of expiration, writing the number associated with the month of expiration on the bottle in a visible area, and placing new products behind old products on the shelf (i.e., rotating stock).

ORDERING AND RECEIVING MEDICATIONS

Pharmacy technicians have a huge role in ordering and maintaining medications in the pharmacy. Although most of this process is completed electronically through computer management software, manual ordering and counts may be necessary at times. Pharmacies use auditing systems to check random medication counts (as determined by the computer). Technicians can verify these counts by taking a scanner, scanning the bar code of the medication in question, and then counting the drug to verify the count.

A **Periodic Automatic Replenishment (PAR) system** is an automated system used to track and maintain levels of medications to be kept at hand in the pharmacy at any given time. This system determines which medications to order for the next shipment based on the quantity at hand and the medication history. PAR levels should be accurate. However, the levels may be off at times. A technician can manually alter the number to reflect the current count. Recalls and expired drugs can affect these counts.

STORAGE REQUIREMENTS

Medication storage is dependent on instructions provided by the manufacturer. If instructions are not provided, the recommended conditions for storage at controlled room temperature, as indicated by USP, are considered to be 20°C to 25°C (68°F to 77°F).

Refrigerated medications should be kept in a medication-only refrigerator at a temperature of 2°C to 8°C (36°F to 46°F). Refrigerator temperature must be checked, verified, and documented daily to ensure that proper storage requirements are maintained.

In general, medications should be stored in their original containers. Some medications need to be stored in special packaging to protect the active drug from light and potential degradation. It is important to maintain proper labeling and affix auxiliary labels to bottles when applicable. Medications should also be stored in the same location, away from heat, sunlight, and humidity. Outdated and expired medications should be removed from the pharmacy and discarded according to pharmacy policy. The pharmacy may receive reimbursement for the medication from the wholesaler.

DRUG REMOVAL

Pharmacy technicians have to keep track of mediations that are leaving the pharmacy for reasons other than being sold to patients. Medications that are expired or recalled can be returned to the distributor.

Recalls can be subdivided into three categories, as outlined in Table 11-1. They are initiated by the manufacturer or the FDA and can be voluntary or involuntary depending on the severity of the situation.

Table 11-1. Medication Recalls

Medication Recalls*	
Class 1 Recall	A situation in which there is a reasonable probability that the use of or exposure to a violative product will cause serious adverse health consequences or death.
Class 2 Recall	A situation in which the use of or exposure to a violative product may cause temporary or medically reversible adverse health consequences or where the probability of serious adverse health consequences is remote.
Class 3 Recall	A situation in which the use of or exposure to a violative product is not likely to cause adverse health consequences.

*As per the U.S. Food and Drug Administration, 2009.

MEDWATCH

After a drug is approved, the FDA oversees phase IV clinical trials that examine long-term side effects of the drug. At this time, additional safety concerns may arise that require attention by the FDA. If dangerous side effects are found, a safer alternative is discovered, or if improper use is detected, that particular medication may be recalled by either the FDA or the manufacturer. In addition, the consumer also has a right to report problems with medications directly to the FDA through a monitoring system called MedWatch. Consumers can submit concerns to the FDA through this online reporting system.

SUMMARY

☐ The National Drug Code, or NDC, is a 10-digit sequence of numbers that identifies the labeler, product, and package size of the medication.

☐ Each medication receives an associated lot number that indicates where and when the medication was processed. This lot number is an important tool that is used to identify medications affected by a recall.

☐ Beyond use dates are determined by the manufacturer and are used to identify the medication expiration date.

☐ The hospital's Pharmacy and Therapeutics (P & T) Committee determines hospital formularies. This committee helps determine medication inclusions based on a variety of factors, including common usage, effectiveness, and cost.

☐ A formulary can be open, meaning that any drug can be prescribed. A formulary can also be closed, meaning that drugs must be selected from a list that is determined by the P & T Committee.

☐ Pharmacy technicians may be responsible for ordering and receiving prescriptions. They may also be responsible for performing cycle counts and maintaining par levels.

☐ Medications should be stored as indicated by the manufacturer. If refrigeration is necessary, a daily refrigerator log should be kept and refrigerator temperatures should be maintained at 2°C to 8°C (36°F to 46°F).

☐ In the event of a recall, the FDA (or the manufacturer) sends a request for the drug to be immediately removed from the pharmacy.

☐ Recalls are subdivided into three categories and are based on the severity of the adverse health effects.

☐ The FDA maintains an online reporting system, called MedWatch, for consumers to report problems with medications.

PHARMACY INVENTORY MANAGEMENT PRACTICE QUESTIONS

1. Which of the following is an example of a Class I recall?

   (A) A drug recall is issued when there is a strong likelihood that the product will cause serious adverse effects or death.
   (B) A drug recall is issued when there is a likelihood of temporary or reversible adverse effects.
   (C) A drug recall is issued when exposure to the product is unlikely to cause adverse drug effects.
   (D) None of the above.

2. The National Drug Code (NDC) contains 10 numbers. The first set of numbers indicates the _____.

   (A) labeler
   (B) product
   (C) quantity
   (D) interactions

3. Who may be responsible for initiating the drug recall process?

   (A) FDA
   (B) DEA
   (C) CDC
   (D) pharmacy

4. True or False: Pharmacy technicians do not participate in medication inventory procedures.

5. What is a PAR?

   (A) a system to determine recalls
   (B) a robot to help fill prescriptions
   (C) an automatic system used to help control inventory
   (D) a computer program that examines potential side effects

6. MedWatch is a monitoring system used by the FDA for consumers to report _____.

   (A) adverse drug reactions
   (B) concerns with pricing
   (C) requests for medication coupons
   (D) discrepancies with pharmacy personnel

7. A beyond use date is used to indicate the _____.

   (A) product expiration
   (B) recall status
   (C) lot number
   (D) NDC number

8. True or False: NDC numbers are the same for each medication within a drug class.

9. Who develops and maintains a hospital's formulary?

    (A) hospital business office
    (B) pharmacy department
    (C) insurance companies
    (D) Pharmacy and Therapeutics (P & T) Committee

10. Pharmacy refrigerators should be maintained at a temperature of _____.

    (A) 36°C to 46°C
    (B) 45°C to 55°C
    (C) 2°C to 8°C
    (D) 10°C to 18°C

ANSWERS EXPLAINED

1. **(A)** The FDA will issue a Class I recall if the use of or exposure to the medication will cause a serious adverse effect.

2. **(A)** The National Drug Code (NDC) is a set of 10 numbers, split into 3 segments, with each segment indicating a specific set of information. The first set of 4–5 numbers identifies the labeler or manufacturer of the drug.

3. **(A)** The FDA oversees the safety and effectiveness of drugs, and it can initiate a recall when there is an issue with safety or contamination. This process may also be initiated by the manufacturer.

4. **False** Pharmacy technicians are greatly involved in this process. They may help order, receive, and maintain inventory.

5. **(C)** The Periodic Automatic Replenishing (PAR) system is an automated system used to track and maintain levels of medication to be kept at hand in the pharmacy at any given time.

6. **(A)** Consumers can use the MedWatch online reporting system to report concerns about medications that they, or their dependents, have taken.

7. **(A)** A beyond use date is indicated on the prescription after reconstitution or compounding. It indicates the product expiration date.

8. **False** Each medication receives a unique NDC number indicating the labeler, product, and package quantity.

9. **(D)** The P & T Committee oversees all aspects of drug therapy, including the availability of drugs.

10. **(C)** Medication-specific refrigerators are monitored by pharmacy personnel and must be maintained at a temperature of 2°C to 8°C (36°F to 46°F).

Pharmacy Billing and Reimbursement

12

KNOWLEDGE DOMAIN 8.0

Pharmacy Billing and Reimbursement **8.75%**

→ Knowledge Area 8.1: Reimbursement policies and plans (e.g., HMOs, PPO, CMS, private plans)
→ Knowledge Area 8.2: Third-party resolution (e.g., prior authorization, rejected claims, plan limitations)
→ Knowledge Area 8.3: Third-party reimbursement systems (e.g., PBM, medication assistance programs, coupons, and self-pay)
→ Knowledge Area 8.4: Health care reimbursement systems (e.g., home health, long-term care, home infusion)
→ Knowledge Area 8.5: Coordination of benefits

LEARNING OBJECTIVES

☐ Understand reimbursement policies and plans.
☐ Be familiar with third-party resolution and systems.
☐ Understand health care reimbursement systems, including home health and home infusion.
☐ Understand coordination of benefits.

In 2013, the annual expenditure for prescription drugs in the United States was $329.2 million according to the IMS Institute for Health Care Informatics. The IMS also reported that patients are paying higher co-pays and deductibles. As prescription growth increases, understanding how to process insurance claims becomes a necessity. Pharmacies bill patients for their medications and deal with insurance issues, including prior authorizations.

REIMBURSEMENT POLICIES AND PLANS

Reimbursement for medications, medical supplies, and services, including Medication Therapy Management (MTM), are received through either private or public insurance or are paid for with cash.

Private Insurance Plans (Managed Care Organizations)

- **Health Maintenance Organizations (HMOs)** usually cover medications in-network and often require generic substitutions.

- **Preferred Provider Organizations (PPOs)** cover medications out-of-network but they will reimburse these at a lower rate than medications in-network. PPOs often require generic substitutions.

Public Insurance Plans (Government Plans)

- **The Centers for Medicare and Medicaid (CMS)** is a federal agency that administers the Medicare program and helps oversee the Medicaid program in conjunction with state governments.

  - **Medicaid:** This is a government insurance program, handled by the states, that offers insurance to individuals with low or no income. Individuals and families must meet state requirements. Having a low income alone does not guarantee Medicaid assistance. Individuals with disabilities may also qualify for this type of assistance.
  - **Medicare:** This is a national social insurance program that guarantees health care to individuals 65 and older. It also provides access to health care for individuals with disabilities and to those who have end-stage renal disease and/or ALS. Medicare can be split into different parts that cover specific services. Medicare Part A (hospital insurance) covers hospital services care, including care in a skilled nursing facility and hospice care. Medicare Part B (medical insurance) covers the patient's outpatient services, medical supplies, and preventive services. Medicare Part C (Medicare Advantage Plan) is a health plan offered by private insurance companies contracted with Medicare to provide Part A and Part B benefits. Medicare Part D (prescription drug coverage) covers outpatient prescription drugs.

- **TRICARE and Military Veterans** offers prescription assistance to families of military personnel. Military veterans receive their prescription benefits through the Veterans Health Administration (VHA).

Other Plans and Policies

- **Worker's compensation** consists of a series of benefits that vary according to state law. However, it generally provides compensation, including medical benefits, to employees injured on the job. These insurance claims are billed directly to the patient's worker's compensation plan.

THIRD-PARTY RESOLUTION

After entering prescription information and insurance information into the computer system, a claim must be sent to the patient's insurance company or other third-party payers. The third party will respond online within moments stating if the claim is paid or has been rejected. This process is called adjudication.

> **Third party:** Another party, besides the patient or pharmacy, that pays for part of, or all of, the medication; usually referred to as an insurer.
>
> **Adjudication:** A term used to refer to the process of paying or denying claims submitted after comparing the claim to the patient's benefit or coverage requirements.
>
> **Co-pay:** A fixed amount paid by the patient after insurance.

If a claim is denied, pharmacy personnel will have to determine the reason and solution, if available, to relay to the patient. Common rejections are due to prior authorizations, plan limitations, and rejected claims.

Prior authorizations are used by insurance companies to prevent improper prescribing of drugs. Each insurance company forms its own prior authorization lists. Medications on this list require physician approval before authorization is granted. This process takes additional time, and patients need to be alerted that they may need to wait 24–48 hours before receiving a response. If a prior authorization is not granted, a patient can still receive the drug, but the patient will have to pay the entire retail cost of the drug. The patient can also contact the prescriber to prescribe an alternate drug.

Rejected claims, or **rejections**, are most commonly seen for medications that are not covered or medications that require prior authorizations. Other reasons may include an incorrect day's supply of the medication, refilling a medication too soon, an incorrect patient identification number, incomplete prescriber information, or an invalid medication quantity.

As a pharmacy technician, you should be aware of **plan limitations**. Insurance companies can limit the quantity of the medication that a patient may receive in a given time. Other limitations can be placed on where the prescription may be filled (retail or mail order). Age limitations may also apply to children or dependents of the cardholder.

If a patient has more than one insurance provider, a coordination of benefits must be determined to provide maximum coverage for the patient. This process includes determining the primary and secondary coverage types and then submitting the claim to the insurance companies in that order. Patients with both private and public insurance coverage must submit their claim to the private plan before submission to the public plan is accepted.

REIMBURSEMENT SYSTEMS

Various third-party reimbursement systems are available. These include Pharmacy Benefits Managers (PBMs), medication assistance programs, coupons, and self-pay.

The **Pharmacy Benefits Manager (PBM)** processes pharmacy claims and acts as the third-party administrator of prescription drug programs for insurance companies.

Medication assistance programs and **coupons** are available for patients who cannot self-pay. Medication assistance programs are provided by state, corporate, pharmaceutical, or private prescription assistance programs to help patients obtain free or low-cost medications. Qualifications may be based on income, disease state, age, or other qualifying factors. Coupons are provided by the pharmaceutical company and allow patients to receive a particular drug for low or no cost for a specific amount of time (one month, multiple months, and so on). These coupons contain a bin and a group number similar to a prescription card, and they are processed the same way.

In other health care practice settings (i.e., home health, long-term care, and home infusion), reimbursement for pharmacy services is handled differently. Reimbursement is usually based off a fee-for-service methodology or an episode-of-care approach. In **fee-for-service methodology**, providers receive reimbursement for services rendered. The provider charges a fee, and the health insurance company pays for their service. Each service has a set price and is known as a charge. In the **episode-of-care approach**, providers receive reimbursement based on the condition they are treating. This method varies from fee-for-service methodology because payment is not given for each individual service.

SUMMARY

☐ Reimbursements for medications and supplies are made through third-party payers. Familiarity with common private and public managed care companies is necessary in order to fill prescriptions and resolve common issues.

☐ Patients with multiple insurance providers may require a coordination of benefits to ensure maximum coverage.

☐ Claim denials may require the attention of pharmacy personnel and/or the provider.

☐ An incorrect patient ID, group number, bin number, or drug are just a few reasons why a claim may be rejected. Patient and drug information, the correct day's supply, and the "refill too soon" error should all be verified in order to fill a prescription successfully.

☐ Information pertaining to prescription rejects, including prior authorizations and prescription updates, should be relayed to patients at drop off.

☐ Reimbursement systems are available to patients to assist with part or all of their prescription cost.

☐ Qualifications for coverage vary and are dependent on the organization that is providing the subsidy.

☐ Medication coupons, provided by pharmaceutical companies, can be input like insurance cards and submitted similarly.

☐ Reimbursements for pharmacy services in health care settings are based on a fee-for-service or an episode-of-care approach. Compensation for services is determined by individual pharmacy encounters or a set of services for a disease state.

PHARMACY BILLING AND REIMBURSEMENT PRACTICE QUESTIONS

1. Which of the following is NOT an example of a claim denial?

   (A) incorrect patient identification number
   (B) incorrect day's supply
   (C) incorrect date of birth
   (D) incorrect label

2. True or False: Prior authorizations may require attention from the provider.

3. Which of the following is NOT a group that administers pharmacy benefits?

   (A) DEA
   (B) HMO
   (C) Medicaid
   (D) PPO

4. Which of the following is NOT an example of a plan limitation?

   (A) patient's age
   (B) quantity of medication
   (C) location of refills at a retail or mail order setting
   (D) All of the above are examples of plan limitations.

5. Coordination of benefits _____.

    (A) helps provide maximum benefits for patients with one insurance provider

    (B) helps provide maximum benefits for patients with more than one insurance provider

    (C) provides patients with an option to purchase another insurance plan

    (D) provides medications to patients at a preset price

6. The part that a customer pays on his or her prescription, after insurance, is called the _____.

    (A) premium

    (B) discount

    (C) co-pay

    (D) coordination of benefits

7. Which of the following is true regarding prior authorizations?

    (A) The insurance company may require the prescriber to call the company to validate the necessity of the medication.

    (B) The patient may have to wait 24–48 hours to receive authorization on a prior authorization request.

    (C) The prior authorization may be denied and, therefore, the medication will not be covered under insurance.

    (D) All of the above.

8. True or False: A worker's compensation claim is billed directly to the patient's worker's compensation plan and not to his or her insurance.

9. The term adjudication means _____.

    (A) the process of filling a prescription from beginning to end

    (B) requesting that the prescriber contact the insurance company to validate the medication's necessity

    (C) a denial of a prescription claim

    (D) the process of paying or denying a claim after it has been submitted to the insurance company

10. True or False: Pharmaceutical companies do not offer prescription assistance programs for selective medications.

ANSWERS EXPLAINED

1. **(D)** An incorrect patient identification number, day's supply, or date of birth can result in a rejection following online submission of a claim. An incorrect prescription label is physically put onto a prescription bottle and is not sent to the insurance company.

2. **True** Prior authorization requests may require a provider to contact the insurance company and verify why the patient needs to take the prescription.

3. **(A)** The DEA is a federal agency that oversees the regulation and scheduling of controlled substances.

4. **(D)** A plan can limit the number of prescriptions for various reasons, including the patient's age (e.g., the plan may not cover the medication for a pediatric population), quantity of medication (e.g., the plan covers only a 30-day supply), and location of refills (e.g., the plan covers refills of chronic medications only at a mail order pharmacy).

5. **(B)** Coordination of benefits is used to determine which insurance provider has primary responsibility and which one has secondary responsibility in paying for the prescription. This system ensures that claims are paid correctly and that patient benefits are maximized.

6. **(C)** The co-pay is a predetermined amount that the patient pays to the pharmacy for the prescription.

7. **(D)** All of the choices are true regarding prior authorizations.

8. **True** A patient's worker's compensation claim is billed directly to the worker's compensation plan for reimbursement.

9. **(D)** Adjudication is the process of paying or denying a prescription claim and is completed in real time via an online claims processor.

10. **False** Pharmaceutical companies *do* offer prescription assistance programs for select medications. The patient must contact the manufacturer directly in order to apply for and receive the assistance.

Pharmacy Information Systems Usage and Application

13

KNOWLEDGE DOMAIN 9.0

Pharmacy Information Systems Usage and Application   10.00%

→ Knowledge Area 9.1: Pharmacy-related computer applications for documenting the dispensing of prescriptions or medication orders (e.g., maintaining the electronic medical record, patient adherence, risk factors, alcohol drug use, drug allergies, side effects)

→ Knowledge Area 9.2: Databases, pharmacy computer applications, and documentation management (e.g., user access, drug database, interface, inventory report, usage reports, override reports, diversion reports)

LEARNING OBJECTIVES

☐ Understand the use of computers and the types of software used, including their functions.

☐ Describe the role of pharmacy information systems in prescription and inventory management.

☐ Understand the advantages and challenges associated with the implementation of pharmacy information systems.

☐ Identify standards and technologies used in the development, management, and implementation of pharmacy information systems.

☐ List the various reports and patient-monitoring functions used in pharmacy practice.

PHARMACY INFORMATION SYSTEMS

Pharmacy information systems (PIS) are complex pharmacy integration systems that allow for prescription and inventory management. These systems vary. However, they are all designed to meet the specific needs of the pharmacy by collecting, processing, reporting, and using information.

Pharmacy information systems should be able to do the following:

- Process data efficiently
- Present information in a simplified form
- Interpret information to identify potential problems

- Use technology to share information
- Provide an action to the user's response
- Provide feedback

Implementing pharmacy information systems has both advantages and challenges. The advantages include:

- Enhanced patient safety
- Increased workflow efficiency
- Improved communication among health care professionals
- Enhanced delivery of patient-sensitive information
- Increased quality of care
- Improved reimbursement procedures

The challenges include:

- The need for continuous support and upgrades to the pharmacy information system
- Barriers in accessing different databases (e.g., databases may vary from one pharmacy to the next)
- Security concerns, including the transmission of patient-sensitive information, user access, and data access
- Alert fatigue due to excessive alerts used in clinical decision support systems (CDS), which may result in pharmacist overrides

Good pharmacy information systems take large amounts of data and process them efficiently. The information generated is used to manage pharmacy resources, determine inventory and supply, request medication refills, or even estimate demand. These systems also improve accountability by capturing pharmacy activity, including inventory, for pharmacy audits.

In order to implement pharmacy information systems, one or more computers, appropriate software, databases, and interfaces are needed. A computer is a machine that stores and processes data according to a set of instructions or programs and then performs tasks based on that input. Different types of computers exist. For example, main computers store large quantities of information. In contrast, dummy computers allow multiples users to access data. Computers contain input devices that help obtain information. These input devices include scanners, keyboards, a mouse, bar codes, and fingerprint recognition devices. Computers also contain output devices, such as the monitor and printers. These output devices are critical for displaying information.

Software is one or more programs used to operate computers. System software, or operation systems, controls the integration of hardware components. Application software, or word processors, accomplishes specific tasks. Application software may consist of individual programs or of larger software systems, such as database management systems.

A database is a collection of information. **Pharmacoinformatics** is the use of information technology to improve medication-related patient health care. One way this field of study has helped improve patient outcomes is by improving drug information support and drug utilization review services. A drug database is a master list of medications. A drug database is dependent on setting and pharmacy usage. In contrast, a pharmacy database is an inventory of pharmacy personnel's biographical and demographic data. For example, personal information pertaining to employees can be kept in this database, including their hiring date, previous employment, qualifications and licensure, salary history, and benefits.

Interfaces are boundaries by which two or more computer systems share information. Pharmacy interfaces are an essential component of pharmacy practice. Without an appropriate system in place, prescription times would be longer, patient records would be inaccessible, and patients would ultimately be frustrated. Two types of pharmacy interfaces exist. The first is a pharmacy-based system. It allows the pharmacy to enter prescriptions that, in turn, are connected to a medical record. The second system, a facility-based system, allows medication orders to be connected to a medical record and pushed to the pharmacy upon request.

STANDARDS AND TECHNOLOGY

The National Council for Prescription Drug Programs (NCPDP) has created a set of standards for the electronic exchange of health information. These standards include:

- Electronic audit requests
- Formulary and benefits
- Prescription and prior authorization transfers
- Codified prescription sig formatting
- Telecommunications
- Medicaid subrogation
- Financial information reporting
- Connectivity operating rules
- SCRIPT

SCRIPT is a standard developed by the NCPDP in order to facilitate the transfer of prescription and medication history information among the pharmacy, the provider, and the computers. This list of standards helps support the exchange of information, including new prescriptions, refill requests, medication history, prior authorization requests, and structured and codified sig codes. Improvements have also been made to drug utilization review alerts, clinical exchanges, allergies, and diagnosis information.

Additionally, the inclusion of various technologies expanded several functions that are provided by pharmacy information systems. The use of bar code technology offered a means of reducing medication errors. Bar code technology can also be used to identify a patient or verify a medication by checking the NDC. These measures are used to assist in processing and delivering medications. Pharmacies have also employed the use of interactive voice response (IVR) systems. These systems are commonly used by many businesses and allow customers to interact with databases to acquire information. The system interacts with people based on prompts, voice responses, or touch-tone responses. Pharmacies commonly rely on IVR technology. Callers can request refills or speak to a staff member, authorized health professionals can call in prescriptions, and prior authorization requests can be started for prescriptions with no remaining refills.

Pharmacy information systems can be used in a variety of ways:

1. Electronic health records
2. Clinical screenings
3. Prescription management
4. Inventory management
5. Patient profiles

6. Medication profiles

7. Report generation

Electronic health records (EHR) contain patient-sensitive information that is transmitted digitally through health information exchanges (HIE). Patient demographics, medication history, laboratory results, medical history, allergies, and billing information can be digitally stored and transferred across electronic interchanges.

Pharmacy information systems are also useful with **clinical screenings**. For example, patient-monitoring functions, also known as clinical decision support systems, help pharmacy personnel analyze and filter data in order to make a clinical decision. The computer system will check for issues and flag or alert the user when an interaction is picked up. Table 13-1 provides examples of these screenings.

Table 13-1. Patient Monitoring Functions

Patient Monitoring Function	Description
Therapeutic duplication	Identifies medications with the same indication or in the same pharmacological drug class
Drug-allergy interactions	Cross-checks the patient record to identify drugs noted as a patient allergy
Drug-drug interactions	Identifies medications that may cause problems if taken simultaneously
Drug-food interactions	Identifies medications and foods that may be problematic if taken simultaneously
Drug-disease interactions	Identifies drugs that may cause problems with a patient's medical condition, age, weight, or other physiological factors
Drug-laboratory test interactions	Detects medication orders that may interfere with specific laboratory tests
Intravenous (IV) compatibility	Checks medication orders for potential problems with physical incompatibilities and stability

Pharmacy information systems provide a means of **prescription management** in both inpatient and outpatient settings. Prescriptions are received via CPOE, e-prescribing, or other means. The computer system matches the prescription order to available pharmaceutical products, locates the patient and prescriber profiles, and dispenses the product accordingly. The pharmacy can interact with the system to track prescriptions by:

- Prescriber information
- Date written
- Controlled/noncontrolled
- Brand/generic drug
- Manufacturer
- Drug class or indication
- Date dispensed
- Pharmacists and technicians involved in prescription processing

The system can also be used to print prescription labels, access clinical information, and interact with similar in-network computer systems to refill or transfer prescriptions, as well as to provide instructions about how the medication should be taken.

Inventory management systems are tedious, time consuming, and difficult to maintain. Pharmacies require continuous inventory assessments and audits to ensure that product is available, being ordered, and that the counts are not off. Pharmacy information systems maintain an internal inventory of all pharmaceutical products. This system can provide alerts when set quantities are not met, reorder products electronically based on past trends or usage, and provide supplier information when necessary.

Patient profiles are personal profiles that contain patient-sensitive information, including the patient's name, birth date, address, and other physiological information. The pharmacy information system can locate a patient's profile by using search parameters, including the patient's last name and birth date.

The **medication profile** is intertwined with the patient profile. The medication profile provides the past prescribing history of all medications, including the prescriber's information and the strength and quantity of the medication prescribed. The operator can check if a patient received the medication from a specific manufacturer. The operator can even determine if a medication has been discontinued or changed. Pharmacists use this profile to perform clinical assessments and determinations on medication appropriateness each time a medication is ordered for the patient.

Pharmacies rely on **generated reports** to determine trends and profit/loss, perform audits, alter inventory, and so on. These reports can be automatically generated, or they can be accessed by the user when needed. Reports can be tracked, stored in the pharmacy interface, sent to another party, or printed to be filed in the pharmacy. Table 13-2 provides examples of reports that are used in pharmacy practice.

Table 13-2. Reports Used in the Pharmacy

Type of Report	Description
Diversion report	A diversion report accounts for significant theft or loss of a controlled substance. This form is then submitted in writing to the appropriate DEA Field Division Office. A DEA form 106 ("Report of Theft or Loss of Controlled Substances") is also filed.
Inventory reports	Inventory reports are used to determine inventory counts based on the section, manufacturer, day/time/year, distributor cost, etc.
Override reports	Override reports are used by pharmacy personnel to determine the pharmacy personnel users that "override" or disregard warnings or safety measures that are employed by the system. These reports can help determine if pharmacy personnel are trying to manipulate the system or even remove medication without an order.
Usage report	Usage reports are an evaluation of patterns and/or trends of medications (e.g., medication usage by quantity or dollar amount).

SUMMARY

☐ Pharmacy information systems employ the use of computers and technology to provide an efficient and safe method of maintaining patient and medication information.

☐ These systems assist pharmacy personnel in processing, filling, and dispensing medications through the use of assisted technologies.

☐ Pharmacy personnel should be familiar with technologies used in the pharmacy and their role in pharmacoinformatics.

PHARMACY INFORMATION SYSTEMS USAGE AND APPLICATION PRACTICE QUESTIONS

1. Which of the following is a database used in pharmacy practice?

    (A) clinical trial database
    (B) product expiration date database
    (C) drug database
    (D) None of the above.

2. The National Council for Prescription Drug Programs (NCPDP) provides standards for the electronic exchange of health information. Which of the following is NOT an example of a standard instituted by the NCPDP?

    (A) SCRIPT
    (B) codified sig reporting
    (C) prescriber demographic reporting
    (D) financial information reporting

3. Which of the following is an example of an output tool?

    (A) keyboard
    (B) mouse
    (C) scanner
    (D) monitor

4. Which of the following statements best describes pharmacoinformatics?

    (A) the integration of information technology to improve patient health care, including medication-related data and knowledge
    (B) the use of information technology to replace a pharmacist's retained knowledge
    (C) the integration of information technology to access patient data
    (D) using pharmacy computer systems to process prescriptions

5. The clinical decision support system contains patient parameters used to assist pharmacists in making clinical decisions. Which of the following is NOT an example of a patient parameter used in this system?

    (A) drug-drug interactions
    (B) drug-vitamin interactions
    (C) food-food interactions
    (D) IV incompatibilities

6. An interface provides a boundary by which information is shared between what two components used in pharmacy information systems?

    (A) printers
    (B) scanners
    (C) computers
    (D) software

7. What type of software system is used to provide integration of hardware components?

    (A) system software
    (B) application software
    (C) printer software
    (D) clinical software

8. What type of information can be saved in a patient's electronic health record (EHR)?

    (A) medical history
    (B) billing information
    (C) allergies
    (D) All of the above.

9. Which of the following is NOT an example of a potential challenge seen when implementing pharmacy information systems?

    (A) the need for continued support
    (B) increased quality of care
    (C) alert fatigue
    (D) security concerns

10. Which of the following is an advantage of using a digital inventory management system?

    (A) The system will reorder products based on a competing pharmacy's usage trends.
    (B) The system will reorder products based on past usage trends.
    (C) The system requires continuous inventory assessments.
    (D) The system is equipped to order medications once a week.

ANSWERS EXPLAINED

1. **(C)** Drug databases are an essential component of any pharmacy information system. They provide the basis for product selection and management. Currently, pharmacy information systems do not incorporate exclusive clinical trial or product expiration date databases. Clinical trials can be searched using an outside database like PubMed (provided by the U.S. National Library of Medicine). Product expiration dates can be verified by searching the drug database and the product's NDC.

2. **(C)** Standards for prescriber demographic reporting have not been instituted by the NCPDP. The prescriber's education and background are typically verified by a governing agency (e.g., state medical board, state nursing board, department of professional regulation, DEA).

3. **(D)** Monitors are a type of output tool used to display information. A keyboard, mouse, and scanner are all examples of input tools used to obtain information.

4. **(A)** Pharmacy information systems are used to integrate information technology into pharmacy practice. Various components are used to achieve this process. The ultimate goal is to improve patient health outcomes. Pharmacoinformatics is not used to replace a pharmacist's retained information. It is not primarily used to access patient data or to just process prescriptions by using a computer.

5. **(C)** Food-food interactions are not tracked by the clinical decision support system. Pharmacies can maintain a record of patient allergies, but a medical practitioner evaluates specific food allergies.

6. **(C)** Interfaces provide a means of communication among two or more computer systems, resulting in an exchange of information. Printers, scanners, and software systems do not use interface boundaries to communicate. Rather, they institute a series of output ports (connections) that allow for the transfer of signals.

7. **(A)** System software allows for the integration of hardware components and is often referred to as the operating system. Application software is used to operate specific tasks. Printer and clinical software can be classified as types of application software.

8. **(D)** The patient's EHR maintains all of the patient's information pertinent to filling a prescription. This information includes the patient's medical history, billing information, and allergies.

9. **(B)** Pharmacy information systems have many challenges and require continued support, training, updates, and maintenance. Pharmacists can develop alert fatigue due to flagged interactions or alerts being displayed. Maintaining secure connections and compliance with HIPAA guidelines are also potential challenges. Ultimately, these systems should assist pharmacy personnel in improving patients' quality of care.

10. **(B)** In manual inventory systems, medications and supplies are tracked on paper and require constant counting to ensure that quantities on hand are correct. The potential for error in manual systems is great. The evolution of digital support systems helps alleviate this issue and provides pharmacy personnel with a means of counting, ordering, and reordering medications easily with the assistance of technology.

Practice Tests

ANSWER SHEET
Practice Test 1

1. Ⓐ Ⓑ Ⓒ Ⓓ
2. Ⓐ Ⓑ Ⓒ Ⓓ
3. Ⓐ Ⓑ Ⓒ Ⓓ
4. Ⓐ Ⓑ Ⓒ Ⓓ
5. Ⓐ Ⓑ Ⓒ Ⓓ
6. Ⓐ Ⓑ Ⓒ Ⓓ
7. Ⓐ Ⓑ Ⓒ Ⓓ
8. Ⓐ Ⓑ Ⓒ Ⓓ
9. Ⓐ Ⓑ Ⓒ Ⓓ
10. Ⓐ Ⓑ Ⓒ Ⓓ
11. Ⓐ Ⓑ Ⓒ Ⓓ
12. Ⓐ Ⓑ Ⓒ Ⓓ
13. Ⓐ Ⓑ Ⓒ Ⓓ
14. Ⓐ Ⓑ Ⓒ Ⓓ
15. Ⓐ Ⓑ Ⓒ Ⓓ
16. Ⓐ Ⓑ Ⓒ Ⓓ
17. Ⓐ Ⓑ Ⓒ Ⓓ
18. Ⓐ Ⓑ Ⓒ Ⓓ
19. Ⓐ Ⓑ Ⓒ Ⓓ
20. Ⓐ Ⓑ Ⓒ Ⓓ
21. Ⓐ Ⓑ Ⓒ Ⓓ
22. Ⓐ Ⓑ Ⓒ Ⓓ
23. Ⓐ Ⓑ Ⓒ Ⓓ
24. Ⓐ Ⓑ Ⓒ Ⓓ
25. Ⓐ Ⓑ Ⓒ Ⓓ
26. Ⓐ Ⓑ Ⓒ Ⓓ
27. Ⓐ Ⓑ Ⓒ Ⓓ
28. Ⓐ Ⓑ Ⓒ Ⓓ
29. Ⓐ Ⓑ Ⓒ Ⓓ
30. Ⓐ Ⓑ Ⓒ Ⓓ

31. Ⓐ Ⓑ Ⓒ Ⓓ
32. Ⓐ Ⓑ Ⓒ Ⓓ
33. Ⓐ Ⓑ Ⓒ Ⓓ
34. Ⓐ Ⓑ Ⓒ Ⓓ
35. Ⓐ Ⓑ Ⓒ Ⓓ
36. Ⓐ Ⓑ Ⓒ Ⓓ
37. Ⓐ Ⓑ Ⓒ Ⓓ
38. Ⓐ Ⓑ Ⓒ Ⓓ
39. Ⓐ Ⓑ Ⓒ Ⓓ
40. Ⓐ Ⓑ Ⓒ Ⓓ
41. Ⓐ Ⓑ Ⓒ Ⓓ
42. Ⓐ Ⓑ Ⓒ Ⓓ
43. Ⓐ Ⓑ Ⓒ Ⓓ
44. Ⓐ Ⓑ Ⓒ Ⓓ
45. Ⓐ Ⓑ Ⓒ Ⓓ
46. Ⓐ Ⓑ Ⓒ Ⓓ
47. Ⓐ Ⓑ Ⓒ Ⓓ
48. Ⓐ Ⓑ Ⓒ Ⓓ
49. Ⓐ Ⓑ Ⓒ Ⓓ
50. Ⓐ Ⓑ Ⓒ Ⓓ
51. Ⓐ Ⓑ Ⓒ Ⓓ
52. Ⓐ Ⓑ Ⓒ Ⓓ
53. Ⓐ Ⓑ Ⓒ Ⓓ
54. Ⓐ Ⓑ Ⓒ Ⓓ
55. Ⓐ Ⓑ Ⓒ Ⓓ
56. Ⓐ Ⓑ Ⓒ Ⓓ
57. Ⓐ Ⓑ Ⓒ Ⓓ
58. Ⓐ Ⓑ Ⓒ Ⓓ
59. Ⓐ Ⓑ Ⓒ Ⓓ
60. Ⓐ Ⓑ Ⓒ Ⓓ

61. Ⓐ Ⓑ Ⓒ Ⓓ
62. Ⓐ Ⓑ Ⓒ Ⓓ
63. Ⓐ Ⓑ Ⓒ Ⓓ
64. Ⓐ Ⓑ Ⓒ Ⓓ
65. Ⓐ Ⓑ Ⓒ Ⓓ
66. Ⓐ Ⓑ Ⓒ Ⓓ
67. Ⓐ Ⓑ Ⓒ Ⓓ
68. Ⓐ Ⓑ Ⓒ Ⓓ
69. Ⓐ Ⓑ Ⓒ Ⓓ
70. Ⓐ Ⓑ Ⓒ Ⓓ
71. Ⓐ Ⓑ Ⓒ Ⓓ
72. Ⓐ Ⓑ Ⓒ Ⓓ
73. Ⓐ Ⓑ Ⓒ Ⓓ
74. Ⓐ Ⓑ Ⓒ Ⓓ
75. Ⓐ Ⓑ Ⓒ Ⓓ
76. Ⓐ Ⓑ Ⓒ Ⓓ
77. Ⓐ Ⓑ Ⓒ Ⓓ
78. Ⓐ Ⓑ Ⓒ Ⓓ
79. Ⓐ Ⓑ Ⓒ Ⓓ
80. Ⓐ Ⓑ Ⓒ Ⓓ
81. Ⓐ Ⓑ Ⓒ Ⓓ
82. Ⓐ Ⓑ Ⓒ Ⓓ
83. Ⓐ Ⓑ Ⓒ Ⓓ
84. Ⓐ Ⓑ Ⓒ Ⓓ
85. Ⓐ Ⓑ Ⓒ Ⓓ
86. Ⓐ Ⓑ Ⓒ Ⓓ
87. Ⓐ Ⓑ Ⓒ Ⓓ
88. Ⓐ Ⓑ Ⓒ Ⓓ
89. Ⓐ Ⓑ Ⓒ Ⓓ
90. Ⓐ Ⓑ Ⓒ Ⓓ

Practice PTCE Test 1

Directions: You will have 1 hour and 50 minutes to complete the following 90 questions. For each question, select the choice that best answers the question, and mark that answer letter on your answer sheet. Remember, this test should be used to help you determine areas that require additional review. Each question represents a particular area of the PTCE blueprint, which can help you pinpoint areas of mastery or concepts that require additional studying. The official PTCE exam uses a scaled score to determine your grade. Only 80 out of 90 questions on the PTCE are scored, and unscored questions are not identified. You should be able to answer about 75 of the questions on this test correctly, averaging an overall percentage of 80% or more on your attempt at this test.

1. How many mL of 70% and 40% alcohol elixirs should be mixed to prepare 300 mL of 60% alcohol?

   (A) 200 mL of 70%, 100 mL of 40%
   (B) 100 mL of 70%, 200 mL of 40%
   (C) 75 mL of 70%, 25 mL of 40%
   (D) 50 mL of 70%, 250 mL of 40%

2. The Poison Prevention Packaging Act of 1970 was created for what reason?

   (A) to ensure that pharmacists provide counseling to patients
   (B) to reduce the amount of unintentional poisoning involving animals
   (C) to reduce accidental poisoning incidences involving children
   (D) to establish two separate drug classes: Rx (prescription) and OTC (over-the-counter)

3. Which of the following is an example of a Class II recall?

   (A) foreign objects that pose a physical hazard
   (B) a label mix-up on a lifesaving drug
   (C) a medication container defect or malfunctioning drug delivery device
   (D) All of the above.

4. The Roman numeral XXXVI is equal to _____.

   (A) 34
   (B) 36
   (C) 26
   (D) 24

5. Many terminally ill patients on pain medications require increasingly higher doses to obtain pain relief. This is known as _____.

   (A) tolerance
   (B) addiction
   (C) dependence
   (D) habituation

6. Which of the following is FALSE?

   (A) Syrups contain sugar, usually to mask the bitter taste of some medications.
   (B) Elixirs contain oil and water and should be shaken well before use.
   (C) Suspensions must be shaken well before use.
   (D) A solution contains a drug that is completely dissolved.

7. Which of the following TPN substrates provides the most calories per gram?

    (A) alcohol
    (B) amino acids
    (C) dextrose
    (D) lipids

8. What is the appropriate form required for a pharmacy to order Schedule II medications from a distributor?

    (A) DEA form 222
    (B) DEA form 41
    (C) DEA form 106
    (D) None of the above.

9. Hydrocortisone 0.5% cream in a 1-ounce tube contains _____.

    (A) hydrocortisone 141.75 mg in 28.35 g of cream
    (B) hydrocortisone 0.4175 g in 100 mg of cream
    (C) hydrocortisone 0.4175 g in 28.35 g of cream
    (D) hydrocortisone 28.35 mg in 141.75 g of cream

10. How many prednisone 5 mg tablets are needed to fill a prescription with the following directions?

    prednisone 5 mg tablets

    take $\frac{1}{2}$ tab PO QID × 2 days

    $\frac{1}{2}$ tab PO TID × 2 days

    $\frac{1}{2}$ tab PO BID × 2 days

    $\frac{1}{2}$ tab PO QD × 2 days

    Then stop

    (A) 5
    (B) 10
    (C) 20
    (D) 30

11. How much Gentamicin 40 mg/mL is needed for a 130 mg dose?

    (A) 2 mL
    (B) 2.25 mL
    (C) 3 mL
    (D) 3.25 mL

12. The four aspects of pharmacokinetics include _____.

    (A) absorption, distribution, mitosis, and excretion
    (B) absorption, distribution, migration, and excretion
    (C) absorption, distribution, metastasis, and excretion
    (D) absorption, distribution, metabolism, and excretion

13. Ibuprofen can be given to a child at a dose of 10 mg/kg. What is the dose for a 44 lb child?

    (A) 200 mg
    (B) 220 mg
    (C) 440 mg
    (D) 968 mg

14. Concentrated sodium chloride solution (23.4%) contains 4 mEq/mL. How much (in mL) is needed to provide 40 mEq of NaCl for a parenteral nutrition admixture?

    (A) 23.4 mL
    (B) 10 mL
    (C) 4 mL
    (D) 40 mL

15. What does "DAW" mean on a written prescription?

    (A) "Take one tablet by mouth once daily."
    (B) "The medication should be taken with food."
    (C) "The brand name medication is to be dispensed as written, no generic substitution."
    (D) It refers to the registration number of the prescriber.

16. Which of the following statements is true?

    (A) LVPs are usually smaller than 100 mL and are infused continuously.
    (B) LVPs are usually greater than 100 mL and are infused intermittently.
    (C) SVPs (IVPBs) are usually smaller than 100 mL and are infused intermittently.
    (D) SVPs (IVPBs) are usually greater than 100 mL and are infused continuously.

17. Drug manufacturers assign drugs a unique identifying number. This is called a National Drug Code (NDC). Which of the following information is NOT indicated by an NDC number?

    (A) manufacturer/distributor
    (B) DEA schedule number
    (C) product code
    (D) package quantity

18. Which federal act was passed to provide for privacy requirements to safeguard identifiable health information?

    (A) Omnibus Budget Reconciliation Act (OBRA '90)
    (B) The Poison Prevention Packaging Act of 1970
    (C) The Food, Drug, and Cosmetic Act (FDC)
    (D) Health Insurance Portability and Accountability Act (HIPAA)

19. Look at the following sig.

    1 tab PO BID AC and HS

    What instructions should be typed on the customer label?

    (A) "Take one capsule by mouth twice a day before meals and at bedtime."
    (B) "Take one tablet by mouth twice a day before meals and at bedtime."
    (C) "Take one tablet by mouth twice a day after meals and at bedtime."
    (D) "Take one capsule by mouth twice a day after meals and at bedtime."

20. Which of the following liquid drug dosage forms contains concentrated sucrose solutions?

    (A) suspension
    (B) elixir
    (C) syrup
    (D) tincture

21. Pharmacy technicians check refrigerators used to hold medications daily and log temperature data. When checking the temperature of a refrigerator, an appropriate range is _____.

    (A) −4° to 14°F
    (B) 36° to 46°F
    (C) 46° to 59°F
    (D) 68° to 77°F

22. Laminar flow hoods need to be certified every _____.

    (A) 3 months
    (B) 6 months
    (C) 1 year
    (D) 2 years

23. How many teaspoons are in 1 ounce?

    (A) 1 teaspoon
    (B) 3 teaspoons
    (C) 6 teaspoons
    (D) 8 teaspoons

24. National health insurance provided to citizens or permanent residents ages 65 years and older is called _____

    (A) Medicare
    (B) Medicaid
    (C) premium
    (D) Pharmacy Benefits Manager

25. A laminar flow hood helps provide a clean working environment needed for compounding. What direction does the air flow in a vertical laminar flow hood?

    (A) from the top of the hood to the bottom
    (B) from the back of the hood to the front
    (C) from the sides of the hood to the top
    (D) from the bottom of the hood to the top

26. Which of the following is NOT a unit-dose item?

    (A) Sucralfate 1 g/10 mL
    (B) Tylenol liquid 325 mg/10 mL
    (C) ibuprofen liquid 2.4 g/120 mL
    (D) Benadryl elixir 12.5 mg/5 mL

27. Most prescriptions, with the exception of controlled substances, are valid for
    _____.

    (A) 6 months or 5 refills
    (B) a 3-month supply because of lower insurance co-pays
    (C) 12 months from the date written
    (D) 12 months from the date filled

28. A medication is to be taken "PC." It should be taken _____.

    (A) in the morning
    (B) in the evening
    (C) before meals
    (D) after meals

29. Oxycodone is a DEA Schedule II drug. This means that the drug has a _____ potential for abuse and _____ accepted medical uses in the United States.

    (A) high; no currently
    (B) low; no currently
    (C) high; currently
    (D) low; currently

30. The Combat Methamphetamine Epidemic Act (CMEA) restricts the sale of which of the following?

    (A) Robitussin
    (B) Delsym
    (C) Sudafed
    (D) Zyrtec

31. HIPAA is a federal law that sets rules and limits on who may view what type of health information?

    (A) electronic
    (B) written
    (C) spoken
    (D) All of the above.

32. What class of drugs is used to treat elevated blood pressure?

    (A) antihistamines
    (B) antihypertensives
    (C) anticoagulants
    (D) antihyperlipidemics

33. If a laminar flow hood is turned off, it must be run for _____ minutes before it can be used again.

    (A) 10
    (B) 20
    (C) 30
    (D) 60

34. A technician must work at least _____ inches inside a laminar flow hood when compounding prescriptions.

    (A) 2
    (B) 6
    (C) 10
    (D) 14

35. The FDA does NOT require which of the following to be on a prescription label?

    (A) drug name
    (B) prescriber name
    (C) drug instructions
    (D) National Drug Code

36. Xanax is listed as a Schedule IV drug in Ohio. Xanax expires after _____ and may have up to _____ refills.

(A) 1 year; no
(B) 6 months; no
(C) 6 months; 5
(D) 1 year; 5

37. Convert 86°F to degrees Celsius.

(A) 20°C
(B) 25°C
(C) 30°C
(D) 35°C

38. The Combat Methamphetamine Epidemic Act places _____ and _____ limits on the over-the-counter sale of products containing pseudoephedrine.

(A) daily, weekly
(B) daily, monthly
(C) weekly, monthly
(D) monthly, yearly

39. How many mL are in 4 L of NS?

(A) 40 mL
(B) 400 mL
(C) 4,000 mL
(D) 40,000 mL

40. A patient weighs 50 kg. What is his weight in lb?

(A) 50 lb
(B) 100 lb
(C) 110 lb
(D) 200 lb

41. A doctor has written a prescription for 10 mL of brand "X" antibiotic suspension to be taken twice daily. How many days will an 8-ounce bottle last?

(A) 10 days
(B) 12 days
(C) 14 days
(D) 16 days

42. HMOs and PPOs are examples of

(A) Pharmacy Benefits Managers
(B) Medication Assistance Programs
(C) Managed Care Organizations
(D) Medication Therapy Management

43. Mixing powders of unequal quantity is called _____.

(A) geometric dilution
(B) spatulation
(C) levigation
(D) emulsion

44. Which regulatory agency could initiate a Class II medication recall?

(A) DEA
(B) ASHP
(C) TJC
(D) FDA

45. Which route of administration is NOT a parenteral route?

(A) intravenous
(B) intradermal
(C) vaginal
(D) oral

46. Which of the following is an autoimmune disease in which the thyroid is overactive and produces excessive amounts of thyroid hormones?

(A) HIV/AIDS
(B) hyperlipidemia
(C) Grave's disease
(D) hypothyroidism

47. If two drugs are taken together and one of them intensifies the action of the other, what type of drug interaction has occurred?

    (A) additive
    (B) synergistic
    (C) potentiated
    (D) antagonistic

48. Which of the following herbal medications can be used to promote relaxation?

    (A) kava
    (B) ginseng
    (C) garlic
    (D) ephedra

49. Which of the following medications is NOT used to treat hyperlipidemia?

    (A) Prilosec
    (B) Zetia
    (C) Caduet
    (D) Zocor

50. The drug name Synthroid is also known as the _____ name.

    (A) chemical
    (B) generic
    (C) brand
    (D) supplier

51. What is the most important step to prevent contamination of an IV product?

    (A) hand washing
    (B) gowns and gloves
    (C) the laminar flow hood
    (D) bleach

52. The percent equivalent of a 1:80 ratio is _____%.

    (A) 1.5
    (B) 1.3
    (C) 1.25
    (D) 1

53. Which of the following dosage forms would NOT be recommended for a patient who has an allergy to alcohol?

    (A) suspension
    (B) ointment
    (C) elixir
    (D) syrup

54. Patients should be instructed to rinse well following corticosteroid use _____.

    (A) due to the potential for candidiasis
    (B) to help relieve headaches
    (C) to prevent future cavities
    (D) to freshen breath

55. What type of drug is metoprolol?

    (A) proton-pump inhibitor (PPI)
    (B) beta blocker
    (C) diuretic
    (D) antihistamine

56. A term used to describe the harmful and undesired effects produced by a medication when taken at normal doses is called

    _____.

    (A) potentiation
    (B) a contraindication
    (C) synergism
    (D) an adverse drug reaction

57. SCRIPT was developed by the NCPDP in order to _____.

    (A) transmit a patient's sensitive information digitally
    (B) transfer prescription and medication history among the pharmacy, the provider, and the computer systems
    (C) help pharmacy personnel analyze and filter through data in order to make a clinical decision
    (D) reduce medication errors by using bar coding technology

58. Which is NOT a violation of HIPAA?

   (A) discussing a patient's information with his or her spouse without the patient's approval
   (B) not asking a patient if he or she would like a HIPAA privacy disclosure
   (C) asking the patient to verify his or her date of birth before picking up his or her prescription
   (D) releasing a patient's records to an unauthorized party

59. Mrs. Smith is picking up an order of drug "X" #50 tablets, which cost her $120. While you're ringing up her order, she asks, "How much does each tablet cost?" What is she being charged for each tablet?

   (A) $1.20
   (B) $1.80
   (C) $2.40
   (D) $2.80

60. What size needle has the largest diameter?

   (A) 24
   (B) 22
   (C) 18
   (D) 16

61. A drug patent lasts _____ years beginning on the _____ date.

   (A) 10; filing
   (B) 10; drug approval
   (C) 20; filing
   (D) 20; drug approval

62. What percent strength of sterile isopropyl alcohol is used to clean a laminar flow hood?

   (A) Do not use isopropyl alcohol.
   (B) 70% isopropyl alcohol
   (C) 95% isopropyl alcohol
   (D) 99% isopropyl alcohol

63. If the manufacturer's expiration date for a drug is 12/18, the drug is considered acceptable to dispense until which date?

   (A) 12/31/18
   (B) 12/01/18
   (C) 12/15/18
   (D) 12/07/18

64. Licensing and general professional oversight of pharmacists and pharmacies are carried out by the _____.

   (A) Department of Professional Regulation
   (B) Federal Drug Administration
   (C) State Board of Pharmacy
   (D) American Society of Health-System Pharmacists (ASHP)

65. Nitroglycerin is provided as a sublingual tablet. This means that the tablet should be dissolved _____.

   (A) in a cup of water
   (B) under the tongue
   (C) in the eye
   (D) in normal saline

66. The type of formulary that allows the pharmacy to obtain all medications that are prescribed is a(n) _____ formulary.

   (A) closed
   (B) patient
   (C) open
   (D) physician

67. The abbreviation "au" means _____.

   (A) right ear
   (B) both ears
   (C) left eye
   (D) both eyes

68. A script is presented for "Zocor 20 mg PO QHS." The pharmacy is currently out of Zocor 20 mg. Which of the following may the pharmacist substitute to fill the order?

    (A) atorvastatin
    (B) simvastatin
    (C) candesartan
    (D) losartan

69. A _____ protects a brand name drug from unauthorized use.

    (A) patent
    (B) copyright
    (C) trademark
    (D) symbol

70. Which clinical trial phase includes 20–100 individuals and tests for safety?

    (A) Phase I
    (B) Phase II
    (C) Phase III
    (D) Phase IV

71. What is the maximum number of refills allowed for a Schedule II medication?

    (A) 0 refills
    (B) 1 refills
    (C) 5 refills
    (D) 12 refills

72. Which of the following is NOT a side effect of the ACE inhibitor lisinopril?

    (A) angioedema
    (B) cough
    (C) rash
    (D) fever

73. There are _____ ounces (oz) in a pound (lb).

    (A) 2
    (B) 8
    (C) 16
    (D) 24

74. Which of the following databases includes a master list of medications?

    (A) drug database
    (B) pharmacy database
    (C) employee database
    (D) system database

75. A certified pharmacy technician must complete _____ hours of continuing education (CE) every _____ year(s).

    (A) 10; 1
    (B) 10; 2
    (C) 20; 1
    (D) 20; 2

76. All of the following drug combinations are at risk for a look-alike/sound-alike error EXCEPT for _____.

    (A) Aciphex and Accupril
    (B) Zebeta and Diabeta
    (C) amoxicillin and cephalexin
    (D) Sinemet and Janumet

77. How would pharmacy personnel identify a medication in a drug recall situation?

    (A) check the medication name
    (B) check the lot number
    (C) check the medication instructions
    (D) look for opened medications

78. Which of the following is an example of "coordination of benefits"?

    (A) submission of a pharmacy claim to a primary insurance payer in order to maximize plan contributions before submitting to a secondary payer
    (B) calling an insurance payer to determine the prescription coverage on a prescription
    (C) submission of a prior authorization request to a third-party payer
    (D) processing an insurance claim through the primary payer only

79. A 70% HCl solution has a strength of 25 mEq/mL. How many mL are needed to prepare 60 mEq?

(A) 1.2 mL
(B) 1.7 mL
(C) 2.1 mL
(D) 2.4 mL

80. Pyxis® and medDISPENSE® are examples of _____.

(A) robotic filling machines
(B) laminar flow hoods
(C) automated dispensing machines
(D) DUR programs

81. Medicare Part _____ covers outpatient prescription drugs.

(A) A
(B) B
(C) C
(D) D

82. Which of the following is NOT an example of a drug interaction?

(A) drug-drug
(B) drug-laboratory
(C) therapeutic duplication
(D) food-environment

83. Which of the following must appear on a written prescription for a controlled substance?

(A) indication
(B) patient medication history
(C) DEA number
(D) patient's social security number

84. A package insert must be dispensed with which of the following?

(A) products containing conjugated estrogen
(B) antihistamines
(C) antifungal ointments
(D) OTC first-aid products

85. Which of the following terms refers to a computer that allows multiple users to access data?

(A) main computer
(B) dummy computer
(C) operating computer
(D) system computer

86. When calculating w/v%, the percentage refers to _____.

(A) mg/100 mL
(B) g/100 mL
(C) mg/100 L
(D) g/100 L

87. On average, how many drops are in 1 mL?

(A) 5 drops
(B) 10 drops
(C) 20 drops
(D) 30 drops

88. Which of the following error prevention strategies may NOT be used when entering a prescription into the computer system?

(A) Verifying the patient's name, address, date of birth, and allergies before inputting the patient's prescription.
(B) Placing the patient's filled medication, stock bottle, and used and original prescription in a pharmacy bin or tray for the pharmacist to perform a drug utilization review.
(C) Using a bar code check system to verify a medication's NDC before filling a prescription.
(D) Making an offer to have the pharmacist counsel the patient.

89. Which of the following is an example of an insurance plan coverage limitation?

    (A) The patient's insurance is not on file.
    (B) The duration of therapy is incorrect.
    (C) The prescriber information is incorrect.
    (D) The wrong person code is listed.

90. Which of the following error prevention strategies is NOT used to reduce medication errors?

    (A) the use of alerts, warnings, and flags in the computer systems
    (B) using independent double checks for high-alert medications
    (C) using nonstandardized sig codes when writing prescriptions
    (D) maintaining proper training procedures, including infection control procedures

ANSWER KEY
Practice Test 1

1. **A**	31. **D**	61. **C**
2. **C**	32. **B**	62. **B**
3. **A**	33. **C**	63. **A**
4. **B**	34. **B**	64. **C**
5. **A**	35. **D**	65. **B**
6. **B**	36. **C**	66. **C**
7. **D**	37. **C**	67. **B**
8. **A**	38. **B**	68. **B**
9. **A**	39. **C**	69. **A**
10. **B**	40. **C**	70. **A**
11. **D**	41. **B**	71. **A**
12. **D**	42. **C**	72. **D**
13. **A**	43. **A**	73. **C**
14. **B**	44. **D**	74. **A**
15. **C**	45. **D**	75. **D**
16. **C**	46. **C**	76. **C**
17. **B**	47. **C**	77. **B**
18. **D**	48. **A**	78. **A**
19. **B**	49. **A**	79. **D**
20. **C**	50. **C**	80. **C**
21. **B**	51. **A**	81. **D**
22. **B**	52. **C**	82. **D**
23. **C**	53. **C**	83. **C**
24. **A**	54. **A**	84. **A**
25. **A**	55. **B**	85. **B**
26. **C**	56. **D**	86. **B**
27. **C**	57. **B**	87. **C**
28. **D**	58. **C**	88. **A**
29. **C**	59. **C**	89. **B**
30. **C**	60. **D**	90. **C**

ANSWERS EXPLAINED

1. **(A)** You will need 200 mL of 70% solution and 100 mL of 40% solution. To answer this question, you need to follow five essential steps:

(STEP 1) Set up your alligation problem using the sample setup below.

Strength of higher strength component (H)		P – L = relative amount of H needed to prepare P
	Desired strength of product (P)	
Strength of lower strength component (L)		H – P = relative amount of L needed to prepare P

70 (H)		P – L = 60 – 40 = 20 parts
	60 (P)	
40 (L)		H – P = 70 – 60 = 10 parts

(STEP 2) Add the part values in the right-hand column together to get the total part value of the product.

$$10 + 20 = 30 \text{ parts}$$

(STEP 3) Divide each part value by the total parts.

The amount of 70% alcohol is $\frac{20}{30}$ of the final product.

The amount of 40% alcohol is $\frac{10}{30}$ of the final product.

(STEP 4) Solve for the volume of alcohol needed for each concentration.

To solve for the volume of 70% alcohol needed:

$$300 \text{ mL} \times \frac{20}{30} = 200 \text{ mL of 70\% alcohol needed}$$

To solve for the volume of 40% alcohol needed:

$$300 \text{ mL} \times \frac{10}{30} = 100 \text{ mL of 40\% alcohol needed}$$

(STEP 5) Check your work to see if your answer makes sense.

When 200 mL of 70% alcohol are mixed with 100 mL of 40% alcohol, the resulting solution is 300 mL of 60% alcohol. Therefore, choice (A)—200 mL of 70%, 100 mL of 40%— is correct. Choice (B) is incorrect because it reverses the mL for 70% and 40%. Choice (C) cannot be the answer because the sum of the respective quantities does not equal the total amount of solution. Choice (D) incorrectly reflects a $\frac{1}{4}$ reduction in the total amount of 70% alcohol solution needed. The total amount of 40% alcohol solution is incorrect in choice (D) as well. (*Knowledge Domain 3.6*)

2. **(C)** The Poison Prevention Packaging Act of 1970 requires childproof packaging on all controlled and most prescription drugs. Containers that are not childproof may be used only if the prescriber or patient requests one. Choice (A) represents the Omnibus Budget Reconciliation Act of 1990 (OBRA '90), which requires that pharmacists offer counseling to Medicaid patients regarding their medications. Choice (B) is incorrect because the Poison Prevention Packaging Act of 1970 does not address packaging regulations for animals. Choice (D) represents the Durham-Humphrey Amendment of 1951, which differentiates between two classes of medications, prescription and over-the-counter medications. This amendment also defines those drugs that must be prescribed by a licensed practitioner. (*Knowledge Domain 6.6*)

3. **(A)** Foreign objects that pose a physical hazard are an example of a Class II recall. This type of recall is defined by the FDA as "a situation in which the use of or exposure to a product may cause temporary or medically reversible adverse health consequences or the probability of serious adverse health consequences is remote." Choice (B) is an example of a Class I recall. This type of recall is defined as "a situation where there is a reasonable probability that the use of or exposure to a product will cause serious adverse health consequences or death." Choice (C) is an example of a Class III recall, which is defined as a situation in which "the use of or exposure to a product is not likely to cause adverse health consequences." Since choices (B) and (C) are not examples of a Class II recall, choice (D) is incorrect as well. (*Knowledge Domain 2.10*)

4. **(B)** The Roman numeral XXXVI is equal to 36. Each X equals 10, each V equals 5, and each I equals 1. Therefore, 10 + 10 + 10 + 5 + 1 = 36. Choice (A) would be correct if the question was asking for the equivalence of XXXIV. Since X equals 10 and IV equals 4, this Roman numeral equals 10 + 10 + 10 + 4 = 34. Choice (C) would be true if the question asked for the equivalence of XXVI. Since X equals 10, V equals 5, and I equals 1, this Roman numeral equals 10 + 10 + 5 + 1 = 26. Choice (D) would be right if the question asked for the equivalence of XXIV. Since X equals 10 and IV equals 4, this Roman numeral equals 10 + 10 + 4 = 24. (*Knowledge Domain 6.2*)

5. **(A)** Tolerance is defined as the need for larger or increased doses to achieve the desired response. Addiction, choice (B), is defined as a pattern of compulsive use, characterized by an overwhelming pattern of drug use and abuse. Dependence, choice (C), is defined as an altered state where continued administration of the drug is necessary to prevent physical and psychological withdrawal. Habituation, choice (D), is defined as becoming accustomed to a behavior or condition, including psychoactive drug use. (*Knowledge Domain 1.5*)

6. **(B)** This statement is false. Elixirs contain alcohol and water, with the alcohol content ranging from 5–40%. All of the other statements are true. (*Knowledge Domain 3.5*)

7. **(D)** Lipids provide the most calories per gram: 9 cal/g. Alcohol is the second highest with 7 cal/g. Amino acids and dextrose are considerably lower. Amino acids provide 4 cal/g and dextrose provides 3.4 cal/g. (*Knowledge Domain 3.6*)

8. **(A)** DEA form 222 can be used to order both Schedule I and Schedule II drugs. DEA form 41, choice (B), is used to return or destroy drugs that are pending DEA approval. DEA form

106, choice (C), is used to report the theft or loss of controlled substances. (*Knowledge Domain 2.4*)

9. **(A)** A percentage weight in weight solution (w/w) is the number of grams of a constituent in 100 grams of mixture. So 0.5% cream is 0.5 grams in 100 grams of mixture. Perform the necessary calculations:

$$\frac{0.5 \text{ g}}{100 \text{ g}} = \frac{x}{28.35 \text{ g}}$$

$$(0.5 \text{ g})(28.35 \text{ g}) = x(100 \text{ g})$$

$$14.175 = 100x$$

$$x = 0.14175 \text{ g}$$

Since no answer contains this amount, convert grams to milligrams:

$$1,000 \text{ mg} = 1 \text{ g}$$

$$0.14175 \times 1,000 = 141.75 \text{ mg}$$

The correct amount is 141.75 mg in 28.35 g of cream, choice (A). (*Knowledge Domain 3.7*)

10. **(B)** To fill this prescription, 10 prednisone 5 mg tablets are needed. To answer this question, solve for how many tabs of QID, TID, BID, and QD are needed:

$$\frac{1}{2} \text{ tab PO QID} \times 2 \text{ days} = 2.5 \times 4 = 10 \text{ mg} \times 2 = 20 \text{ mg} = 4 \text{ tabs}$$

$$\frac{1}{2} \text{ tab PO TID} \times 2 \text{ days} = 2.5 \times 3 = 7.5 \text{ mg} \times 2 = 15 \text{ mg} = 3 \text{ tabs}$$

$$\frac{1}{2} \text{ tab PO BID} \times 2 \text{ days} = 2.5 \times 2 = 5 \text{ mg} \times 2 = 10 \text{ mg} = 2 \text{ tabs}$$

$$\frac{1}{2} \text{ tab PO QD} \times 2 \text{ days} = 2.5 \times 1 = 2.5 \text{ mg} \times 2 = 5 \text{ mg} = 1 \text{ tab}$$

$$4 \text{ tabs} + 3 \text{ tabs} + 2 \text{ tabs} + 1 \text{ tab} = 10 \text{ tablets}$$

The answer is 10 tablets. (*Knowledge Domain 6.3*)

11. **(D)**

$$\frac{40 \text{ mg}}{1 \text{ mL}} = \frac{130 \text{ mg}}{x}$$

$$40x = 130$$

$$x = 3.25 \text{ mL}$$

The answer is 3.25 mL, choice (D). (*Knowledge Domain 6.3*)

12. **(D)** The four aspects of pharmacokinetics include absorption, distribution, metabolism, and excretion. The acronym ADME can be used to remember this process. Choice (A) is wrong because mitosis is not a part of pharmacokinetics. Choices (B) and (C) mistakenly include "migration" and "metastasis," respectively, instead of "metabolism." (*Knowledge Domain 1.2*)

13. **(A)** The correct dose is 200 mg. Since 1 kg = 2.2 lb:

$$\frac{1 \text{ kg}}{2.2 \text{ lb}} = \frac{x}{44 \text{ lb}}$$

$$2.2x = 44$$

$$x = 20 \text{ kg}$$

Therefore:

$$\frac{10 \text{ mg}}{1 \text{ kg}} \times 20 \text{ kg} = 200 \text{ mg dose}$$

220 mg, choice (B), reflects an error in the conversion calculation of lb to kg. When dividing 44 lb by 2.2 lb, 22 kg is mistakenly the answer, rather than 20 kg:

$$10 \text{ mg} \times 22 \text{ kg} = 220 \text{ mg dose}$$

Choice (C), 440 mg, reflects more than double the dose of ibuprofen that should be given to a 20 kg child. Choice (D), 968 mg, reflects more than quadruple the dose of ibuprofen that should be given to a 20 kg child. (*Knowledge Domain 6.3*)

14. **(B)** If NaCl = 4 mEq/ml, then:

$$\frac{4 \text{ mEq}}{1 \text{ mL}} = \frac{40 \text{ mEq}}{x}$$

Cross multiply and solve for *x*:

$$x = 10 \text{ mL}$$

The correct amount is 10 mL, choice (B). (*Knowledge Domain 3.6*)

15. **(C)** DAW is an acronym for the phrase "dispense as written." Choice (A) is an example of the prescription "signa" and indicates the directions for use and the administration route. Choice (B) is an example of an auxiliary label that is applied to the prescription container. The prescriber's registration number, choice (D), is referred to as the Drug Enforcement Agency (DEA) number. (*Knowledge Domain 6.2*)

16. **(C)** Small-volume parenterals, or SVPs, are packaged products that are either directly administered to a patient or added to another parenteral formulation. They are available in solutions of 100 mL or less. Choice (A) is incorrect because LVPs, or large-volume parenterals, are intravenous solutions packaged in containers holding 100 mL or more. They are generally infused continuously because of their large volume and slow infusion rate. Choice (B) is incorrect because large-volume parenterals are generally infused continuously, not intermittently. Choice (D) is incorrect because small-volume parenterals are packaged products that are generally available in solutions less than 100 mL. They can be introduced into the ongoing LVP or put into a minibag and used as a piggyback on the LVP intermittently. (*Knowledge Domain 3.5*)

17. **(B)** The question asks for which information is NOT indicated by an NDC number, like the one below:

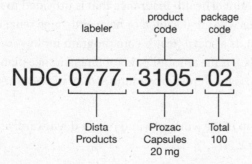

The manufacturer/distributor number, choice (A), can be located by looking at the first set of numbers on the NDC code. The product code, choice (C), can be determined by looking at the second set of numbers on the NDC code. The package quantity, choice (D), can be determined by looking at the third set of numbers on the NDC code. Therefore, the DEA schedule number, choice (B), is the correct answer because this is the only piece of information listed in the answer choices that cannot be deciphered by looking at the NDC. (*Knowledge Domain 7.1*)

18. **(D)** Choice (D) is correct because the Health Insurance Portability and Accountability Act provides for privacy requirements to safeguard identifiable health information. Choice (A) is incorrect because the Omnibus Budget Reconciliation Act of 1990 was enacted to provide three main components: drug utilization review (DUR), record-keeping requirements, and an offer to counsel all Medicaid patients. Choice (B) is incorrect because the Poison Prevention Packaging Act of 1970 requires the use of child-resistant packaging on most prescription and over-the-counter medications and hazardous materials. Choice (C) is incorrect because the Food, Drug, and Cosmetic Act grants authority to the Food and Drug Administration (FDA) to oversee the safety of drugs, foods, and cosmetics. (*Knowledge Domain 2.8*)

19. **(B)** The label should advise the customer to take one tablet by mouth twice a day before meals and at bedtime. Choice (A) is incorrect because "tab" refers to a tablet, not a capsule. Capsule is the incorrect dosage form. Choice (C) is incorrect because the sig "ac" refers to "before meals," not "after meals." Choice (D) contains the same errors as choices (A) and (C). (*Knowledge Domain 6.5*)

20. **(C)** Syrups are concentrated sucrose solutions where sugar is used to mask the taste of the medication. Suspensions, choice (A), are prepared when solid particles are dispersed but not completely dissolved in the solvent. Elixirs, choice (B), are sweetened liquids that contain concentrations of alcohol. Tinctures, choice (D), are alcoholic solutions of nonvolatile substances. (*Knowledge Domain 1.4*)

21. **(B)** *USP* <797> defines the temperature range of 36° to 46° F as "cold." When in this range, the temperature is maintained thermostatically. Choice (A) is the appropriate temperature range for a freezer. Choice (C) is a temperature range that the *USP* <797> defines as "cool." Choice (D) is an appropriate temperature range for working areas. (*Knowledge Domain 7.4*)

22. **(B)** Laminar flow hoods should be certified every 6 months. (*Knowledge Domain 3.1*)

23. **(C)** One ounce is equal to 30 mL. One teaspoon is equal to 5 mL. Therefore, $\frac{30}{5}$ = 6 teaspoons, choice (C). (*Knowledge Domain 6.2*)

24. **(A)** Medicare is a national health insurance that is provided to individuals ages 65 years and older. Individuals who are disabled or have end-stage renal disease may also qualify. Medicaid, choice (B), is a social health care program for low- or no-income individuals. A premium, choice (C), is the amount paid for an insurance plan. The Pharmacy Benefits Manager, choice (D), is the third-party administrator of prescription services. (*Knowledge Domain 8.1*)

25. **(A)** Air enters the top of the work area and moves downward, as described in choice (A). (*Knowledge Domain 2.11*)

26. **(C)** 2.4 g/120 mL refers to the quantity of ibuprofen in 120 mL of ibuprofen solution. This quantity is too large to be taken at one time. Instead, it refers to the total quantity to be

dispensed for the prescription. Sucralfate, choice (A), and Tylenol, choice (B), can each be compounded or purchased in a 10 mL one-time use dose. Benadryl, choice (D), can be compounded or purchased in a 5 mL one-time use dose. (*Knowledge Domain 3.7*)

27. **(C)** A majority of noncontrolled prescriptions are valid for 12 months from the date written. Choice (A) is wrong because although laws vary from state to state, some states may place limitations on Schedule III and IV controlled substances. Choice (B) is incorrect because insurance does not determine the validity of a prescription. Choice (D) is wrong because prescription filling laws are determined from the date the prescription is written, not the fill date. (*Knowledge Domain 7.1*)

28. **(D)** A medication that is "PC" should be taken after meals. In the morning, choice (A), is written as "AM." In the evening, choice (B), is written as "PM." Before meals, choice (C), is written as "AC." (*Knowledge Domain 6.2*)

29. **(C)** Oxycodone has a high potential for abuse and currently accepted medical uses in the United States. Choice (A) is the definition of a Schedule I drug. Choice (B) is not an appropriate definition of a scheduled drug. Choice (D) is the definition of a Schedule IV drug. (*Knowledge Domain 1.6*)

30. **(C)** Sudafed contains the active ingredient pseudoephedrine, which is restricted by the CMEA. None of the other drugs are restricted by the CMEA. (*Knowledge Domain 2.7*)

31. **(D)** All types of health information are protected under the HIPAA privacy act. (*Knowledge Domain 2.8*)

32. **(B)** Antihypertensives treat high blood pressure. Antihistamines, choice (A), treat allergies. Anticoagulants, choice (C), work to prevent the clotting of blood. Antihyperlipidemics, choice (D), lower lipid levels. (*Knowledge Domain 1.6*)

33. **(C)** A laminar flow hood should run for at least 30 minutes to reestablish air flow. (*Knowledge Domain 2.11*)

34. **(B)** All sterile compounding inside the hood should take place at least 6 inches inside the hood. (*Knowledge Domain 3.6*)

35. **(D)** The drug name, prescriber name, and drug instructions can all be found on the prescription label. The national drug code is not found on the prescription label. (*Knowledge Domain 6.5*)

36. **(C)** Federal law states that Schedule III through Schedule V medications may be refilled up to 5 times in 6 months. (*Knowledge Domain 6.1*)

37. **(C)** $°C = (°F - 32) \times \frac{5}{9}$; $°C = (86 - 32) \times \frac{5}{9} = 54 \times \frac{5}{9} = 30°C$ (*Knowledge Domain 7.4*)

38. **(B)** The Combat Methamphetamine Epidemic Act (CMEA) places a maximum limit of 3.6 g/day and 9 g/month of base product. (*Knowledge Domain 2.7*)

39. **(C)** 1 L = 1,000 mL. Therefore, 4 L = 4,000 mL. (*Knowledge Domain 6.3*)

40. **(C)** 1 kg = 2.2 lb. Therefore, 50 kg × 2.2 = 110 lb. (*Knowledge Domain 6.3*)

41. **(B)** 1 oz = 30 mL and 8 oz = 240 mL. The patient is taking 20 mL a day. So the bottle will last $\frac{240}{20} = 12$ days. (*Knowledge Domain 6.1*)

42. **(C)** Health Maintenance Organizations (HMOs) and Preferred Provider Organizations (PPOs) are both examples of Managed Care Organizations that provide reimbursement for medications, medical supplies, and services. Pharmacy Benefits Managers process pharmacy claims and act as the third-party administrator of prescription drug programs for insurance companies. A Medication Assistance Program is provided through state, corporate, pharmaceutical, or private prescription assistance programs to help patients obtain medications at free or low-cost. Medication Therapy Management is a term used to describe medical services, provided by pharmacists, used to optimize drug therapy and improve patient outcomes. *(Knowledge Domain 8.1)*

43. **(A)** Geometric dilution is used when mixing powders of unequal quantity. Spatulation, choice (B), involves mixing powders with a spatula. Levigation, choice (C), is a technique used to reduce particle size by triturating with a solvent. A mixture of two drugs that are normally immiscible is an emulsion, choice (D). *(Knowledge Domain 6.4)*

44. **(D)** The FDA and/or the manufacturer may initiate recalls on medications. *(Knowledge Domain 7.5)*

45. **(D)** Intravenous, intradermal, and vaginal are all parenteral routes. Sublingual (oral) is an enteral route. *(Knowledge Domain 1.4)*

46. **(C)** Grave's disease results in the overproduction of thyroid hormones. HIV/AIDS, choice (A), is an infection caused by the human immunodeficiency virus. Choice (B) is incorrect because hyperlipidemia causes elevated lipid levels in the blood. Hypothyroidism, choice (D), causes an underactive thyroid, so this is incorrect. *(Knowledge Domain 1.6)*

47. **(C)** A potentiated interaction is an interaction that occurs when one drug intensifies the activity of another drug. An additive interaction, choice (A), is an interaction that results when two drugs given in combination have an effect equal to the sum of the individual effects. A synergistic interaction, choice (B) is an interaction where two drugs that are taken together produce greater effects than when they are taken separately. An antagonist interaction, choice (D), happens when drugs given in combination cause a decreased, or diminished, effect in one or more drugs. *(Knowledge Domain 1.3)*

48. **(A)** Kava has properties that cause relaxation and may be taken to relieve anxiety. Ginseng, choice (B), is used for its stimulant effects. Garlic, choice (C), is rich in antioxidants and is used for its cardioprotective effects. Ephedra, choice (D), is a supplement that has been banned in the United States but has noted uses for nasal congestion, weight loss, and the ability to increase energy. *(Knowledge Domain 1.6)*

49. **(A)** Prilosec belongs to a class of medications known as proton-pump inhibitors. It is used to treat gastroesophageal reflux disease (GERD) and other conditions resulting in excess stomach acid. *(Knowledge Domain 1.6)*

50. **(C)** Synthroid is the brand name of this drug. Choice (A) is incorrect because it refers to the atomic structure of the drug. Choice (B) is incorrect because Synthroid is not the generic name of this drug. The generic name for Synthroid is levothyroxine. Choice (D) is incorrect because Synthroid does not refer to the name of the drug supplier. *(Knowledge Domain 1.1)*

51. **(A)** Hand washing is an easy, aseptic technique to remove disease-causing bacteria. *(Knowledge Domain 3.1)*

52. **(C)** Percent is defined as parts per 100:

$$\frac{1}{80} = \frac{x}{100}$$

$$\frac{100}{80} = x$$

$$x = 1.25$$

The answer is 1.25, choice (C). (*Knowledge Domain 6.3*)

53. **(C)** An elixir is a solution of sucrose and hydroalcoholic liquids. This should be avoided in patients with an alcohol allergy. A suspension, ointment, or syrup would all be acceptable for a patient with an alcohol allergy. A suspension contains a solid (with a small particle size) dispersed in a liquid. An ointment contains an active drug in an ointment (oleaginous) base. A syrup contains sucrose and water. (*Knowledge Domain 1.4*)

54. **(A)** Inhaled corticosteroids can depress your immune system. This can lead to an increased chance for thrush to form and accumulate in the oral cavity. (*Knowledge Domain 1.5*)

55. **(B)** Metoprolol is a beta blocker that is used in the treatment of hypertension. Examples of proton-pump inhibitors (PPIs), choice (A), are omeprazole and esomeprazole. PPIs are used in the treatment of GERD and excess stomach acid. Diuretics, choice (C), include triamterene and furosemide. They are used in the treatment of hypertension. Antihistamines, choice (D), may include loratadine and diphenhydramine, which are used in the treatment of allergies. (*Knowledge Domain 1.6*)

56. **(D)** An adverse drug reaction is a term used to describe an unintended side effect. A reaction that occurs when one drug intensifies the activity of another drug is called potentiation, choice (A). A contraindication, choice (B), is the possibility of unwanted side effects. A contraindication is a reason why a patient should not take a particular medication. In a synergism reaction, choice (C), two drugs that are taken together produce greater effects than when either drug is taken separately. (*Knowledge Domain 1.5*)

57. **(B)** SCRIPT is a standard developed by the NCPDP to facilitate the transfer of prescription and medication history information among the pharmacy, the provider, and the computer systems. Choice (A) is an example of how the electronic health record (EHR) is transmitted digitally through the health information exchange (HIE). Choice (C) is a description of the clinical decision support system. Choice (D) is an example of technology incorporated into the pharmacy information system. (*Knowledge Domain 9.1*)

58. **(C)** Pharmacy personnel must verify patient information before allowing the person to pick up his or her prescription. Choice (A) is wrong because patient information may not be discussed with a spouse without written consent of the patient. Choice (B) is incorrect because all patients must be informed of their right to receive a HIPAA privacy disclosure. Choice (D) is incorrect because this is a direct violation of HIPAA. Patient records may be shared only with authorized individuals, and each instance must be documented. (*Knowledge Domain 4.1*)

59. **(C)** To figure out the cost per tablet, you need to take the total cost and divide it by the number of tablets. In this case, $\frac{120 \text{ dollars}}{50 \text{ tablets}} = \$2.40$. (*Knowledge Domain 8.3*)

60. **(D)** The smaller the size of the needle, the larger the diameter. (*Knowledge Domain 3.5*)

61. **(C)** A drug patent is valid for 20 years beginning on the date the application was originally filed. (*Knowledge Domain 1.1*)

62. **(B)** The *USP* has found that sterile 70% isopropyl alcohol is the best concentration to use when disinfecting a laminar flow hood. (*Knowledge Domain 3.1*)

63. **(A)** The drug is considered valid until the last day of that month. (*Knowledge Domain 7.1*)

64. **(C)** The State Board of Pharmacy oversees the regulation of pharmacists, technicians, and interns. (*Knowledge Domain 2.13*)

65. **(B)** The term *sublingual* means to dissolve "under the tongue." (*Knowledge Domain 6.2*)

66. **(C)** Open formularies allow for all medications to be prescribed. A closed formulary, choice (A), limits the medications that are prescribed to those on the formulary. Choice (B), patient formulary, is incorrect because there are no patient-specific formularies. Choice (D) does not accurately answer the question. (*Knowledge Domain 7.2*)

67. **(B)** The abbreviation "au" refers to both ears. The abbreviation "ad" is used to indicate the right ear. The abbreviation "os" is used to indicate the left eye. The abbreviation "ou" refers to both eyes. (*Knowledge Domain 6.2*)

68. **(B)** Simvastatin is the generic therapeutic equivalent for the brand name drug Zocor. Atorvastatin, choice (A), is the generic therapeutic equivalent for the brand name drug Lipitor. Candesartan, choice (C), is the generic therapeutic equivalent for the brand name drug Atacand. Losartan, choice (D), is the generic therapeutic equivalent for the brand name drug Cozaar. (*Knowledge Domain 1.2*)

69. **(A)** A patent is a right granted to an entity and prohibits others from copying or selling that product for a set period of time. A copyright, choice (B), gives an entity the right to copy, print, and use material. A trademark, choice (C), is a proprietary term that represents a company or an organization. Choice (D) does not answer the question. (*Knowledge Domain 1.1*)

70. **(A)** Phase I clinical trials include 20–100 individuals, may take several months, and are the phase when testing safety begins. Phase II clinical trials include 100–500 participants, may take months to years, and are the phase when an emphasis is made on efficacy while still testing for safety. Phase III clinical trials include several thousand participants, may take several years, and are the phase when testing focuses on dosing while still looking at safety and efficacy. Phase IV clinical trials are performed after the product is on the market and focus on long-term side effects. (*Knowledge Domain 1.1*)

71. **(A)** Schedule II medications are not refillable. The patient must present a new hard copy of a prescription to receive more of the medication. (*Knowledge Domain 6.2*)

72. **(D)** ACE inhibitors have the potential to cause angioedema, cough, and rash. These are important counseling points that should be emphasized by the pharmacist. Fever is not one of lisinopril's side effects. (*Knowledge Domain 1.5*)

73. **(C)** There are 16 ounces in 1 pound. (*Knowledge Domain 6.3*)

74. **(A)** A drug database provides a master list of medications that are used in that particular setting. Pharmacy database, choice (B), is incorrect because it provides an inventory of the pharmacy personnel's biographical and demographic data. Choices (C) and (D) are not separate databases that are maintained by the pharmacy. (*Knowledge Domain 9.2*)

75. **(D)** To maintain certification through the Pharmacy Technician Certification Board, a pharmacy technician must complete 20 CE hours every 2 years. (*Knowledge Domain 2.13*)

76. **(C)** Amoxicillin and cephalexin are not included on the Institute for Safe Medication Practices' list of look-alike/sound-alike drug names. (*Knowledge Domain 4.4*)

77. **(B)** In a recall situation, the pharmacy would be provided with the specific lot number(s) affected. (*Knowledge Domain 7.5*)

78. **(A)** A coordination of benefits ensures that the amount paid by plans is maximized by determining the respective payment responsibilities. (*Knowledge Domain 8.5*)

79. **(D)** In order to solve this problem, set up a proportion, and solve for x.

$$\frac{25 \text{ mEq}}{1 \text{ mL}} = \frac{60 \text{ mEq}}{x}$$
$$x = 2.4 \text{ mL}$$

The answer is 2.4 mL, choice (D). (*Knowledge Domain 3.6*)

80. **(C)** These automated dispensing machines are located on units throughout a hospital and are stocked with medications specific to each unit's needs. (*Knowledge Domain 6.7*)

81. **(D)** Medicare Part D covers outpatient prescription drugs. Medicare Part A covers hospital services. Medicare Part B covers outpatient services. Medicare Part C is a Medicare Advantage Plan that allows private insurance companies to provide Medicare benefits. (*Knowledge Domain 8.1*)

82. **(D)** A food-environment allergy occurs when the safety and quality of food is affected by the environment. Drug interactions can affect the activity of another drug (drug-drug). Medication administration can affect a laboratory result (drug-laboratory). Drug interactions also can occur when one drug reacts with another that has a similar interaction (therapeutic duplication). (*Knowledge Domain 1.3*)

83. **(C)** The prescriber's DEA number is required to be present on all controlled substances. (*Knowledge Domain 6.5*)

84. **(A)** A package insert provides additional information about a drug and is included with most drug packaging or containers. Some medications are regulated and require PPIs; these include medications containing estrogen. (*Knowledge Domain 4.2*)

85. **(B)** A dummy computer allows multiple users to access data. Choice (A), a main computer, is used to store large amounts of data. Choices (C) and (D) are not names used when addressing computer access for multiple users. (*Knowledge Domain 9.2*)

86. **(B)** w/v% refers to g/100 mL. (*Knowledge Domain 3.6*)

87. **(C)** On average, 20 drops are equivalent to 1 mL. (*Knowledge Domain 6.1*)

88. **(A)** Verifying a patient's personal information is an essential error prevention strategy employed *before* data entry of the prescription. For example, there may be multiple

patients with the same name, but different dates of birth, within the same household (e.g., John Smith, Sr., John Smith, Jr.). Choices (B), (C), and (D) are all examples of error prevention strategies that are used *during* the fill process and patient pickup procedures. (*Knowledge Domain 4.1*)

89. **(B)** An insurance company can limit the amount of tablets filled within a time frame. The other options are common examples of insurance rejections. (*Knowledge Domain 8.2*)

90. **(C)** Nonstandardized sig codes should *not* be used when writing prescriptions due to the possibility that they will be misinterpreted. (*Knowledge Domain 5.3*)

ANSWER SHEET
Practice Test 2

1. Ⓐ Ⓑ Ⓒ Ⓓ
2. Ⓐ Ⓑ Ⓒ Ⓓ
3. Ⓐ Ⓑ Ⓒ Ⓓ
4. Ⓐ Ⓑ Ⓒ Ⓓ
5. Ⓐ Ⓑ Ⓒ Ⓓ
6. Ⓐ Ⓑ Ⓒ Ⓓ
7. Ⓐ Ⓑ Ⓒ Ⓓ
8. Ⓐ Ⓑ Ⓒ Ⓓ
9. Ⓐ Ⓑ Ⓒ Ⓓ
10. Ⓐ Ⓑ Ⓒ Ⓓ
11. Ⓐ Ⓑ Ⓒ Ⓓ
12. Ⓐ Ⓑ Ⓒ Ⓓ
13. Ⓐ Ⓑ Ⓒ Ⓓ
14. Ⓐ Ⓑ Ⓒ Ⓓ
15. Ⓐ Ⓑ Ⓒ Ⓓ
16. Ⓐ Ⓑ Ⓒ Ⓓ
17. Ⓐ Ⓑ Ⓒ Ⓓ
18. Ⓐ Ⓑ Ⓒ Ⓓ
19. Ⓐ Ⓑ Ⓒ Ⓓ
20. Ⓐ Ⓑ Ⓒ Ⓓ
21. Ⓐ Ⓑ Ⓒ Ⓓ
22. Ⓐ Ⓑ Ⓒ Ⓓ
23. Ⓐ Ⓑ Ⓒ Ⓓ
24. Ⓐ Ⓑ Ⓒ Ⓓ
25. Ⓐ Ⓑ Ⓒ Ⓓ
26. Ⓐ Ⓑ Ⓒ Ⓓ
27. Ⓐ Ⓑ Ⓒ Ⓓ
28. Ⓐ Ⓑ Ⓒ Ⓓ
29. Ⓐ Ⓑ Ⓒ Ⓓ
30. Ⓐ Ⓑ Ⓒ Ⓓ

31. Ⓐ Ⓑ Ⓒ Ⓓ
32. Ⓐ Ⓑ Ⓒ Ⓓ
33. Ⓐ Ⓑ Ⓒ Ⓓ
34. Ⓐ Ⓑ Ⓒ Ⓓ
35. Ⓐ Ⓑ Ⓒ Ⓓ
36. Ⓐ Ⓑ Ⓒ Ⓓ
37. Ⓐ Ⓑ Ⓒ Ⓓ
38. Ⓐ Ⓑ Ⓒ Ⓓ
39. Ⓐ Ⓑ Ⓒ Ⓓ
40. Ⓐ Ⓑ Ⓒ Ⓓ
41. Ⓐ Ⓑ Ⓒ Ⓓ
42. Ⓐ Ⓑ Ⓒ Ⓓ
43. Ⓐ Ⓑ Ⓒ Ⓓ
44. Ⓐ Ⓑ Ⓒ Ⓓ
45. Ⓐ Ⓑ Ⓒ Ⓓ
46. Ⓐ Ⓑ Ⓒ Ⓓ
47. Ⓐ Ⓑ Ⓒ Ⓓ
48. Ⓐ Ⓑ Ⓒ Ⓓ
49. Ⓐ Ⓑ Ⓒ Ⓓ
50. Ⓐ Ⓑ Ⓒ Ⓓ
51. Ⓐ Ⓑ Ⓒ Ⓓ
52. Ⓐ Ⓑ Ⓒ Ⓓ
53. Ⓐ Ⓑ Ⓒ Ⓓ
54. Ⓐ Ⓑ Ⓒ Ⓓ
55. Ⓐ Ⓑ Ⓒ Ⓓ
56. Ⓐ Ⓑ Ⓒ Ⓓ
57. Ⓐ Ⓑ Ⓒ Ⓓ
58. Ⓐ Ⓑ Ⓒ Ⓓ
59. Ⓐ Ⓑ Ⓒ Ⓓ
60. Ⓐ Ⓑ Ⓒ Ⓓ

61. Ⓐ Ⓑ Ⓒ Ⓓ
62. Ⓐ Ⓑ Ⓒ Ⓓ
63. Ⓐ Ⓑ Ⓒ Ⓓ
64. Ⓐ Ⓑ Ⓒ Ⓓ
65. Ⓐ Ⓑ Ⓒ Ⓓ
66. Ⓐ Ⓑ Ⓒ Ⓓ
67. Ⓐ Ⓑ Ⓒ Ⓓ
68. Ⓐ Ⓑ Ⓒ Ⓓ
69. Ⓐ Ⓑ Ⓒ Ⓓ
70. Ⓐ Ⓑ Ⓒ Ⓓ
71. Ⓐ Ⓑ Ⓒ Ⓓ
72. Ⓐ Ⓑ Ⓒ Ⓓ
73. Ⓐ Ⓑ Ⓒ Ⓓ
74. Ⓐ Ⓑ Ⓒ Ⓓ
75. Ⓐ Ⓑ Ⓒ Ⓓ
76. Ⓐ Ⓑ Ⓒ Ⓓ
77. Ⓐ Ⓑ Ⓒ Ⓓ
78. Ⓐ Ⓑ Ⓒ Ⓓ
79. Ⓐ Ⓑ Ⓒ Ⓓ
80. Ⓐ Ⓑ Ⓒ Ⓓ
81. Ⓐ Ⓑ Ⓒ Ⓓ
82. Ⓐ Ⓑ Ⓒ Ⓓ
83. Ⓐ Ⓑ Ⓒ Ⓓ
84. Ⓐ Ⓑ Ⓒ Ⓓ
85. Ⓐ Ⓑ Ⓒ Ⓓ
86. Ⓐ Ⓑ Ⓒ Ⓓ
87. Ⓐ Ⓑ Ⓒ Ⓓ
88. Ⓐ Ⓑ Ⓒ Ⓓ
89. Ⓐ Ⓑ Ⓒ Ⓓ
90. Ⓐ Ⓑ Ⓒ Ⓓ

PRACTICE TEST 2

Practice PTCE Test 2

Directions: You will have 1 hour and 50 minutes to complete the following 90 questions. For each question, select the choice that best answers the question, and mark that answer letter on your answer sheet. Remember, this test should be used to help you determine areas that require additional review. Each question represents a particular area of the PTCE blueprint, which can help you pinpoint areas of mastery or concepts that require additional studying. The official PTCE exam uses a scaled score to determine your grade. Only 80 out of 90 questions on the PTCE are scored, and unscored questions are not identified. You should be able to answer about 75 of the questions on this test correctly, averaging an overall percentage of 80% or more on your attempt at this test.

1. The retail price of a prescription is based on the Average Wholesale Price (AWP) plus a markup and dispensing fee. Using the table below, determine the retail price for 30 tablets if a bottle of 100 tablets has an AWP of $56.79 and a markup of 7%.

AWP	Dispensing Fee
$0–$5.00	$3.00
$5.01–$10.00	$4.00
$10.01–$20.00	$5.00
$20.01 and up	$6.00

(A) $21.23
(B) $22.69
(C) $23.23
(D) $24.14

2. Prior authorization requests require that _____.

(A) physicians seek approval from the insurance provider to prescribe a specific medication
(B) insurance companies seek approval from the physician in order to cover a specific medication
(C) pharmacies seek approval from the physician to dispense a specific medication
(D) patients seek prior approval from the pharmacy in order to fill a specific medication

3. Zetia is indicated for the treatment of _____.

(A) hypertension
(B) gout
(C) rheumatoid arthritis
(D) hyperlipidemia

4. A resource that contains official standards, including monographs pertaining to drug substances, dosage forms, and pharmaceutical ingredients, is the _____.

   (A) *United States Pharmacopeia-National Formulary (USP-NF)*
   (B) *United States Pharmacopeia Drug Information Volume 1 (USP-DI Vol. 1)*
   (C) *United States Pharmacopeia Drug Information Volume 2 (USP-DI Vol. 2)*
   (D) Remington's *The Science and Practice of Pharmacy*

5. Which of the following dosage forms bypasses the digestive system?

   (A) elixir
   (B) suspension
   (C) sublingual tablet
   (D) ointment

6. You receive a prescription from Dr. Jameson for a controlled substance. The doctor's DEA number is AJ7234035. Should the prescription be filled?

   (A) Yes, the DEA number is valid.
   (B) Yes, a DEA number is not needed on a prescription written for a controlled substance.
   (C) No, the DEA number is invalid.
   (D) No, the second letter of the DEA number does not match the first letter in the doctor's last name.

7. According to the Controlled Substances Act, which of the following drugs is classified as a controlled substance?

   (A) warfarin (Coumadin)
   (B) tramadol (Ultram)
   (C) minocycline (Minocin, Soldyne)
   (D) mometasone (Nasonex)

8. A prescription for a controlled substance must include which of the following statements on the label?

   (A) "Caution: State law prohibits the sale of this drug to any person"
   (B) "Caution: Federal law prohibits the transfer of this drug to any person other than the patient for whom it was prescribed"
   (C) "Caution: State law prohibits the sale of this drug to any person other than the patient for whom it was prescribed"
   (D) "Caution: State law prohibits the sale of this drug"

9. Which of the following nasal corticosteroids is available over-the-counter?

   (A) Omnaris
   (B) Zetonna
   (C) Flonase
   (D) Rhinocort

10. Which auxiliary label should be placed onto a prescription vial containing metronidazole (Flagyl)?

   (A) "Refrigerate"
   (B) "Shake before use"
   (C) "Do not drink alcohol"
   (D) "Take with food"

11. Which of the following prescription medications should NOT be handled by a pharmacy technician who is pregnant?

   (A) famotidine
   (B) furosemide
   (C) fexofenadine
   (D) finasteride

12. How many mg of magnesium sulfate are in 3 mL of a 50% solution?

   (A) 1,000 mg
   (B) 1,500 mg
   (C) 1,750 mg
   (D) 2,000 mg

13. How many mL of a 2% (w/v) solution are needed to make 8 oz of a 1:200 solution?

   (A) 15 mL
   (B) 30 mL
   (C) 60 mL
   (D) 80 mL

14. What is the antibiotic classification of the drug azithromycin (Zithromax)?

   (A) tetracycline
   (B) penicillin
   (C) macrolide
   (D) cephalosporin

15. Which type of laminar flow hood is used in the preparation of chemotherapeutic agents?

   (A) horizontal flow hood
   (B) vertical flow hood
   (C) upright flow hood
   (D) aseptic flow hood

16. The acronym NDC is used when identifying a drug product. It also relays information pertaining to the manufacturer and the medication package size. What does the acronym NDC stand for?

   (A) Nationwide Drug Carrier
   (B) National District Code
   (C) Nationwide District Code
   (D) National Drug Code

17. Sodium lauryl sulfate is an example of an emulsifier used in the formulation of compounded sterile preparations. Which of the following best describes the addition of an emulsifier in solution?

   (A) It is used to create a uniform concentration of an active drug in solution.
   (B) It is used to help stabilize a solution against degradation.
   (C) It is used to prevent oxidation of the component drug.
   (D) It is used to help adjust a formulation to an appropriate isotonicity.

18. What is the maximum amount of continuing education (CE) hours that may be earned toward recertification by completing an in-service project or training under the direction of a pharmacist?

   (A) 1
   (B) 2
   (C) 5
   (D) 10

19. In the NDC number 0084-6571-10, what does the number 0084 indicate?

   (A) package size
   (B) product strength
   (C) manufacturer
   (D) dosage form

20. How many 250 mg capsules are needed to prepare 75 mL of a 1% solution?

   (A) 1 capsule
   (B) 2 capsules
   (C) 3 capsules
   (D) 4 capsules

21. Which of the following patient service principles should NOT be used by pharmacy personnel when dealing with a patient's complaint?

   (A) Avoid passing judgment on the patient.
   (B) Provide accurate information to the patient.
   (C) Maintain a positive attitude toward the patient.
   (D) Provide a follow-up survey to gauge the patient's feedback.

22. Which government agency enforces the Controlled Substances Act?

   (A) DEA
   (B) OSHA
   (C) FDA
   (D) CDC

23. CCXI is equal to _____.

   (A) 209
   (B) 210
   (C) 211
   (D) 212

24. What is the minimum sensitivity reading on a Class A prescription balance?

   (A) 2 mg
   (B) 6 mg
   (C) 8 mg
   (D) 10 mg

25. A pharmacy technician is filling out a controlled medication order on a DEA 222 form. Which copy of the paper form is kept by the pharmacy?

   (A) top copy
   (B) middle copy
   (C) bottom copy
   (D) top and bottom copies

26. What is the brand name of the drug rabeprazole?

   (A) Aciphex
   (B) Nexium
   (C) Prilosec
   (D) Protonix

27. Nitrostat 0.4 mg is exempt from the child-resistant cap requirement according to which pharmacy-specific law?

   (A) Poison Prevention Packaging Act of 1970
   (B) Isotretinoin Safety and Risk Management Act of 2004
   (C) Combat Methamphetamine Epidemic Act of 2005
   (D) Health Insurance Portability and Accountability Act of 1996

28. How many tablets should be dispensed, given the following order?

   prednisone 5 mg sig:
   ii tabs PO TID × 2 days
   ii tabs PO BID × 2 days
   i tab PO TID × 2 days
   ii tabs PO QD × 2 days
   i tab PO QD × 2 days
   Then stop

   (A) 22 tablets
   (B) 30 tablets
   (C) 32 tablets
   (D) 38 tablets

29. Laminar flow hoods should _____.

   (A) be cleaned from top to bottom and from side to side to avoid contact and contamination of the HEPA filter
   (B) be cleaned from top to bottom and from back to front to avoid contact and contamination of the HEPA filter
   (C) be cleaned in any direction to avoid contact and contamination of the HEPA filter
   (D) not be cleaned

30. The convex or concave curve located at the top of a volume of liquid in a graduated cylinder is known as a(n) _____.

   (A) levigation
   (B) meniscus
   (C) ointment
   (D) troches

31. Which of the following reports is NOT commonly found in a pharmacy information system?

   (A) physician report
   (B) usage report
   (C) diversion report
   (D) override report

32. Which of the following is NOT a solid dosage form?

(A) powder
(B) capsule
(C) suspension
(D) suppository

33. A patient receives a prescription for an otic preparation. Where is an otic product instilled?

(A) in the eye
(B) in the nose
(C) in the rectum
(D) in the ear

34. A medication is to be kept at room temperature. What is the appropriate temperature range for this medication?

(A) –4°F to 14°F
(B) 36°F to 46°F
(C) 68°F to 77°F
(D) 90°F to 110°F

35. What is the maximum number of refills permitted for a Class III prescription according to federal law?

(A) 0 refills
(B) 1 refill
(C) 5 refills in 6 months
(D) 11 refills in 12 months

36. All of the following are classified as high-alert medications by the Institute for Safe Medication Practices (ISMP) EXCEPT _____.

(A) metformin
(B) warfarin
(C) midazolam
(D) ampicillin

37. How may a pharmacy technician participate in OBRA '90?

(A) by asking the pharmacist to come over and counsel a patient who has questions about his or her prescription
(B) by counseling a patient on how to take a medication appropriately
(C) by calling the doctor to verify how a patient should use his or her inhaler
(D) by asking the pharmacist questions that the patient has and relaying the answers back to the patient

38. Nonaqueous solutions, such as a capsule without water, have a maximum beyond use date (BUD) of no later than _____.

(A) 14 days
(B) 30 days
(C) 6 months
(D) 1 year

39. Which of the following statements best describes the electronic health record (EHR)?

(A) It is an automated system of transmitting prescription data among the prescriber, the pharmacy, and the third-party payer.
(B) It is an automated system used to increase the efficiency of work flow.
(C) It is an automated system used to provide for warnings, flags, and alerts during drug utilization review (DUR).
(D) It is an automated system that uses bar code technology to assist in reducing medication errors.

40. A patient is requesting that her Class IV prescription be transferred to a pharmacy that does not share the same online database. What is the maximum number of times a Class IV prescription can be transferred to this pharmacy?

(A) 1 transfer
(B) 2 transfers
(C) 5 transfers
(D) unlimited transfers

41. A list of medications from which a prescriber may prescribe in a given setting is known as a(n) _____.

   (A) reconciliation
   (B) formulary
   (C) therapeutic equivalent
   (D) adjudication

42. Which of the following is NOT a strategy used to decrease the potential for expired drugs to be on pharmacy shelves?

   (A) using colored stickers to indicate the month of expiration
   (B) placing medications with similar drug names away from each other
   (C) writing the month of expiration on the stock bottle
   (D) placing new products behind old products on the shelves

43. Which of the following forms is required to order mephylphenidate (Ritalin)?

   (A) DEA 224
   (B) DEA 222
   (C) DEA 106
   (D) DEA 41

44. Why was the Health Insurance Portability and Accountability Act (HIPAA) of 1996 created?

   (A) to reduce accidental poisoning involving children
   (B) to provide a safe working environment
   (C) to make sure that patients receive counseling about their medication
   (D) to ensure that all patient information is safeguarded

45. Which of the following error prevention strategies is used to avoid variation or complexity?

   (A) the use of electronic processing software
   (B) the integration of a computer with the pharmacy register
   (C) the use of a scanner to match the NDC of the selected drug to the profiled medication
   (D) the use of preprinted prescription blanks containing frequently prescribed medications

46. Needles used to prepare intravenous solutions are discarded by _____.

   (A) throwing the used needles into the trash can
   (B) placing the used needles into a sharps container
   (C) recapping the needles and tossing them into the trash can
   (D) recapping the needles and placing them into a sharps container

47. What is the therapeutic equivalent for Claritin?

   (A) diphenhydramine
   (B) cetirizine
   (C) loratadine
   (D) fexofenadine

48. Counting trays should be _____

   (A) tossed, and new trays purchased, every 6 months
   (B) labeled to be used with hazardous medications
   (C) made of glass
   (D) kept in the compounding area

49. What type of prescriptions may NOT be prescribed over the phone?

   (A) Class II prescriptions
   (B) Class III prescriptions
   (C) Class IV prescriptions
   (D) noncontrolled prescriptions

50. When a prescription for an inhaler is dispensed, a patient package insert (PPI) _____.

 (A) must be included the first time the prescription is dispensed
 (B) must be included every time the prescription is dispensed
 (C) does not need to be included with this medication
 (D) should be included only at the patient's request

51. A formulation record should include which of the following sets of information for each compound listed?

 (A) the name, the strength and the dose of the compounded medication, the name and the strength of each ingredient used, a list of equipment used, and a mixing process (if applicable)
 (B) the name, the strength, and the manufacturer of each compounded medication, the name of each ingredient used, and a list of equipment used
 (C) the name and the strength of the compounded medication, and a list of equipment used
 (D) the name of the compounded medication, and the name and the strength of each ingredient used

52. Which instrument is used to grind tablets into fine powders?

 (A) spatula and ointment slab
 (B) electronic balance and spatula
 (C) stir rod and beaker
 (D) mortar and pestle

53. According to federal law, how long should Schedule II prescriptions be kept in the pharmacy?

 (A) 1 year
 (B) 2 years
 (C) 5 years
 (D) 7 years

54. Which of the following is an example of a patient assistance program?

 (A) a company that administers a drug benefit program
 (B) the portion of the price of a medication that a patient is required to pay
 (C) a set amount that must be paid by the patient before the insurer will cover any costs
 (D) a manufacturer-sponsored prescription drug program

55. Which of the following vitamins is fat-soluble?

 (A) vitamin A
 (B) vitamin B12
 (C) vitamin B6
 (D) vitamin C

56. What is the minimum weighable quantity for a Class A prescription balance?

 (A) 6 mg
 (B) 120 mg
 (C) 6 mL
 (D) 120 mL

57. Which measuring device would be the most appropriate for dispensing liquid for an infant?

 (A) oral syringe
 (B) medication cup
 (C) oral dropper
 (D) teaspoon

58. Which of the following is a long-acting insulin?

 (A) insulin glulisine
 (B) insulin aspart
 (C) insulin glargine
 (D) insulin lispro

59. A sig states that a medication should be taken QID. The medication should be taken _____ a day.

   (A) once
   (B) twice
   (C) three times
   (D) four times

60. Which of the following elements is NOT necessary when implementing a pharmacy information system?

   (A) computer
   (B) software
   (C) telephone
   (D) fax machine

61. A woman comes to the pharmacy to pick up a prescription for her 15-year-old daughter. At pickup, the woman is informed that her insurance plan rejected her insurance claim. After further review, the pharmacy technician notices that the rejection claim indicates that the person code is incorrect. What should the pharmacy technician do?

   (A) verify the person code and reprocess the claim
   (B) ask the pharmacist to call the insurance company
   (C) tell the patient that the medication is not covered
   (D) ask the patient to call her insurance company

62. How many gallons are contained in 240 pints?

   (A) 10 gallons
   (B) 20 gallons
   (C) 30 gallons
   (D) 40 gallons

63. According to federal law, who may perform the final check for all prescriptions processed and filled in the pharmacy?

   (A) pharmacy technician
   (B) pharmacist
   (C) physician
   (D) pharmacy intern

64. Knowledge of which of the following can best assist a pharmacy technician in preventing medication data entry errors?

   (A) the brand and generic names of medications
   (B) insurance input codes
   (C) the physician's phone number
   (D) the pharmacy's hours of operation

65. How much dextrose is in 1,000 mL of D10W?

   (A) 100 g
   (B) 1,000 g
   (C) 100 mg
   (D) 1,000 mg

66. Which of the following pieces of information is NOT required in order to fill a prescription in an institutional pharmacy?

   (A) the patient's name
   (B) the prescriber's information
   (C) insurance information
   (D) the manufacturer's information

67. *USP* <797> guidelines state that personnel must wash their fingers, hands, wrists, and arms up to the elbow for what minimum time frame?

   (A) 15 seconds
   (B) 30 seconds
   (C) 1 minute
   (D) 2 minutes

68. Why should medication stock be rotated in a pharmacy?

   (A) to ensure that short-dated medications are used first
   (B) to ensure that long-dated medications are used first
   (C) to ensure that the pharmacy supply is maximized
   (D) to ensure that the stock is facing properly

69. Which of the following best describes information that should be included on unit-dose packaged medications?

   (A) the medication name, the strength, the manufacturer's name, the NDC, the lot number, and the expiration date
   (B) the medication name, the strength, the manufacturer's name, the NDC, the lot number, and the instructions for patient use
   (C) the medication name, the strength, and the instructions for patient use
   (D) the medication name, the strength, and the manufacturer's name

70. Which of the following agencies accredits health care services, including hospitals and long-term care facilities?

   (A) State Board of Pharmacy
   (B) The Joint Commission
   (C) Centers for Medicare and Medicaid
   (D) Drug Enforcement Agency

71. Misbranded drugs may include
   _____.

   (A) labels containing misleading information
   (B) medications in containers packed under unsanitary conditions
   (C) unsafe color additives
   (D) containers made from hazardous or poisonous substances

72. A physician orders an IV drip rate of a medication to be infused at 15 mL/hr for a total of 36 hours. What is the total volume of medication to be administered?

   (A) 240 mL
   (B) 480 mL
   (C) 540 mL
   (D) 615 mL

73. Which FDA recall classification is the least severe?

   (A) Class I
   (B) Class II
   (C) Class III
   (D) Class IV

74. The doctor has prescribed antihistamine drops to treat seasonal allergy symptoms. The directions state 1–2 gtts os TID. What should be typed on the prescription label?

   (A) Instill 1–2 drops in each eye three times a day.
   (B) Instill 1–2 drops in the right eye three times a day.
   (C) Instill 1–2 drops in the left eye three times a day.
   (D) Instill 1–2 drops in the left ear three times a day.

75. The pharmacy should complete which of the following steps after receiving an alert from the FDA about a drug recall from a specific manufacturer?

(A) pull the offending drug from pharmacy shelves and, if deemed appropriate, call patients taking this medication to inform them of the significant medication problem

(B) pull the offending drug from pharmacy shelves but do not contact patients taking this medication until it is time for the next mediation refill

(C) continue to use the offending drug until stock runs out but do not order more for future fills

(D) continue to use the offending drug but post an alert in the pharmacy for patients to see information about the significant medication problem

76. Which of the following is an angiotensin II receptor blocker (ARB)?

(A) metoprolol
(B) lisinopril
(C) lovastatin
(D) candesartan

77. The expiration date of a bottle reads 9/19. What is the last day the medication may be used?

(A) 09/01/2019
(B) 09/30/2019
(C) 10/01/2019
(D) 08/31/2019

78. The Combat Methamphetamine Act of 2005 was enacted to regulate over-the-counter sales of which of the following substances?

(A) dextromethorphan
(B) pseudoephedrine
(C) guaifenesin
(D) phenylephrine

79. The pharmacy receives a prescription for 500 mL of 15% solution "X." The pharmacy carries 30% and 5% stock solutions. How much of the 30% and 5% solutions, respectively, should be used to mix this order?

(A) 100 mL of 30% solution, 400 mL of 5% solution
(B) 200 mL of 30% solution, 300 mL of 5% solution
(C) 300 mL of 30% solution, 200 mL of 5% solution
(D) 400 mL of 30% solution, 100 mL of 5% solution

80. What volume of a 125 mg/mL injectable should be drawn up for a 275 mg dose?

(A) 1.4 mL
(B) 2.2 mL
(C) 2.8 mL
(D) 3.1 mL

81. Aseptic manipulations in a laminar flow hood should be prepared at least _____ inches within the hood.

(A) 2
(B) 6
(C) 10
(D) 12

82. Online processing of a claim to determine payment is called a(n) _____.

(A) formulary
(B) co-pay
(C) deductible
(D) adjudication

83. What is the color of the "C" stamped on controlled substance prescriptions and manufacturer bottles?

(A) green
(B) blue
(C) red
(D) black

84. A patient receives her medication at 1800 military hours. At what standard time did she receive her medication?

(A) 9:00 P.M.
(B) 6:00 P.M.
(C) 9:00 A.M.
(D) 6:00 A.M.

85. What should a pharmacy technician do if he or she receives an incomplete prescription order?

(A) Call the prescriber to inquire about the missing information.
(B) Ask the patient, and fill in the missing information.
(C) Refuse to fill the prescription.
(D) Fill the prescription using information from a previous fill.

86. Which organization accredits continuing education for pharmacists and pharmacy technicians?

(A) State Board of Pharmacy
(B) Accreditation Council for Pharmacy Education
(C) American Society of Health-System Pharmacists
(D) American Pharmacists Association®

87. Capsules and tablets are counted in multiples of what number?

(A) 2
(B) 3
(C) 5
(D) 10

88. What is the technical name for the stem of a needle?

(A) shaft
(B) bevel
(C) hub
(D) lumen

89. Which of the following is NOT an advantage of bar coding technology?

(A) It ensures that the patient receives the correct drug.
(B) It ensures that the correct dose is given to the patient.
(C) It ensures that the patient receives the medication at the best cost.
(D) It ensures that the correct patient receives the dose.

90. What is the term for "solid particles dispersed in a liquid medium"?

(A) suspension
(B) emulsion
(C) elixir
(D) solution

1. **C**	31. **A**	61. **A**
2. **A**	32. **C**	62. **C**
3. **D**	33. **D**	63. **B**
4. **A**	34. **C**	64. **A**
5. **C**	35. **C**	65. **A**
6. **C**	36. **D**	66. **C**
7. **B**	37. **A**	67. **B**
8. **B**	38. **C**	68. **A**
9. **C**	39. **A**	69. **A**
10. **C**	40. **A**	70. **B**
11. **D**	41. **B**	71. **A**
12. **B**	42. **B**	72. **C**
13. **C**	43. **B**	73. **C**
14. **C**	44. **D**	74. **C**
15. **B**	45. **D**	75. **A**
16. **D**	46. **B**	76. **D**
17. **A**	47. **C**	77. **B**
18. **C**	48. **B**	78. **B**
19. **C**	49. **A**	79. **B**
20. **C**	50. **B**	80. **B**
21. **D**	51. **A**	81. **B**
22. **A**	52. **D**	82. **D**
23. **C**	53. **B**	83. **C**
24. **B**	54. **D**	84. **B**
25. **C**	55. **A**	85. **C**
26. **A**	56. **B**	86. **B**
27. **A**	57. **A**	87. **C**
28. **C**	58. **C**	88. **A**
29. **B**	59. **D**	89. **C**
30. **B**	60. **D**	90. **A**

ANSWERS EXPLAINED

1. **(C)** First determine the cost for 30 tablets by setting up a proportion:

$$\frac{100 \text{ tablets}}{\$56.79} = \frac{30 \text{ tablets}}{x}$$

$$100x = 1,703.70$$

$$x = 17.037 \approx \$17.04$$

   Then calculate the cost of the tablets with the markup:

$$\$17.04 \times 0.07 = \$1.19 \text{ markup}$$

   Now determine the dispensing fee. Since the AWP is $17.04, the dispensing fee is $5.00. Add all the costs together:

$$\$17.04 + \$1.19 + \$5.00 = \$23.23$$

   The answer is $23.23. (*Knowledge Domain 6.1*)

2. **(A)** Prior authorization requests are used by insurance providers to ensure that medications are prescribed appropriately and to reduce costs. Prior authorization requests are sent to the prescriber to validate the necessity of a specific medication in order for the insurance provider to approve coverage of that medication. (*Knowledge Domain 8.2*)

3. **(D)** Zetia is a medication used to treat hyperlipidemia by inhibiting intestinal absorption of cholesterol. (*Knowledge Domain 1.6*)

4. **(A)** The *United States Pharmacopeia-National Formulary (USP-NF)* is the official compendium of drug information from the United States Pharmacopeial Convention. It includes official monographs of information about drug substances and dosage forms, pharmaceutical ingredients, and drug standards and specifications. The *United States Pharmacopeia Drug Information Volume 1 (USP-DI Vol. 1)* provides drug information aimed at the health professional, including label and off-label uses and drug monographs. The *United States Pharmacopeia Drug Information Volume 2 (USP-DI Vol. 2)* provides medical advice for the patient, including simplified monographs. Remington's *The Science and Practice of Pharmacy* is a text covering an array of topics, including pharmaceutics, pharmacodynamics, pharmacokinetics, pharmaceutical manufacturing, and pharmacy practice. (*Knowledge Domain 2.15*)

5. **(C)** Sublingual tablets bypass the digestive system because they diffuse into the bloodstream. Elixirs and suspensions are ingested and follow the gastrointestinal tract before entering the bloodstream. Ointments are used topically for local administration and therefore are not systemically absorbed. (*Knowledge Domain 1.4*)

6. **(C)** The validity of a DEA number is determined by first adding the 1st, 3rd, and 5th numbers together (in this case, 7 + 3 + 0 = 10). Next add the 2nd, 4th, and 6th numbers together (2 + 4 + 3 = 9) and then multiply that sum by two (9 × 2 = 18). Now add both sets of numbers, and check the number in the ones position (10 + 18 = 28). The number in the ones position should match the last number in the DEA number. The second letter in the DEA should also match the first letter of the prescriber's last name. In this example, the number in the ones position does not match the last number in the calculated number. Therefore, this is an invalid DEA number. The second letter (J) does match the first letter

of the prescriber's last name, but the DEA number has already been invalidated because of the incorrect last number. (*Knowledge Domain 2.5*)

7. **(B)** Tramadol (Ultram) is classified as a Schedule IV controlled substance under the Controlled Substances Act. Warfarin (Coumadin), minocycline (Minocin, Soldyne), and mometasone (Nasonex) are not classified as controlled substances under the Controlled Substances Act. (*Knowledge Domain 1.1*)

8. **(B)** Controlled prescriptions must include the following statement on the prescription label "Caution: Federal law prohibits the transfer of this drug to any person other than the patient for whom it was prescribed." Choices (A), (C), and (D) are all incorrect because this statement is a federal law, not a state law. In addition, the correct statement should not reference the "sale" but, rather, the "transfer" of the drug. (*Knowledge Domain 7.5*)

9. **(C)** Flonase is approved for the over-the-counter treatment of hay fever. Omnaris, Zetonna, and Rhinocort are prescription nasal sprays indicated for the treatment of allergic rhinitis. (*Knowledge Domain 1.6*)

10. **(C)** Metronidazole (Flagyl) is an antibiotic used to treat anaerobic bacterial infections. The concomitant consumption of alcohol while taking metronidazole can produce a disulfiram-like reaction, resulting in tachycardia, flushing, and hypotension. (*Knowledge Domain 1.5*)

11. **(D)** Finasteride (Proscar, Propecia) is a pregnancy category X drug, indicating that, in clinical studies, this drug has been shown to cause abnormal effects and risks to the human fetus. Famotidine (Pepcid), furosemide (Lasix), and fexofenadine (Allegra) are not categorized as pregnancy category X drugs and may be handled by a pharmacy technician during her pregnancy. (*Knowledge Domain 6.4*)

12. **(B)** A proportion can be used to solve this problem:

$$\frac{50 \text{ g}}{100 \text{ mL}} = \frac{x}{3 \text{ mL}}$$

$$100x = 150$$

$$x = 1.5 \text{ g}$$

Since none of the answer choices are in grams (g), we must convert this answer to milligrams (mg):

$$\frac{1,000 \text{ mg}}{1 \text{ g}} = \frac{x}{1.5 \text{ g}}$$

$$x = 1,500 \text{ mg}$$

The answer is 1,500 mg. (*Knowledge Domain 3.6*)

13. **(C)** This problem can be solved using the following equation: (IS)(IV) = (FS)(FV). The initial strength (IS) is 2%. You must solve for the initial volume (IV). The final strength (FS) is 1:200. The strength is presented as a ratio in this problem and should be converted to a percentage. To convert to a percentage, you must first realize that 1:200 is a ratio written as $\frac{1}{200}$. Multiply $\frac{1}{200}$ by 100 to get 0.5%. The final volume (FV) is 8 oz, which

is the same as 240 mL $\left(\dfrac{1 \text{ oz}}{30 \text{ mL}} = \dfrac{8 \text{ oz}}{x}\right)$. Now plug the numbers into the equation, and solve for x:

$$(2\%)(x \text{ mL}) = (0.5\%)(240 \text{ mL})$$

$$2x \text{ mL} = 120 \text{ mL}$$

$$x = 60 \text{ mL}$$

The answer is 60 mL. (*Knowledge Domain 3.6*)

14. **(C)** Azithromycin (Zithromax) is classified as a macrolide antibiotic. (*Knowledge Domain 1.6*)

15. **(B)** Vertical flow hoods are used to prepare cytotoxic or hazardous drugs. Horizontal flow hoods, choice (A), are used to prepare aseptic preparations. Choices (C) and (D) are not common names of flow hoods used in pharmacy practice. (*Knowledge Domain 3.5*)

16. **(D)** The acronym NDC stands for National Drug Code. (*Knowledge Domain 7.1*)

17. **(A)** An emulsifier is used to create a uniform concentration of an active drug in solution. Choice (B) is the definition of a pH buffer. Choice (C) is the definition of an antioxidant. Choice (D) is the definition of a tonicity agent. (*Knowledge Domain 3.5*)

18. **(C)** The Pharmacy Technician Certification Board (PTCB) specifies that up to 5 out the 20 required continuing education hours may be earned by completing an in-service project or by training under the direct supervision of a pharmacist. (*Knowledge Domain 2.13*)

19. **(C)** The first set of numbers in a National Drug Code (NDC) identifies the labeler, defined as the manufacturer or the distributor of the drug. The second set of numbers identifies the product, and the third set identifies the package size. (*Knowledge Domain 7.1*)

20. **(C)** First set up a proportion to find the number of milligrams required:

$$\frac{1 \text{ g}}{100 \text{ mL}} = \frac{x}{75 \text{ mL}}$$

$$100x = 75$$

$$x = 0.75 \text{ g} = 750 \text{ mg}$$

Then set up another proportion to find the number of capsules needed:

$$\frac{250 \text{ mg}}{1 \text{ capsule}} = \frac{750 \text{ mg}}{x}$$

$$250x = 750$$

$$x = 3$$

The answer is 3 capsules. (*Knowledge Domain 3.7*)

21. **(D)** A follow-up survey may be provided by the pharmacy to collect data regarding patient satisfaction, but it is *not* an example of a patient service principle that may be used when speaking with a patient. When dealing with a patient's complaint, pharmacy personnel should avoid passing judgment, provide accurate information to the patient, and maintain a positive attitude toward the patient. (*Knowledge Domain 5.5*)

22. **(A)** The Drug Enforcement Agency (DEA) enforces the Controlled Substances Act. Choice (B) is incorrect because OSHA, the Occupational Safety and Health Administration, is a federal agency that regulates workplace safety and health. Choice (C) is incorrect because the FDA assures the safety and efficacy of drugs, foods, medical devices, and other biological products. Choice (D) is incorrect because the Centers for Disease Control and Research (CDC) supports health promotion, awareness, and preparedness. (*Knowledge Domain 2.11*)

23. **(C)** C equals 100, X equals 10, and I equals I. Therefore, CCXI = 100 + 100 + 10 + 1 = 211. (*Knowledge Domain 6.1*)

24. **(B)** The minimum sensitivity reading required to move the pointer on the scale is 6 mg. (*Knowledge Domain 3.5*)

25. **(C)** The bottom form is kept by the pharmacy and will be used to notate receipt of the medications ordered. The top copy, choice (A), is forwarded to the supplier. The middle copy, choice (B), is forwarded to the special agent in charge of the Drug Enforcement Administration in the local area of the supplier. The top and bottom copies, choice (D), are not both kept by the pharmacy. (*Knowledge Domain 2.3*)

26. **(A)** Aciphex is the brand name for rabeprazole. Nexium, choice (B), is the brand name for esomeprazole. Prilosec, choice (C), is the brand name for omeprazole. Protonix, choice (D), is the brand name for pantoprazole. (*Knowledge Domain 1.1*)

27. **(A)** The Poison Prevention Packaging Act of 1970 has some exemptions to the child-resistant packaging requirement. These exemptions including effervescent aspirin, oral contraceptives, sublingual nitroglycerin, and hormone replacement therapy. The Isotretinoin Safety and Risk Management Act of 2004, choice (B), was enacted to restrict the use of isotretinoin (Accutane). The Combat Methamphetamine Epidemic Act of 2005, choice (C), places restrictions on products containing pseudoephedrine, ephedrine, and/or phenylpropanolamine. The Health Insurance Portability and Accountability Act of 1996, choice (D), places safeguards on all protected health information (PHI). (*Knowledge Domain 6.6*)

28. **(C)**

$$ii \text{ tabs PO TID} \times 2 \text{ days}: 2 \times 3 = 6 \times 2 = 12 \text{ tablets}$$
$$ii \text{ tabs PO BID} \times 2 \text{ days}: 2 \times 2 = 4 \times 2 = 8 \text{ tablets}$$
$$i \text{ tab PO TID} \times 2 \text{ days}: 1 \times 3 = 3 \times 2 = 6 \text{ tablets}$$
$$ii \text{ tabs PO QD} \times 2 \text{ days}: 2 \times 1 = 2 \times 2 = 4 \text{ tablets}$$
$$i \text{ tab PO QD} \times 2 \text{ days}: 1 \times 1 = 1 \times 2 = 2 \text{ tablets}$$
$$12 + 8 + 6 + 4 + 2 = 32 \text{ tablets}$$

The answer is 32 tablets, choice (C). (*Knowledge Domain 6.3*)

29. **(B)** A laminar flow hood should be cleaned using 70% isopropyl alcohol and a lint-free towel, starting at the top of the walls and working toward the bottom. Then the hood floor should be cleaned from the back to the front. (*Knowledge Domain 2.11*)

30. **(B)** A meniscus is the curved surface that appears at the top of a volume of liquid in a graduated cylinder. Levigation, choice (A), is the process of grinding a powder through the incorporation of a liquid. Ointment, choice (C), is a water in oil (w/o) emulsion. Troches, choice (D), are a tablet designed to be dissolved in the mouth. (*Knowledge Domain 3.7*)

31. **(A)** Pharmacies use reports to determine trends and profit/loss, to perform audits, and to alter inventory. Physician reports are not commonly found in pharmacy information systems. Usage reports evaluate patterns and/or trends. Diversion reports are used when reporting a significant theft or loss of a controlled substance. Override reports can be used to determine specific users who override or disregard warnings or safety measures employed by the system. (*Knowledge Domain 9.2*)

32. **(C)** A suspension is an example of a liquid dosage form where the active ingredient is dispersed in the liquid vehicle. Powders, capsules, and suppositories are all examples of solid dosage forms. (*Knowledge Domain 3.5*)

33. **(D)** Otic = ear; ophthalmic = eye; nasal = nose; and rectal = rectum. (*Knowledge Domain 1.4*)

34. **(C)** Medications kept at room temperature should be maintained at temperatures of 68°F to 77°F. Medications that need to be frozen are maintained at temperatures of −4°F to 14°F. Refrigerated medications are maintained at temperatures of 36°F to 46°F. Medications should not be kept at temperatures exceeding those of room temperature. (*Knowledge Domain 7.4*)

35. **(C)** Class III, IV, and V prescriptions may be refilled up to 5 times in 6 months. (*Knowledge Domain 6.2*)

36. **(D)** Ampicillin is not classified as a high-alert medication as indicated by the Institute for Safe Medication Practices (ISMP). Oral hypoglycemics (e.g., metformin), anticoagulants (e.g., warfarin), and intravenous sedative agents (e.g., midazolam) are all listed by ISMP for their potential to cause patient harm when used in error. (*Knowledge Domain 4.5*)

37. **(A)** A pharmacy technician may ask the patient if he or she has any questions about the prescription. According to OBRA '90, the pharmacist would need to come over in order to counsel the patient about the medication. A pharmacy technician should not call the doctor to confirm any aspect of the patient's therapy. In addition, a pharmacy technician should not reiterate the patient's concerns to the pharmacist; the pharmacist should speak to the patient directly. (*Knowledge Domain 2.9*)

38. **(C)** Nonaqueous solutions have a beyond use date of no later than 6 months. Oral solutions containing water have a beyond use date of no later than 14 days. Topical solutions containing water have a beyond use date of no later than 30 days. (*Knowledge Domain 3.4*)

39. **(A)** The electronic health record (EHR) is a digital version of a patient's chart that can be shared among the prescriber, the pharmacy, and the third-party payer. (*Knowledge Domain 9.1*)

40. **(A)** Class III and Class IV prescriptions may be transferred only 1 time when a transfer to a pharmacy that does not share a real-time online database is requested. If the pharmacy does share an online database, the prescription may be refilled as many times as needed or until the prescription expires or the refills are out. (*Knowledge Domain 2.3*)

41. **(B)** A formulary is a list of medications from which a prescriber may prescribe in a given setting. Reconciliation is the process of identifying an accurate list of medications that a patient is taking. A therapeutic equivalent is a term used to describe drug products that are pharmaceutical equivalents and have similar clinical effects when given to patients.

Adjudication is the process of submitting an online insurance claim in order to determine the payer's financial responsibility. (*Knowledge Domain 7.2*)

42. **(B)** It is true that medications with similar drug names (e.g. look-alike/sound-alike drugs) should not be placed next to each other on a pharmacy shelf. This, however, is an example of an error prevention strategy, not an example of a strategy used to prevent finding expired drugs on pharmacy shelves. Using colored stickers that indicate the month of expiration, writing the month of expiration on pharmacy stock bottles, and placing new stock bottles behind old stock bottles (e.g., rotating stock) are all common strategies used to prevent expired products from being found on pharmacy shelves. (*Knowledge Domain 7.3*)

43. **(B)** The purchasing and returning of outdated Class II medications are made using a DEA 222 form. A DEA 224 form is used by a pharmacy looking to dispense controlled substances. A DEA 106 form is used to report lost or stolen substances. A DEA 41 form is used to document the destruction of controlled substances. (*Knowledge Domain 2.4*)

44. **(D)** The Health Insurance Portability and Accountability Act of 1996 institutes privacy safeguards for all protected health information (PHI). The Poison Prevention Packaging Act of 1970 was enacted in response to a growing number of accidental poisonings in children. This act identifies household and drug products that require child-resistant containers. The Occupational Safety and Health Administration (OSHA) requires employees to be protected from hazardous chemicals. Facilities must implement infection prevention and control procedures. The Omnibus Budget Reconciliation Act (OBRA) places expectations on the pharmacist by imposing counseling obligations, prospective drug utilization review, and record-keeping mandates. (*Knowledge Domain 6.6*)

45. **(D)** The use of preprinted prescription blanks with commonly used protocols or frequently prescribed medications is an example of a standardization technique used to avoid variation or complexity. Electronic processing software is an example of automation and computerization. Fail-safe constraints, such as the integration of pharmacy computers with the pharmacy register, may be implemented as an error prevention strategy. Pharmacies may also use forcing functions to provide a stop in the system, requiring verification before proceeding to fill the prescription. An example of this would be the use of a scanner to match the selected medication to the profiled medication. (*Knowledge Domain 5.3*)

46. **(B)** Used needles should be placed into a sharps container without recapping. The recapping of needles can result in a finger prick and is an unnecessary step to take before disposing of the needle into a sharps container. (*Knowledge Domain 5.2*)

47. **(C)** Loratadine is the therapeutic equivalent for Claritin. Diphenhydramine is the therapeutic equivalent for Benadryl. Cetirizine is the therapeutic equivalent for Zyrtec. Fexofenadine is the therapeutic equivalent for Allegra. (*Knowledge Domain 1.2*)

48. **(B)** Counting trays that are used to count antibiotics or hazardous medications should be labeled and should only be used for counting those specific medications. General counting trays can be used to count all other medications. Counting trays are not made of glass. They are typically made of plastic or metal to avoid accidental breakage. Counting trays should be kept in an accessible area, typically the pharmacy filling area. They should not be kept in the compounding area of the pharmacy. (*Knowledge Domain 3.1*)

49. **(A)** Class II prescriptions must be presented in person or sent in electronically (check with your state laws) and therefore may not be prescribed over the phone. Class III, Class IV, and noncontrolled prescriptions may all be called into the pharmacy by the prescriber. (*Knowledge Domain 6.2*)

50. **(B)** Federal law mandates that a patient package insert (PPI) must always be dispensed with select medications, including oral contraceptives, hormone replacement therapy, and inhalers. (*Knowledge Domain 4.2*)

51. **(A)** A formulation record contains the "recipe" for all compounded medications. Each recipe contains the name, the strength and the dose of the compounded medication, the name and strength of each ingredient used, a list of equipment used, and a mixing process (if applicable). (*Knowledge Domain 3.3*)

52. **(D)** A mortar and pestle are used to grind tablets or granules into a fine powder. A spatula may be used in conjunction with an ointment slab to mix ointments. A spatula may be used on an electronic balance to transfer a compound to be weighed. A stirring rod is used in a beaker to mix an aqueous solution. (*Knowledge Domain 3.5*)

53. **(B)** Federal law mandates that Schedule II prescriptions must be maintained in the pharmacy for at least 2 years. (*Knowledge Domain 2.6*)

54. **(D)** The drug manufacturer sponsors patient assistance programs in order to receive medications that are not typically covered by insurance. A company that administers a drug benefit program is referred to as a Pharmacy Benefits Manager. The portion of the price of a medication that a patient is required to pay is called a co pay. A set amount that must be paid by the patient before the insurer will cover any costs is known as a deductible. (*Knowledge Domain 8.3*)

55. **(A)** Fat-soluble vitamins can be recalled using the acronym "ADEK," referring to vitamins A, D, E, and K. (*Knowledge Domain 1.6*)

56. **(B)** The minimum weighable quantity for a Class A prescription balance is 120 mg. The prescription balance is used to measure mass, not volume, and has a minimum sensitivity reading of 6 mg. (*Knowledge Domain 3.5*)

57. **(A)** The oral syringe is most appropriate when dispensing liquid for an infant because the caregiver can draw up the correct amount of medication into the syringe. A measuring cup would not be appropriate because an infant is not able to drink from a cup. An oral dropper is difficult to use, and the caregiver may not accurately count the number of drops given to the child. A teaspoon is a household unit of measure that should not be used when dosing a patient. (*Knowledge Domain 6.6*)

58. **(C)** Insulin glargine (Lantus, Toujeo) is classified as a long-acting insulin. Insulin glulisine (Apridra), insulin aspart (Humalog), and insulin lispro (Novolog) are all classified as rapid-acting insulin. (*Knowledge Domain 1.4*)

59. **(D)** QID is an acronym meaning "four times a day." QD means every day, BID refers to twice a day, and TID means three times a day. (*Knowledge Domain 6.2*)

60. **(D)** A pharmacy information system does not require the use of a fax machine when being implemented. A computer, software, a database, and a telephone interface are all necessary for a pharmacy information system. (*Knowledge Domain 9.2*)

61. **(A)** An insurance claim rejection, resulting in a person code error, may be fixed by verifying the person code and reprocessing the claim. (*Knowledge Domain 8.2*)

62. **(C)** This problem can be solved by setting up a proportion:

$$\frac{1 \text{ gallon}}{8 \text{ pints}} = \frac{x \text{ gallons}}{240 \text{ pints}}$$

$$8x = 240$$

$$x = 30$$

The answer is 30 gallons. (*Knowledge Domain 6.3*)

63. **(B)** The final check, which includes a comprehensive drug utilization review, must be performed only by a licensed pharmacist. (*Knowledge Domain 6.4*)

64. **(A)** A comprehensive knowledge of brand and generic medication names can assist a pharmacy technician in identifying medications. Having this knowledge also lessens the chance of potential interpretation errors. (*Knowledge Domain 6.2*)

65. **(A)** This problem may be solved by setting up a proportion. Recall that D10W is a solution containing 10% dextrose in water:

$$\frac{10 \text{ g}}{100 \text{ mL}} = \frac{x}{1,000 \text{ mL}}$$

$$100x = 10,000$$

$$x = 100$$

The answer is 100 g. (*Knowledge Domain 3.6*)

66. **(C)** Institutional pharmacies do not process insurance information; this is typically handled by the hospital's business office. Pharmacies need the patient's name, the prescriber's information, and the manufacturer's information in order to process the prescription. (*Knowledge Domain 8.4*)

67. **(B)** *USP* <797> suggests that all personnel thoroughly wash their hands, nails, and arms up to the elbow using an antiseptic cleansing agent for 30 seconds. Hands should be dried with a lint-free towel. (*Knowledge Domain 2.11*)

68. **(A)** Medication stock is rotated in order to minimize stock loss by placing short-date medications near the front of the shelf and long-date medications at the back of the shelf. (*Knowledge Domain 7.3*)

69. **(A)** Unit-dose packaged medications should include the medication name, the strength, the manufacturer's name, the NDC, the lot number, and the expiration date. They may also include bar coding technology to identify the medication. They do not include instructions for patient use. (*Knowledge Domain 6.5*)

70. **(B)** The Joint Commission accredits health care agencies, including hospitals and long-term care facilities. The State Board of Pharmacy is responsible for licensing pharmacists and technicians, where applicable by law. The Centers for Medicare and Medicaid administer Medicare and Medicaid services. The Drug Enforcement Agency oversees the Controlled Substances Act. (*Knowledge Domain 2.13*)

71. **(A)** Misbranded drugs are those that contain labeling that is false or misleading or those for which the labeling fails to contain pertinent information. (The name and address of the manufacturer, the name of the drug, the packer's or distributor's name, the weight of active ingredients per dose, the lot number, and the expiration date are all information required on a label.) Adulterated drugs may be prepared or stored in unsanitary conditions. Additionally, adulterated drugs can contain unsafe color additives. They may also be within containers composed of poisonous substances that can cause contamination. (*Knowledge Domain 2.12*)

72. **(C)** This problem can be solved by setting up a proportion:

$$\frac{15 \text{ mL}}{1 \text{ hr}} = \frac{x}{36 \text{ hr}}$$

$$x = 540$$

The answer is 540 mL. (*Knowledge Domain 3.6*)

73. **(C)** The FDA classifies recalls according to severity. Class III recalls are not likely to cause adverse health consequences. Class I recalls are initiated when the likelihood of causing an adverse health consequence, or even death, is possible. Class II recalls are initiated when the use of a product may cause temporary health problems and the probability of a serious adverse health consequence is minimal. The FDA currently classifies recalls based on one of three categories and does not recognize a Class IV recall. (*Knowledge Domain 2.10*)

74. **(C)** The sig "1–2 gtts os TID" can be translated to mean "Instill 1–2 drops in the left eye three times a day." Os refers to the left eye, ou means both eyes, and od means the right eye. (*Knowledge Domain 6.2*)

75. **(A)** Upon receipt of a drug recall, pharmacy staff should pull the offending drug from pharmacy shelves immediately and contact patients who are taking this medication. The offending drug should not be left on pharmacy shelves nor should it be used to fill additional prescriptions. In addition, an attempt to order additional quantities of the offending drug should be avoided. (*Knowledge Domain 5.4*)

76. **(D)** Angiotensin II receptor blockers (ARB) are used to treat hypertension by causing vasodilation. These agents, also known as angiotensin antagonists, can be recognized by the suffix "-sartan" and are often referred to as "sartans." An example of an ARB is candesartan. Metoprolol is a beta receptor agonist used in the treatment of hypertension. Beta receptor blockers, also knows as beta blockers, are often recognized by the suffix "-olol." Lisinopril is an ACE inhibitor used to treat hypertension. ACE inhibitors can be recognized by the suffix "-pril." Lovastatin is an HMG-CoA reductase inhibitor used in the treatment of hyperlipidemia. HMG-CoA reductase inhibitors are often recognized by the suffix "-statin" and are often referred to as "statins." (*Knowledge Domain 1.6*)

77. **(B)** Medication bottles are assumed to expire at the end of the month unless otherwise stated. (*Knowledge Domain 7.1*)

78. **(B)** The Combat Methamphetamine Act of 2005 was enacted to regulate the sale of products containing pseudoephedrine, ephedrine, and phenylpropanolamine. (*Knowledge Domain 2.7*)

79. **(B)** This problem can be solved by using an alligation. Set up a tic-tac-toe grid as follows:

30 (H)		10 (P – L)
	15 (P)	
5 (L)		15 (H – P)

STEP 1 Set up an allegation placing 30 into the top left corner and 5 into the bottom left corner. The final preparation concentration is placed into the middle.

STEP 2 Determine the number of parts by subtracting as indicated above.

STEP 3 Add the number of parts together to determine the total number of parts:

$$10 + 15 = 25 \text{ total parts}$$

STEP 4 Set up a proportion to determine the quantity needed of each solution:

$$30\%: \frac{10}{25} = \frac{x}{500 \text{ mL}}$$

$$25x = 5{,}000$$

$$x = 200 \text{ mL}$$

$$5\%: \frac{15}{25} = \frac{x}{500 \text{ mL}}$$

$$25x = 7{,}500$$

$$x = 300 \text{ mL}$$

The answer is 200 mL of 30% solution and 300 mL of 5% solution. (*Knowledge Domain 3.6*)

80. **(B)** This problem can be solved by setting up a proportion:

$$\frac{125 \text{ mg}}{1 \text{ mL}} = \frac{275 \text{ mg}}{x}$$

$$125x = 275$$

$$x = 2.2$$

The answer is 2.2 mL. (*Knowledge Domain 6.3*)

81. **(B)** Aseptic manipulations should be prepared at least 6 inches within a laminar flow hood in order to avoid contamination with air located outside of the hood. (*Knowledge Domain 3.6*)

82. **(D)** The online processing of a claim to determine payment is called an adjudication. This process is completed in real time and provides an accurate determination of co-pays for the patient. Formularies are a list of available medications that can be used in a variety of settings. A co-pay is a fixed amount that a patient pays for his or her medication or service. A deductible is the amount a patient pays for health care services before the insurer will pay for these services. (*Knowledge Domain 8.2*)

83. **(C)** The "C" stamped or printed on controlled substance prescriptions and manufacturer bottles is red in color. (*Knowledge Domain 2.3*)

84. **(B)** Military time can be converted to standard time by subtracting 1200 for military times 1300 and larger (e.g., 1800 – 1200 = 6:00 P.M.). Military times less than 1300 can similarly be converted by adding 1200 to the military time. (*Knowledge Domain 6.1*)

85. **(C)** Pharmacy technicians should refuse to fill incomplete prescriptions and bring the prescription to the attention of the pharmacist. Pharmacy technicians should never contact the prescriber directly to verify a prescription. Pharmacy technicians should never fill the script based on past trends or the patient's recollection. (*Knowledge Domain 4.1*)

86. **(B)** The Accreditation Council for Pharmacy Education oversees providers of continuing education for both pharmacists and pharmacy technicians. The State Board of Pharmacy oversees the licensing of pharmacists and pharmacy technicians. The American Society of Health-System Pharmacists represents pharmacists in a variety of settings. It serves to improve medication use and enhance patient safety. The American Pharmacists Association® is a national organization consisting of pharmacists, pharmacy interns, pharmacy students, and pharmacy technicians. It aims to promote the pharmacy itself and the voice of pharmacy. (*Knowledge Domain 2.13*)

87. **(C)** Capsules and tablets are typically counted in multiples of 5 when using a counting tray. (*Knowledge Domain 6.4*)

88. **(A)** The shaft is the stem of the needle that provides the overall length. The bevel is the angled surface at the top of the needle. The hub is the portion of the needle that attaches to the syringe. The lumen is the hollow center of the needle. (*Knowledge Domain 3.5*)

89. **(C)** Bar coding technology is not used to identify cost-saving strategies at this time. Verification of the correct drug, correct dose, and correct patient are all ways that bar coding technology is implemented to improve patient outcome and enhance patient safety. (*Knowledge Domain 9.2*)

90. **(A)** A suspension is a liquid dosage form where the active ingredient, most commonly a solid particle, is dispersed in a liquid vehicle. An emulsion is a mixture of two or more liquids that are immiscible. An elixir is a hydroalcoholic solution containing water and alcohol. A solution is a liquid dosage form where the active ingredient is dissolved in the liquid medium. (*Knowledge Domain 3.5*)

Appendixes

Appendix A:
Top 200 Brand Name Drugs

Brand Name	Generic Name	Classification and Use
Abilify	aripiprazole	Antipsychotic
Aciphex	rabeprazole	gastric antisecretory and GERD
Actonel	risedronate	Bisphosphonate
Actos	pioglitazone	Antidiabetic
Adderall XR	amphetamine and dextroamphetamine	Stimulant
Advair Diskus	fluticasone and salmeterol	Topical corticosteroid and bronchodilator combination
Aleve	naproxen	Nonsteroidal anti-inflammatory
Allegra	fexofenadine	Antihistamine
Allegra-D	fexofenadine and pseudoephedrine	Antihistamine and decongestant combination
Altace	ramipril	Antihypertensive
Amaryl	glimepiride	Antidiabetic
Ambien	zolpidem	Anxiolytics and sedatives and hypnotics
Amoxil	amoxicillin	Antibiotic
Ancef	cefazolin	Antibiotic
Aricept	donepezil	Neurodegenerative agent
Ativan	lorazepam	Anxiolytics and sedatives and hypnotics
Atropen	atropine	Antimuscarinic
Atrovent	ipratropium bromide	Bronchodilator
Augmentin	amoxicillin and clavulanate	Antibiotic
Avodart	dutasteride	Antitestosterone
Bactrim	trimethoprim and sulfamethoxazole	Antibiotic
Bactroban	mupirocin	Topical antibiotic
Bayer	aspirin	Nonsteroidal anti-inflammatory and antiplatelet
Benadryl	diphenhydramine	Antihistamine
Benicar	olmesartan	Antihypertensive
Biaxin	clarithromycin	Antibiotic

Brand Name	Generic Name	Classification and Use
Bystolic	nebivolol	Antihypertensive
Caduet	amlodipine and atorvastatin	Antihypertensive and hypolipidemic
Calan	verapamil	Antihypertensive and antiarrhythmic
Calciferol	ergocalciferol	Vitamin derivative
Catapres	clonidine	Antihypertensive
Celebrex	celecoxib	Nonsteroidal anti-inflammatory
Celexa	citalopram	Antidepressant
Cialis	tadalafil	PDE-5 inhibitor
Cipro	ciprofloxacin	Antibiotic
Claforan	cefotaxime	Antibiotic
Claritin	loratadine	Antihistamine
Claritin-D 24 Hour	loratadine and pseudoephedrine	Antihistamine and decongestant combination
Colace	docusate sodium	Laxative
Combivent Respimat	ipratropium bromide and albuterol	Bronchodilator combination
Compazine	prochlorperazine	Antiemetic
Concerta	methylphenidate ER	Stimulant
Cordarone	amiodarone	Antiarrhythmic
Coreg	carvedilol	Antihypertensive
Cortizone 10	hydrocortisone	Topical corticosteroid
Coumadin	warfarin	Anticoagulant
Cozaar	losartan	Antihypertensive
Crestor	rosuvastatin	Hypolipidemic
Cymbalta	duloxetine	Antidepressant
Decadron	dexamethasone	Systemic adrenal corticosteroid
Delsym	dextromethorphan	Antitussive
Deltasone	prednisone	Systemic adrenal corticosteroid
Desyrel	trazodone	Antidepressant
Detrol LA	tolterodine	Nonvascular smooth muscle relaxant
Diflucan	fluconazole	Antifungal
Diovan	valsartan	Antihypertensive
Diovan HCT	valsartan and hydrochlorothiazide	Antihypertensive and diuretic combination
Diprivan	propofol	General anesthetic and sedative and hypnotic
Dobutrex	dobutamine	Inotrope
Dopastat	dopamine	Inotrope and pressor
Duragesic	fentanyl	Opioid analgesic
Effexor	venlafaxine	Antidepressant
Elavil	amitriptyline	Antidepressant
Epogen	epoetin alpha	Growth factor
Flexeril	cyclobenzaprine	Skeletal muscle relaxant

Brand Name	Generic Name	Classification and Use
Flomax	tamsulosin	Alpha blocker
Flonase	fluticasone	Topical corticosteroid
Flovent HFA	fluticasone	Inhaled corticosteroid
FluMist	influenza vaccine live	Vaccine
Fluzone	inactivated influenza vaccine	Vaccine
Focalin XR	dexmethylphenidate	Stimulant
Fosamax	alendronate	Bisphosphonate
Glucophage	metformin	Antidiabetic
Humalog	insulin lispro	Antidiabetic
Humulin N	insulin NPH (human)	Antidiabetic
Humulin R	insulin regular (human)	Antidiabetic
Hydrodiuril	hydrochlorothiazide	Diuretic
Imitrex	sumatriptan	Antimigraine and central vasoconstrictor
Inderal	propanolol	Antihypertensive
Ismo	isosorbide mononitrate	Antianginal
Isordil	isosorbide dinitrate	Antianginal
Januvia	sitagliptin	Antidiabetic
Keflex	cephalexin	Antibiotic
Klonopin	clonazepam	Anxiolytics and sedatives and hypnotics
Lamasil	terbinafine	Topical antifungal
Lanoxin	digoxin	Inotrope
Lantus	insulin glargine	Antidiabetic
Lasix	furosemide	Diuretic
Levaquin	levofloxacin	Antibiotic
Levemir	insulin detemir	Antidiabetic
Lexapro	escitalopram	SSRI antidepressant
Lipitor	atorvastatin	Hypolipidemic
Loestrin	ethinyl estradiol and norethindrone	Contraceptive
Lotensin	benazepril	Antihypertensive
Lotrel	amlodipine and benazepril	Antihypertensive
Lovaza	omega-3-acid ethyl esters	Hypolipidemic
Lovenox	enoxaparin	Anticoagulant
Lunesta	eszopiclone	Anxiolytics and sedatives and hypnotics
Lyrica	pregabalin	Anticonvulsant
Maxzide	triamterene and hydrochlorothiazide	Diuretic
Medrol	methylprednisolone	Systemic adrenal corticosteroid
Micro-K	potassium chloride	Electrolyte
Micronase	glyburide	Antidiabetic

Brand Name	Generic Name	Classification and Use
Miralax	polyethylene glycol 3350	Laxative
Mobic	meloxicam	Nonsteroidal anti-inflammatory
Motrin	ibuprofen	Nonsteroidal anti-inflammatory
MS Contin	morphine	Opioid analgesic
Namenda	memantine	Neurodegenerative agent
Narcan	naloxone	Opioid antagonist
Nasonex	mometasone furoate	Topical corticosteroid
Neosporin	neomycin and polymixin B and bacitracin	Topical antibiotic
Neurontin	gabapentin	Anticonvulsant
Nexium	esomeprazole	gastric antisecretory and GERD
Nitrostat	nitroglycerin	Antianginal
Norvasc	amlodipine	Antihypertensive
NuvaRing	etonogestrel and ethinyl estradiol	Contraceptive
Os-Cal	calcium carbonate	Vitamin derivative
Oxycontin	oxycodone	Opioid analgesic
Paxil	paroxetine	Antidepressant
Pepcid AC	famotidine	gastric antisecretory and GERD
Pepto Bismol	bismuth subsalicylate	gastric antisecretory and GERD
Percocet	oxycodone and acetaminophen	Opioid analgesic and analgesic combination
Phenergan	promethazine	Antihistamine
Phenergan with Codeine	promethazine and codeine	Antitussive combination
Plavix	clopidogrel	Anticoagulant
Pradaxa	dabigatran etexilate	Anticoagulant
Pravachol	pravastatin	Hypolipidemic
Premarin	conjugated estrogens	Female sex hormone
Prevacid 24-Hour	lansoprazole	gastric antisecretory and GERD
Prilosec	omeprazole	gastric antisecretory and GERD
Prinizide	lisinopril and hydrochlorothiazide	Antihypertensive and diuretic combination
Pristiq	desvenlafaxine	Antidepressant
Protonix	pantoprazole	gastric antisecretory and GERD
Prozac	fluoxetine	Antidepressant
Qvar	beclomethasone	Topical corticosteroid
Restoril	temazepam	Anxiolytics and sedatives and hypnotics
Rhinocort	budesonide	Topical corticosteroid
Robitussin	guiafenesin	Expectorant
Rocaltrol	calcitriol	Vitamin derivative

Brand Name	Generic Name	Classification and Use
Rocephin	ceftriaxone	Antibiotic
Senokot	senna	Laxative
Seroquel	quetiapine	Antipsychotic
Singulair	montelukast	Immune modulator
Solu-Cortef	hydrocortisone	Systemic adrenal corticosteroid
Soma	carisoprodol	Skeletal muscle relaxant
Spiriva HandiHaler	tiotropium bromide	Bronchodilator
St. John's Wort	*Hypericum perforatum*	Antidepressant (non-FDA approved)
Sublimaze	fentanyl	Opioid analgesic
Suboxone	buprenorphine and naloxone	Opioid analgesic and opioid antagonist combination
Sudafed	pseudoephedrine	Decongestant
Sudafed PE	phenylephrine	Pressor and vasoconstrictor
Symbicort	budesonide and formoterol	Topical corticosteroid and bronchodilator combination
Synthroid	levothyroxine	Thyroid agent
Tamiflu	oseltamivir	Antiviral
Tenormin	atenolol	Antihypertensive
Toprol XL	metoprolol succinate	Antihypertensive
Toradol	ketorolac	Nonsteroidal anti-inflammatory
Tricor	fenofibrate	Hypolipidemic
Tylenol	acetaminophen	Analgesic and Antipyretic
Tylenol with Codeine	acetaminophen and codeine	Opioid analgesic and analgesic combination
Ultram	tramadol	Opioid analgesic
Valium	diazepam	Anxiolytics and sedatives and hypnotics
Valtrex	valacyclovir	Antiviral
Vancocin	vancomycin	Antibiotic
Ventolin	albuterol	Bronchodilator
Versed	midazolam	Anxiolytics and sedatives and hypnotics
Vesicare	solifenacin	Nonvascular smooth muscle relaxant
Viagra	sildenafil	Vasodilator
Vicodin	hydrocodone and acetaminophen	Opioid analgesic and analgesic combination
Vytorin	ezetimibe and simvastatin	Hypolipidemic
Vyvanse	lisdexamfetamine	Stimulant
Wellbutrin	bupropion	Antidepressant
Xalatan	latanoprost	Topical prostaglandin analog
Xanax	alprazolam	Anxiolytics and sedatives and hypnotics
Xarelto	rivaroxaban	Anticoagulant

Brand Name	Generic Name	Classification and Use
Xopenex	levalbuterol	Bronchodilator
Xylocaine	lidocaine	Local anesthetic
Yaz	ethinyl estradiol and drospirenone	Contraceptive
Zantac	ranitidine	gastric antisecretory
Zestril	lisinopril	Antihypertensive
Zetia	ezetimibe	Hypolipidemic
Zithromax	azithromycin	Antibiotic
Zocor	simvastatin	Hypolipidemic
Zofran	ondansetron	Antiemetic
Zoloft	sertraline	Antidepressant
Zosyn	piperacillin and tazobactam	Antibiotic
Zovirax	acyclovir	Antiviral
Zyloprim	allopurinol	Gout
Zyprexa	olanzepine	Antipsychotic
Zyrtec	cetirizine	Antihistamine
	echinacea*	Immune stimulator
	ferrous sulfate*	Iron preparation
	Ginkgo biloba*	Stimulant
	green tea*	Anti-inflammatory and antioxidant
	heparin*	Anticoagulant
	magnesium sulfate*	Electrolyte
	penicillin*	Antibiotic
	potassium chloride*	Electrolyte
	triamcinolone*	Topical corticosteroid
	vitamin D3*	Vitamin derivative

*No brand name formulation is currently available.

**Note that the Pharmacy Technician Certification Board does not endorse any one list of the top 200 brand name drugs because this information is constantly being updated. However, this list should provide you with a general idea of some of the most common brand name drugs that you should be familiar with.

Appendix B: Top 200 Brand Name Drugs by Classification

Classification and Use	Brand Name	Generic Name
Alpha blocker	Flomax	tamsulosin
Analgesic and antipyretic	Tylenol	acetaminophen
Antianginal	Ismo	isosorbide mononitrate
Antianginal	Isordil	isosorbide dinitrate
Antianginal	Nitrostat	nitroglycerin
Antiarrhythmic	Cordarone	amiodarone
Antibiotic	Amoxil	amoxicillin
Antibiotic	Ancef	cefazolin
Antibiotic	Augmentin	amoxicillin and clavulanate
Antibiotic	Bactrim	trimethoprim and sulfamethoxazole
Antibiotic	Biaxin	clarithromycin
Antibiotic	Cipro	ciprofloxacin
Antibiotic	Claforan	cefotaxime
Antibiotic	Keflex	cephalexin
Antibiotic	Levaquin	levofloxacin
Antibiotic	Rocephin	ceftriaxone
Antibiotic	Vancocin	vancomycin
Antibiotic	Zithromax	azithromycin
Antibiotic	Zosyn	piperacillin and tazobactam
Antibiotic		penicillin*
Anticoagulant	Coumadin	warfarin
Anticoagulant	Lovenox	enoxaparin
Anticoagulant	Plavix	clopidogrel
Anticoagulant	Pradaxa	dabigatran etexilate
Anticoagulant	Xarelto	rivaroxaban
Anticoagulant		heparin*
Anticonvulsant	Lyrica	pregabalin
Anticonvulsant	Neurontin	gabapentin
Antidepressant	Celexa	citalopram
Antidepressant	Cymbalta	duloxetine
Antidepressant	Desyrel	trazodone
Antidepressant	Effexor	venlafaxine
Antidepressant	Elavil	amitriptyline

Classification and Use	Brand Name	Generic Name
Antidepressant	Paxil	paroxetine
Antidepressant	Pristiq	desvenlafaxine
Antidepressant	Prozac	fluoxetine
Antidepressant (non-FDA approved)	St. John's Wort	*Hypericum perforatum*
Antidepressant	Wellbutrin	bupropion
Antidepressant	Zoloft	sertraline
Antidiabetic	Actos	pioglitazone
Antidiabetic	Amaryl	glimepiride
Antidiabetic	Glucophage	metformin
Antidiabetic	Humalog	insulin lispro
Antidiabetic	Humulin N	insulin NPH (human)
Antidiabetic	Humulin R	insulin regular (human)
Antidiabetic	Januvia	sitagliptin
Antidiabetic	Lantus	insulin glargine
Antidiabetic	Levemir	insulin detemir
Antidiabetic	Micronase	glyburide
Antiemetic	Compazine	prochlorperazine
Antiemetic	Zofran	ondansetron
Antifungal	Diflucan	fluconazole
Antihistamine	Allegra	fexofenadine
Antihistamine	Benadryl	diphenhydramine
Antihistamine	Claritin	loratadine
Antihistamine	Phenergan	promethazine
Antihistamine	Zyrtec	cetirizine
Antihistamine and decongestant combination	Allegra-D	fexofenadine and pseudoephedrine
Antihistamine and decongestant combination	Claritin-D 24 Hour	loratadine and pseudoephedrine
Antihypertensive	Altace	ramipril
Antihypertensive	Benicar	olmesartan
Antihypertensive	Bystolic	nebivolol
Antihypertensive	Catapres	clonidine
Antihypertensive	Coreg	carvedilol
Antihypertensive	Cozaar	losartan
Antihypertensive	Diovan	valsartan
Antihypertensive	Inderal	propanolol
Antihypertensive	Lotensin	benazepril
Antihypertensive	Lotrel	amlodipine and benazepril
Antihypertensive	Norvasc	amlodipine
Antihypertensive	Tenormin	atenolol
Antihypertensive	Toprol XL	metoprolol succinate
Antihypertensive	Zestril	lisinopril

Classification and Use	Brand Name	Generic Name
Antihypertensive and antiarrhythmic	Calan	verapamil
Antihypertensive and diuretic combination	Diovan HCT	valsartan and hydrochlorothiazide
Antihypertensive and diuretic combination	Prinizide	lisinopril and hydrochlorothiazide
Antihypertensive and hypolipidemic	Caduet	amlodipine and atorvastatin
Anti-inflammatory and antioxidant		green tea*
Antimigraine and central vasoconstrictor	Imitrex	sumatriptan
Antimuscarinic	Atropen	atropine
Antipsychotic	Abilify	aripiprazole
Antipsychotic	Seroquel	quetiapine
Antipsychotic	Zyprexa	olanzepine
Antitestosterone	Avodart	dutasteride
Antitussive	Delsym	dextromethorphan
Antitussive combination	Phenergan with Codeine	promethazine and codeine
Antiviral	Tamiflu	oseltamivir
Antiviral	Valtrex	valacyclovir
Antiviral	Zovirax	acyclovir
Anxiolytics and sedatives and hypnotics	Ambien	zolpidem
Anxiolytics and sedatives and hypnotics	Ativan	lorazepam
Anxiolytics and sedatives and hypnotics	Klonopin	clonazepam
Anxiolytics and sedatives and hypnotics	Lunesta	eszopiclone
Anxiolytics and sedatives and hypnotics	Restoril	temazepam
Anxiolytics and sedatives and hypnotics	Valium	diazepam
Anxiolytics and sedatives and hypnotics	Versed	midazolam
Anxiolytics and sedatives and hypnotics	Xanax	alprazolam
Bisphosphonate	Actonel	risedronate
Bisphosphonate	Fosamax	alendronate
Bronchodilator	Atrovent	ipratropium bromide
Bronchodilator	Spiriva HandiHaler	tiotropium bromide
Bronchodilator	Ventolin	albuterol
Bronchodilator	Xopenex	levalbuterol
Bronchodilator combination	Combivent Respimat	ipratropium bromide and albuterol

Classification and Use	Brand Name	Generic Name
Contraceptive	Loestrin	ethinyl estradiol and norethindrone
Contraceptive	NuvaRing	etonogestrel and ethinyl estradiol
Contraceptive	Yaz	ethinyl estradiol and drospirenone
Decongestant	Sudafed	pseudoephedrine
Diuretic	Hydrodiuril	hydrochlorothiazide
Diuretic	Lasix	furosemide
Diuretic	Maxzide	triamterene and hydrochlorothiazide
Electrolyte	Micro-K	potassium chloride
Electrolyte		magnesium sulfate*
Electrolyte		potassium chloride*
Expectorant	Robitussin	guiafenesin
Female sex hormone	Premarin	conjugated estrogens
gastric antisecretory	Pepcid AC	famotidine
gastric antisecretory	Pepto Bismol	bismuth subsalicylate
gastric antisecretory	Zantac	ranitidine
gastric antisecretory and GERD	Aciphex	rabeprazole
gastric antisecretory and GERD	Nexium	esomeprazole
gastric antisecretory and GERD	Prevacid 24-Hour	lansoprazole
gastric antisecretory and GERD	Prilosec	omeprazole
gastric antisecretory and GERD	Protonix	pantoprazole
General anesthetic and sedative and hypnotic	Diprivan	propofol
Gout	Zyloprim	allopurinol
Growth factor	Epogen	epoetin alpha
Hypolipidemic	Crestor	rosuvastatin
Hypolipidemic	Lipitor	atorvastatin
Hypolipidemic	Lovaza	omega-3-acid ethyl esters
Hypolipidemic	Pravachol	pravastatin
Hypolipidemic	Tricor	fenofibrate
Hypolipidemic	Vytorin	ezetimibe and simvastatin
Hypolipidemic	Zetia	ezetimibe
Hypolipidemic	Zocor	simvastatin
Immune modulator	Singulair	montelukast
Immune stimulator		echinacea*
Inhaled corticosteroid	Flovent HFA	fluticasone
Inotrope	Dobutrex	dobutamine
Inotrope	Lanoxin	digoxin
Inotrope and pressor	Dopastat	dopamine

Classification and Use	Brand Name	Generic Name
Iron preparation		ferrous sulfate*
Laxative	Colace	docusate sodium
Laxative	Miralax	polyethylene glycol 3350
Laxative	Senokot	senna
Local anesthetic	Xylocaine	lidocaine
Neurodegenerative agent	Aricept	donepezil
Neurodegenerative agent	Namenda	memantine
Nonsteroidal anti-inflammatory	Aleve	naproxen
Nonsteroidal anti-inflammatory	Celebrex	celecoxib
Nonsteroidal anti-inflammatory	Mobic	meloxicam
Nonsteroidal anti-inflammatory	Motrin	ibuprofen
Nonsteroidal anti-inflammatory	Toradol	ketorolac
Nonsteroidal anti-inflammatory and antiplatelet	Bayer	aspirin
Nonvascular smooth muscle relaxant	Detrol LA	tolterodine
Nonvascular smooth muscle relaxant	Vesicare	solifenacin
Opioid analgesic	Duragesic	fentanyl
Opioid analgesic	MS Contin	morphine
Opioid analgesic	Oxycontin	oxycodone
Opioid analgesic	Sublimaze	fentanyl
Opioid analgesic	Ultram	tramadol
Opioid analgesic and analgesic combination	Percocet	oxycodone and acetaminophen
Opioid analgesic and analgesic combination	Tylenol with Codeine	acetaminophen and codeine
Opioid analgesic and analgesic combination	Vicodin	hydrocodone and acetaminophen
Opioid analgesic and opioid antagonist combination	Suboxone	buprenorphine and naloxone
Opioid antagonist	Narcan	naloxone
PDE-5 inhibitor	Cialis	tadalafil
PDE-5 inhibitor	Viagra	sildenafil
Pressor and vasoconstrictor	Sudafed PE	phenylephrine
Skeletal muscle relaxant	Flexeril	cyclobenzaprine
Skeletal muscle relaxant	Soma	carisoprodol
SSRI antidepressant	Lexapro	escitalopram
Stimulant	Adderall XR	amphetamine and dextroamphetamine
Stimulant	Concerta	methylphenidate ER
Stimulant	Focalin XR	dexmethylphenidate
Stimulant	Vyvanse	lisdexamfetamine
Stimulant		*Ginkgo biloba**
Systemic adrenal corticosteroid	Decadron	dexamethasone

Classification and Use	Brand Name	Generic Name
Systemic adrenal corticosteroid	Deltasone	prednisone
Systemic adrenal corticosteroid	Medrol	methylprednisolone
Systemic adrenal corticosteroid	Solu-Cortef	hydrocortisone
Thyroid agent	Synthroid	levothyroxine
Topical antibiotic	Bactroban	mupirocin
Topical antibiotic	Neosporin	neomycin and polymixin B and bacitracin
Topical antifungal	Lamasil	terbinafine
Topical corticosteroid	Cortizone 10	hydrocortisone
Topical corticosteroid	Flonase	fluticasone
Topical corticosteroid	Nasonex	mometasone furoate
Topical corticosteroid	Qvar	beclomethasone
Topical corticosteroid	Rhinocort	budesonide
Topical corticosteroid		triamcinolone*
Topical corticosteroid and bronchodilator combination	Advair Diskus	fluticasone and salmeterol
Topical corticosteroid and bronchodilator combination	Symbicort	budesonide and formoterol
Topical prostaglandin analog	Xalatan	latanoprost
Vaccine	FluMist	influenza vaccine live
Vaccine	Fluzone	inactivated influenza vaccine
Vitamin derivative	Calciferol	ergocalciferol
Vitamin derivative	Os-Cal	calcium carbonate
Vitamin derivative	Rocaltrol	calcitriol
Vitamin derivative		vitamin D3*

*No brand name formulation is currently available.

**Note that the Pharmacy Technician Certification Board does not endorse any one list of the top 200 brand name drugs because this information is constantly being updated. However, this list should provide you with a general idea of some of the most common brand name drugs that you should be familiar with.

Appendix C: Commonly Refrigerated Prescription Medications

Brand Name	Generic Name
Amoxil*	amoxicillin
Apidra	insulin glulisine
Augmentin*	amoxicillin and clavulanic
Avonex	interferon beta-1a
Benzamycin gel	erythromycin and benzoyl peroxide
Byetta	exenatide
Ceclor*	cefaclor
Ceftin*	cefuroxime axetil
Cipro	ciprofloxacin
Combipatch	estradiol and norethindrone
DDAVP	desmopressin
Duac	clindamycin and benzoyl peroxide
Duricef*	cefadroxil
Enbrel	etanercept
Epogen	epoetin alfa
Foradil	formoterol
Forteo	teriparatide
Humalog	insulin aspart
Humira	adalimumab
Humulin N	NPH insulin
Humulin R	regular insulin
Iletin	insulin
Infergen	interferon alfacon-1
Kaletra	lopinavir and ritonavir
Keflex*	cephalexin
Kineret	anakinra
Lantus	insulin glargine
Levemir	insulin detemir
Miacalcin	calcitonin
Neulasta	pegfilgrastim
Neupogen	filgrastim
Novolin N	NPH insulin
Novolin R	regular insulin

Brand Name	Generic Name
Novolog	insulin lispro
NuvaRing	etonogestrel and ethinyl estradiol vaginal ring
Phenergan suppository	promethazine
Procrit	epoetin alfa
Rebetron	interferon alfa-2b and ribavirin
Suprax	cefixime
Tamiflu*	oseltamivir
V-Cillin K*	penicillin V potassium
Veetids*	penicillin V
Vibramycin	doxycycline
Victoza	liraglutide
Viroptic	trifluridine
Xalatan	latanoprost
Zithromax*	azithromycin

*Indicates anti-infective therapy that may require refrigeration after reconstitution

Appendix D: Vitamins

Common Name	Alternate Name	Function in the Body
Vitamin A	Retinol	Essential for vision, bone growth, and skin; antioxidant
Vitamin B complex	Comprised of B-1, B-2, B-3, B-5, B-6, B-7, and B-12	Helps convert food into energy
Vitamin B1	Thiamine	Helps convert food into energy; coenzyme is used in the production of ATP
Vitamin B2	Riboflavin	Helps convert food into energy
Vitamin B3	Niacin	Helps convert food into energy; aids in the conversion of carbohydrates into energy; increases good cholesterol
Vitamin B5	Pantothenic acid	Helps convert food into energy; aids in the synthesis of fatty acids and cholesterol
Vitamin B6	Pyridoxine	May reduce the risk of heart disease; aids in the production of RBCs; plays a role in the production of key indicators that are essential to sleep, mood, and appetite
Vitamin B7	Biotin	Bone and hair growth; helps to synthesize glucose and covert food into energy
Vitamin B9	Folate	Synthetic folic acid is used in pregnancy to prevent spinal cord and brain defects
Vitamin B12	Cobalamin	May reduce the risk of heart disease; aids in the production of new cells while also encouraging the normal growth of cells; protects nerve cells; aids in the production of RBCs
Vitamin C	Ascorbic acid	Helps to produce collagen, serotonin, and norepinephrine; antioxidant
Vitamin D	Calciferol	Helps maintain normal levels of calcium and phosphorous; essential for teeth and bones
Vitamin E	Alpha-tocopherol	Antioxidant; essential for nerve function
Vitamin K	Phylloquinone	Essential in the blood-clotting cascade

Appendix E: Common Over-the-Counter Products

Brand Name	Generic Name	Classification
Abreva	docosanol	Cold sores
Afrin	oxymetazoline	Nasal decongestant
Aleve	naproxen	Anti-inflammatory
Allegra	fexofenadine	Antihistamine
Alli	orlistat	Weight loss
Benadryl	diphenhydramine	Antihistamine, sleep aid
Benefiber	wheat dextrin	Constipation
Bonine	meclizine	Nausea, motion sickness
Caladryl	calamine lotion	Topical anti-itch
Chlor-Trimeton	chlorpheniramine	Antihistamine
Citrucel	methylcellulose	Bulk laxative
Claritin	loratadine	Antihistamine
Clearasil	benzoyl peroxide	Acne
Colace	docusate	Stool softener
Cortizone	hydrocortisone	Topical corticosteroid
Debrox	carbamide peroxide	Earwax removal
Delsym	dextromethorphan	Antitussive
Dramamine	dimenhydrenate	Nausea, motion sickness
Dulcolax	bisacodyl	Stimulant laxative
Ecotrin	aspirin (enteric coated)	Anti-inflammatory
Emetrol	dextrose, levulose, phosphoric acid	Antiemetic
Excedrin	acetaminophen and aspirin and caffeine	Analgesic, anti-inflammatory, diuretic
Fibercon	polycarbophil	Laxative
Fleet suppositories	glycerin	Laxative
Flonase	fluticasone nasal	Corticosteroid used in allergic rhinitis
Gas-X, Phazyme	simethicone	Antiflatulent
Gyne-Lotrimin-3, Gyne-Lotrimin-7	clotrimazole	Vaginal antifungal
Immodium A-D	loperamide	Antidiarrheal

Brand Name	Generic Name	Classification
Ivy Dry	benzyl alcohol	Uroshiol-induced contact dermatitis
Kaopectate	bismuth subsalicylate	Antidiarrheal
Lactaid	lactase	Lactose intolerance
Lamisil AT	terbinafine	Topical antifungal
Lotrimin AF	clotrimazole	Topical antifungal
Maalox	magnesium and aluminum and simethicone	Heartburn, antacid
Melatonin	melatonin	Sleep aid
Metamucil	psyllium fiber	Fiber laxative
Miralax	polyethylene glycol 3350	Osmotic laxative
Monistat-3, Monistat-7	miconazole	Vaginal antifungal
Motrin, Advil	ibuprofen	Anti-inflammatory
Murine, Artificial Tears	artificial tears	Ocular lubricant
Mylanta	magnesium and aluminum and simethicone	Heartburn, antacid
Naphcon-A	naphazoline and pheniramine	Ocular antihistamine and decongestant
Nasacort	triamcinolone	Corticosteroid used in allergic rhinitis
Nasalcrom	cromolyn sodium	Nasal antihistamine
Neosporin	neomycin and bacitracin and polymyxin	Topical antibiotic
Nexium	esomeprazole	GERD
Nix	permethrin	Topical scabicide
NoDoz	caffeine	Stimulant
Ocean	normal saline	Nasal moisturizer
Orajel	benzocaine	Topical anesthetic
OxyClean	salicylic acid	Acne
Pepcid	famotidine	Antiulcer
Pepto-bismol	bismuth subsalicylate	Indigestion, antidiarrheal
Peroxyl Oral Cleanser	hydrogen peroxide	Oral antiseptic
Phillip's Milk of Magnesia	magnesium hydroxide	Constipation
Plan B	levonorgestrol	Emergency contraceptive
Polysporin	bacitracin and polymyxin	Topical antibiotic
Prevacid OTC	lansoprazole	GERD
Prilosec OTC	omeprazole	GERD
RID	piperonyl and pyrethrins	Pediculicide
Robitussin, Mucinex	guaifenesin	Expectorant
Rogaine	minoxidil	Hair growth
Rolaids	calcium and magnesium	Antacid
Senokot	senna	Laxative
Sudafed	pseudoephedrine	Decongestant

Brand Name	Generic Name	Classification
Sudafed PE	phenylephrine	Decongestant
Tagamet	cimetidine	Antacid
Tinactin	tolnaftate	Topical antifungal
Tums	calcium carbonate	Antacid
Tylenol	acetaminophen	Analgesic
Vagistat-1, Vagistat-3	miconazole	Vaginal antifungal
Visine Allergy	nephazoline and pheniramine	Ocular antihistamine
Zanfel	Polyethylene granules	Uroshiol-induced contact dermatitis
Zantac 75	ranitidine	Antiulcer
Zostrix	capsaicin	Topical neuralgia
Zyrtec	cetirizine	Antihistamine

Appendix F: Commonly Used Pharmacy Abbreviations

Pharmacy technicians must be able to identify pharmacy abbreviations. Check your knowledge using this list of common pharmacy abbreviations. The use of these abbreviations, as well as the placement of periods and capitalization, varies. Refer to ISMP's list of error-prone abbreviations located in Appendix G.

Each of the following tables list common abbreviations in the left column and the definitions of those abbreviations in the right column. Test your knowledge by covering the definitions. Do you remember what the abbreviations mean?

Table F-1. Frequency

Abbreviation	Definition
AC	Before meals
PC	After meals
AM	Morning
PM	Evening
HS	At nighttime
Q	Every
Q __ H	Every __ hour(s)
QD	Every day
BID	Twice a day
TID	Three times a day
QID	Four times a day
PRN	As needed

Table F-2. Formulation

Abbreviation	Definition
amp	Ampule
cap	Capsule
elix	Elixir
inj	Injection
IUD	Intrauterine device
lot	Lotion
loz	Lozenge
MDI	Metered-dose inhaler
supp	Suppository
susp	Suspension
syr	Syrup
tab	Tablet
tbsp	Tablespoon
tinct	Tincture
TPN	Total parenteral nutrition
tsp	Teaspoon
ung, oint.	Ointment

Table F-3. Route of Administration

Abbreviation	Definition
ad	Right ear
as	Left ear
au	Both ears
IM	Intramuscular
IV	Intravenous
IVP	Intravenous push
IVPB	Intravenous piggyback
od	Right eye
os	Left eye
ou	Both eyes
PO	By mouth
PR	Rectal
PV	Vaginal
subq, SC	Subcutaneous
top	Topical

Table F-4. Units

Abbreviation	Definition
cc	Cubic centimeter
fl oz	Fluid ounce
g or G	Gram
gal	Gallon
gr	Grain
kg	Kilogram
L	Liter
lb	Pound
mcg	Microgram
mg	Milligram
mL	Milliliter
oz	Ounce
pt	Pint
qt	Quart

Table F-5. Other

Abbreviation	Definition
aa	Of each
c	With
disp	Dispense
Div	Divide
non rep	Do not repeat
NR	No refills
Rx	Prescription
S	Without
sig	Label, write
ss	One-half
ud	As directed

Appendix G: Institute for Safe Medication Practices's (ISMP's) List of Error-Prone Abbreviations, Symbols, and Dose Designations

The use of pharmacy abbreviations, acronyms, and symbols may be misinterpreted due to ambiguities, which could result in significant patient safety concerns. These errors are often reported to the Institute for Safe Medication Practices National Medication Errors Reporting Program (ISMP MERP). ISMP maintains the voluntary practitioner error-reporting program to learn more about these errors and share information learned with the health care community. Examples of these errors include those made when prescribing, transcribing, dispensing, and administering medications/vaccines. ISMP has argued that these abbreviations, acronyms, and symbols should be avoided in all medical communications, including written communications, telephone/verbal communications, computer-generated labels and storage bin labels, computer order entry screens, and medication administration records. Examples of these dose designations, medication abbreviations, and symbols can be found in the following table.

Institute for Safe Medication Practices

ISMP's List of *Error-Prone Abbreviations, Symbols*, and *Dose Designations*

The abbreviations, symbols, and dose designations found in this table have been reported to ISMP through the ISMP National Medication Errors Reporting Program (ISMP MERP) as being frequently misinterpreted and involved in harmful medication errors. They should **NEVER** be used when communicating medical information. This includes internal communications, telephone/verbal prescriptions, computer-generated labels, labels for drug storage bins, medication administration records, as well as pharmacy and prescriber computer order entry screens.

Abbreviations	Intended Meaning	Misinterpretation	Correction
μg	Microgram	Mistaken as "mg"	Use "mcg"
AD, AS, AU	Right ear, left ear, each ear	Mistaken as OD, OS, OU (right eye, left eye, each eye)	Use "right ear," "left ear," or "each ear"
OD, OS, OU	Right eye, left eye, each eye	Mistaken as AD, AS, AU (right ear, left ear, each ear)	Use "right eye," "left eye," or "each eye"
BT	Bedtime	Mistaken as "BID" (twice daily)	Use "bedtime"
cc	Cubic centimeters	Mistaken as "u" (units)	Use "mL"
D/C	Discharge or discontinue	Premature discontinuation of medications if D/C (intended to mean "discharge") has been misinterpreted as "discontinued" when followed by a list of discharge medications	Use "discharge" and "discontinue"
IJ	Injection	Mistaken as "IV" or "intrajugular"	Use "injection"
IN	Intranasal	Mistaken as "IM" or "IV"	Use "intranasal" or "NAS"
HS	Half-strength	Mistaken as bedtime	Use "half-strength" or "bedtime"
hs	At bedtime, hours of sleep	Mistaken as half-strength	
IU**	International unit	Mistaken as IV (intravenous) or 10 (ten)	Use "units"
o.d. or OD	Once daily	Mistaken as "right eye" (OD-oculus dexter), leading to oral liquid medications administered in the eye	Use "daily"
OJ	Orange juice	Mistaken as OD or OS (right or left eye); drugs meant to be diluted in orange juice may be given in the eye	Use "orange juice"
Per os	By mouth, orally	The "os" can be mistaken as "left eye" (OS-oculus sinister)	Use "PO," "by mouth," or "orally"
q.d. or QD**	Every day	Mistaken as q.i.d., especially if the period after the "q" or the tail of the "q" is misunderstood as an "i"	Use "daily"
qhs	Nightly at bedtime	Mistaken as "qhr" or every hour	Use "nightly"
qn	Nightly or at bedtime	Mistaken as "qh" (every hour)	Use "nightly" or "at bedtime"
q.o.d. or QOD**	Every other day	Mistaken as "q.d." (daily) or "q.i.d. (four times daily) if the "o" is poorly written	Use "every other day"
q1d	Daily	Mistaken as q.i.d. (four times daily)	Use "daily"
q6PM, etc.	Every evening at 6 PM	Mistaken as every 6 hours	Use "daily at 6 PM" or "6 PM daily"
SC, SQ, sub q	Subcutaneous	SC mistaken as SL (sublingual); SQ mistaken as "5 every;" the "q" in "sub q" has been mistaken as "every" (e.g., a heparin dose ordered "sub q 2 hours before surgery" misunderstood as every 2 hours before surgery)	Use "subcut" or "subcutaneously"
ss	Sliding scale (insulin) or ½ (apothecary)	Mistaken as "55"	Spell out "sliding scale;" use "one-half" or "½"
SSRI	Sliding scale regular insulin	Mistaken as selective-serotonin reuptake inhibitor	Spell out "sliding scale (insulin)"
SSI	Sliding scale insulin	Mistaken as Strong Solution of Iodine (Lugol's)	
i/d	One daily	Mistaken as "tid"	Use "1 daily"
TIW or tiw	3 times a week	Mistaken as "3 times a day" or "twice in a week"	Use "3 times weekly"
U or u**	Unit	Mistaken as the number 0 or 4, causing a 10-fold overdose or greater (e.g., 4U seen as "40" or 4u seen as "44"); mistaken as "cc" so dose given in volume instead of units (e.g., 4u seen as 4cc)	Use "unit"
UD	As directed ("ut dictum")	Mistaken as unit dose (e.g., diltiazem 125 mg IV infusion "UD" misinterpreted as meaning to give the entire infusion as a unit [bolus] dose)	Use "as directed"

Dose Designations and Other Information	Intended Meaning	Misinterpretation	Correction
Trailing zero after decimal point (e.g., 1.0 mg)**	1 mg	Mistaken as 10 mg if the decimal point is not seen	Do not use trailing zeros for doses expressed in whole numbers
"Naked" decimal point (e.g., .5 mg)**	0.5 mg	Mistaken as 5 mg if the decimal point is not seen	Use zero before a decimal point when the dose is less than a whole unit
Abbreviations such as mg. or mL. with a period following the abbreviation	mg mL	The period is unnecessary and could be mistaken as the number 1 if written poorly	Use mg, mL, etc. without a terminal period

ISMP's List of *Error-Prone Abbreviations, Symbols,* and *Dose Designations* (continued)

Dose Designations and Other Information	Intended Meaning	Misinterpretation	Correction
Drug name and dose run together (especially problematic for drug names that end in "l" such as Inderal40 mg; Tegretol300 mg)	Inderal 40 mg Tegretol 300 mg	Mistaken as Inderal 140 mg Mistaken as Tegretol 1300 mg	Place adequate space between the drug name, dose, and unit of measure
Numerical dose and unit of measure run together (e.g., 10mg, 100mL)	10 mg 100 mL	The "m" is sometimes mistaken as a zero or two zeros, risking a 10- to 100-fold overdose	Place adequate space between the dose and unit of measure
Large doses without properly placed commas (e.g., 100000 units; 1000000 units)	100,000 units 1,000,000 units	100000 has been mistaken as 10,000 or 1,000,000; 1000000 has been mistaken as 100,000	Use commas for dosing units at or above 1,000, or use words such as 100 "thousand" or 1 "million" to improve readability

Drug Name Abbreviations	Intended Meaning	Misinterpretation	Correction
To avoid confusion, do not abbreviate drug names when communicating medical information. Examples of drug name abbreviations involved in medication errors include:			
APAP	acetaminophen	Not recognized as acetaminophen	Use complete drug name
ARA A	vidarabine	Mistaken as cytarabine (ARA C)	Use complete drug name
AZT	zidovudine (Retrovir)	Mistaken as azathioprine or aztreonam	Use complete drug name
CPZ	Compazine (prochlorperazine)	Mistaken as chlorpromazine	Use complete drug name
DPT	Demerol-Phenergan-Thorazine	Mistaken as diphtheria-pertussis-tetanus (vaccine)	Use complete drug name
DTO	Diluted tincture of opium, or deodorized tincture of opium (Paregoric)	Mistaken as tincture of opium	Use complete drug name
HCl	hydrochloric acid or hydrochloride	Mistaken as potassium chloride (The "H" is misinterpreted as "K")	Use complete drug name unless expressed as a salt of a drug
HCT	hydrocortisone	Mistaken as hydrochlorothiazide	Use complete drug name
HCTZ	hydrochlorothiazide	Mistaken as hydrocortisone (seen as HCT250 mg)	Use complete drug name
MgSO4**	magnesium sulfate	Mistaken as morphine sulfate	Use complete drug name
MS, MSO4**	morphine sulfate	Mistaken as magnesium sulfate	Use complete drug name
MTX	methotrexate	Mistaken as mitoxantrone	Use complete drug name
PCA	procainamide	Mistaken as patient controlled analgesia	Use complete drug name
PTU	propylthiouracil	Mistaken as mercaptopurine	Use complete drug name
T3	Tylenol with codeine No. 3	Mistaken as liothyronine	Use complete drug name
TAC	triamcinolone	Mistaken as tetracaine, Adrenalin, cocaine	Use complete drug name
TNK	TNKase	Mistaken as "TPA"	Use complete drug name
ZnSO4	zinc sulfate	Mistaken as morphine sulfate	Use complete drug name

Stemmed Drug Names	Intended Meaning	Misinterpretation	Correction
"Nitro" drip	nitroglycerin infusion	Mistaken as sodium nitroprusside infusion	Use complete drug name
"Norflox"	norfloxacin	Mistaken as Norflex	Use complete drug name
"IV Vanc"	intravenous vancomycin	Mistaken as Invanz	Use complete drug name

Symbols	Intended Meaning	Misinterpretation	Correction
ʒ ♏	Dram Minim	Symbol for dram mistaken as "3" Symbol for minim mistaken as "mL"	Use the metric system
x3d	For three days	Mistaken as "3 doses"	Use "for three days"
> and <	Greater than and less than	Mistaken as opposite of intended; mistakenly use incorrect symbol; "< 10" mistaken as "40"	Use "greater than" or "less than"
/ (slash mark)	Separates two doses or indicates "per"	Mistaken as the number 1 (e.g., "25 units/10 units" misread as "25 units and 110" units)	Use "per" rather than a slash mark to separate doses
@	At	Mistaken as "2"	Use "at"
&	And	Mistaken as "2"	Use "and"
+	Plus or and	Mistaken as "4"	Use "and"
°	Hour	Mistaken as a zero (e.g., q2° seen as q 20)	Use "hr," "h," or "hour"
Φ or ⌀	zero, null sign	Mistaken as numerals 4, 6, 8, and 9	Use 0 or zero, or describe intent using whole words

**These abbreviations are included on The Joint Commission's "minimum list" of dangerous abbreviations, acronyms, and symbols that must be included on an organization's "Do Not Use" list, effective January 1, 2004. Visit www.jointcommission.org for more information about this Joint Commission requirement.

© ISMP 2013. Permission is granted to reproduce material with proper attribution for internal use within healthcare organizations. Other reproduction is prohibited without written permission from ISMP. Report actual and potential medication errors to the ISMP National Medication Errors Reporting Program (ISMP MERP) via the Web at www.ismp.org or by calling 1-800-FAIL-SAF(E).

www.ismp.org

Appendix H:
Important Math Conversions to Remember

Table H-1. Avoirdupois (Household)

Liquid Measurements	Weight Measurements
– 1 cc is synonymous with 1 mL (1 cc = 1 mL)	– 1 gr = 65 mg
– 5 mL = 1 tsp	– 1 kg = 2.2 lbs
– 15 ml = 1 tbsp (the same as saying 3 tsp = 1 tbsp)	– 1 lb = 454 grams
– 30 mL = 1 oz (the same as saying 2 tbsp = 1 oz)	– 1 oz = 28.35 grams
– 480 mL = 1 pt (the same as saying 16 oz = 1 pt)	– 16 oz = 1 lb
– 2 pt = 1 qt	
– 3,785 mL = 1 gal (the same as saying 4 qt = 1 gal)	

Table H-2. Metric System

- 1 liter = 1,000 milliliters
- 1 kilogram = 1,000 grams
- 1 gram = 1,000 milligrams
- 1 milligram = 1,000 micrograms
- ss = one-half

Table H-3. Other

- insulin U-100 = 100 IU and mL (100 international units and mL)

- ophthalmic and otic drops are assumed to be 20 gtts and mL unless stated otherwise

- $°F = (°C \times \frac{9}{5}) + 32$

- $°C = (°F - 32) \times \frac{5}{9}$

- I = 1

- V = 5

- X = 10

- L = 50

- C = 100

- D = 500

- M = 1,000

Appendix I:
References

Academy of Managed Care Pharmacy. "Drug Utilization Review," last modified in November 2009. http://www.amcp.org and WorkArea and DownloadAsset.aspx?id=9296

American Journal of Health-System Pharmacy. "Introduction to the New Prescription Drug Labeling by the Food and Drug Administration," 2007; 64(23):2488–2494.

American Society of Hospital Pharmacists. "ASHP Technical Assistance Bulletin on Compounding Nonsterile Products in Pharmacies," *American Journal of Hospital Pharmacy*, 1994, 51:1441–1448.

Chaffee, Bruce, and Josephine Bonasso. "Strategies for Pharmacy Integration and Pharmacy Information System Interfaces, Part 1: History and Pharmacy Integration Options," *American Journal of Health-System Pharmacy* 61, no. 5, 502–506.

Chaffee, Bruce, and Josephine Bonasso. "Strategies for Pharmacy Integration and Pharmacy Information System Interfaces, Part 2: Scope of Work and Technical Aspects of Interfaces," *American Journal of Health-System Pharmacy* 61, no. 5, 506–514.

Institute for Safe Medication Practices. "ISMP List of High-Alert Medications in Acute Care Settings," last modified in 2014. http://www.ismp.org/Tools/highalertmedications.pdf

Institute for Safe Medication Practices. "ISMP List of High-Alert Medications in Community/ Ambulatory Health Care," last modified in 2011. http://www.ismp.org/communityRx/tools and highAlert-community.pdf

National Council for Presciption Drug Programs. "EPrescribing Fact Sheet," last retrieved April 23, 2015. https://www.ncpdp.org/NCPDP/media/pdf/EprescribingFactSheet.pdf

National Council for Prescription Drug Programs. "Standards Information," last retrieved April, 23, 2015. https://www.ncpdp.org/Standards/Standards-Info

Riffkin, Rebecca. "Americans Rate Nurses Highest on Honesty, Ethical Standards," Gallup, last modified December 18, 2014. http://www.gallup.com/poll/180260/americans-rate-nurses-highest-honesty-ethical-standards.aspx

Shrewsbury, Robert P. "Excipients Used in Pharmaceutical Compounding," The Pharmaceutics and Compounding Laboratory :: Resources," last modified in 2015. http://pharmlabs.unc.edu/appendix_resources.htm.

Substance Abuse and Mental Health Services Administration, "Drug Abuse Warning Network, 2011: National Estimates of Drug-Related Emergency Department Visits," last modified in 2013. http://www.samhsa.gov/data/sites/default/files/DAWN2k11ED/DAWN2k11ED/DAWN2k11ED.pdf.

The Pharmacy Technician Certification Board. (2014). Certification Guidelines and Requirements: A Candidate Guidebook. Washington D.C. http://ptcb.org

U.S. Consumer Product Safety Commission. "Poison Prevention Packaging: A Guide for Health Care Professionals," last modified in 2005. http://www.cpsc.gov/pagefiles/113945/384.pdf

U.S. Drug Enforcement Administration. "Drug Scheduling," last retrieved May 5, 2015. www.dea.gov/druginfo/ds.shtml

U.S. Food and Drug Administration. "Background and Definitions," last modified in 2009. http://www.fda.gov/Safety/Recalls/ucm165546.htm

U.S. Food and Drug Administration. "CPG Sec. 420.100 Adulteration of Drugs Under Section 501(b) and 501(c) of the Act. *Direct Reference Seizure Authority for Adulterated Drugs under Section 501(b)," last modified May 1, 1992. www.fda.gov/ICECI/ComplianceManuals/CompliancePolicyGuidanceManual/ucm074367.htm

U.S. Food and Drug Administration. "Labeling Requirements—Misbranding," last modified March 11, 2015. www.fda.gov/MedicalDevices/DeviceRegulationandGuidance/Overview/DeviceLabeling/GeneralDeviceLabelingRequirements/ucm052190.htm

U.S. Food and Drug Administration. "Product-Specific Recommendations for Generic Drug Development," last modified November 4, 2015. http://www.fda.gov/Drugs/GuidanceComplianceRegulatoryInformation/Guidances/ucm075207.htm

U.S. Food and Drug Administration. "Sulfanilamide Disaster," last modified October 7, 2012. www.fda.gov/aboutfda/whatwedo/history/productregulation/sulfanilamidedisaster/default.htm

U.S. Food and Drug Administration. "The Current Over-the-Counter Medication Label: Take a Look," last modified December 17, 2014. http://www.fda.gov/drugs/resourcesforyou/ucm133411.htm

U.S. Government Publishing Office. "General Administrative Requirements. 45 C.F.R. § 160.103 (2000)," last modified January 25, 2013. http://www.ecfr.gov/cgi-bin/text-idx?SID=128171e810d2f66d37c119fe90729f95&mc=true&node=se45.1.160_1103&rgn=div8

United States Pharmacopeial Convention. "Pharmaceutical compounding—nonsterile preparations (revision bulletin chapter 795)," *The United States Pharmacopeia, 27th Rev., and the National Formulary. 22nd edition*, Rockville, MD: United States Pharmacopeial Convention, 2013. http://www.usp.org/sites/default/files/usp_pdf/EN/gc795.pdf

United States Pharmacopeial Convention. "Pharmaceutical compounding—sterile preparations (general information chapter 797)," *The United States Pharmacopeia, 27th Rev., and the National Formulary. 22nd edition*, Rockville, MD: United States Pharmacopeial Convention, 2004. 2350-2370.

Van Dusen, Virgil, PharmacyTimes.com. "A Review of Federal Legislation Affecting Pharmacy Practice," last modified December 1, 2006. http://www.pharmacytimes.com/publications/issue/2006/2006-12/2006-12-6154#sthash.2NH7ru0F.dpuf

http://www.medscape.com/pharmacists

http://pharmlabs.unc.edu/appendix_resources.htm

Index

Pharmacy Technician Certification Exam
  information for the, 3–4
  recertification, 7
  test-taking strategies, 5–6
Pharmacy-based system, 193
Phosphodiesterase (PDE) inhibitors, 77
Physicians' Desk Reference®, 100t
Plan limitations, 187
Plasminogen activators, 50
Poison Prevention Packaging Act (PPPA) of
  1970, 94–95
Potassium-sparing diuretics, 49–50
Potentiated interaction, 34
Preferred Provider Organizations (PPOs),
  186
Prescriber errors, 135t
Prescription(s)
  calculations for, 160–165
  drug labeling requirements, 89
  entry into computer system, 167–170
  label, 168–169
  management, 194
  preparing the, 170–172
  receiving, 156 157
  steps to fill a, 155
  translating the, 159–160
  transmission methods, 156–157
Prevention strategies, 146–147
Priapism, 77
Prior authorization, 187
Product expiration date, 180
Professional standards, 99
Prospective drug utilization review
  (ProDUR), 95
Protozoa, 38
Psoriasis, treatment of, 56t
Psychotherapy, 80
Pulverization, 120
Pure Food and Drug Act of 1906, 88

Q

Quality assurance guidelines, 150–151
Quality-related event (QRE), 147–148
Quinolones, 42t

R

Rashes, treatment of, 54t–56t

Recalls
  classification of, 98
  medication, 181–182
  quality assurance, 150–151
  stems used in, 32
Recertification, pharmacy technician, 7
Reimbursement systems, 187
Remington's, *The Science and Practice of
  Pharmacy*, 100
Reproductive agents, 71–73
Rescue inhalers, 73
Resources, pharmacy, 99–100
Respiratory agents, 73–76
Respiratory syncytial virus (RSV), 47
Restricted drug programs and provisions,
  Isotretinoin Safety and Risk Management
  Act of 2004, 96–97
Rheumatoid arthritis, treatment of, 67, 70t
Rhinitis, treatment of, 57t, 74t
Risk Evaluation and Mitigation Strategies
  (REMS), 54, 97

S

Safety cabinet, biological, 111
Safety strategies, 140–141
Schizophrenia, treatment of, 81t
Sedative agents, 35
Shingles, 47
Side effects, defined, 33
Skeletal medications, 66–71
Skin redness and itching, treatment of,
  54t–56t
Skin wounds, treatment of, 55t
Smoking cessation agents, 82, 83t
Solution, 33t
Spatulation, 120
Spirit(s), 33t
State Board of Pharmacy, 149t
Statins, 50
Sterile compounding process
  handling and disposal, 108–109
  risk levels, 108t
  safety, 106–108
Stool softener, 65t
Strokes, agents to prevent, 53t
Suppository, 33t
Surface area calculations, 128

2016.
3/17; 2x Rad 3/17
4/19 4x " 9/18